MALIGNANT GROWTH

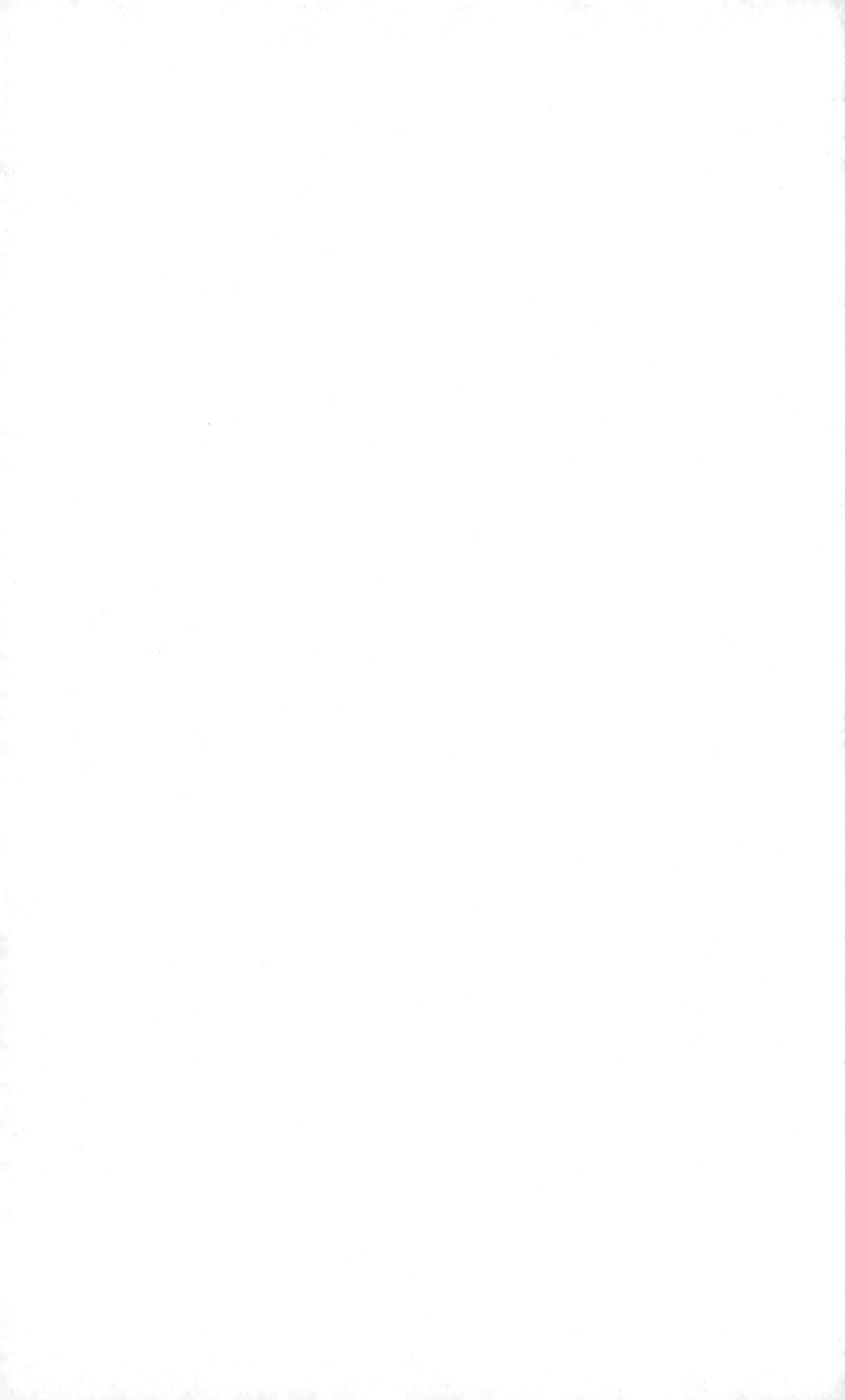

MALIGNANT GROWTH

CREATING THE MODERN CANCER RESEARCH ESTABLISHMENT 1875–1915

ALAN I MARCUS

THE UNIVERSITY OF ALABAMA PRESS
TUSCALOOSA

The University of Alabama Press
Tuscaloosa, Alabama 35487-0380
uapress.ua.edu

Typeface: Scala Pro

Cover image: Rendering of a malignant cell; courtesy of 123RF.com, © lightwise
Cover design: David Nees

Library of Congress Cataloging-in-Publication Data

Names: Marcus, Alan I, 1949– author.
Title: Malignant growth : creating the modern cancer research establishment, 1875–1915 / Alan I Marcus.
Description: Tuscaloosa : The University of Alabama Press, [2018] | Includes bibliographical references and index.
Identifiers: LCCN 2017038244| ISBN 9780817319793 (cloth) | ISBN 9780817391775 (ebook)
Subjects: LCSH: Cancer—Research—History—19th century. | Cancer—Research—History—20th century.
Classification: LCC RC275 .M37 2018 | DDC 362.19699/40072—dc23
LC record available at https://lccn.loc.gov/2017038244

To Jean, my partner in everything; I fail way too often to tell her how much I admire, adore, and appreciate her.

CONTENTS

ACKNOWLEDGMENTS

I incurred many debts as I researched and wrote this book. The fine, underappreciated Iowa State University Library gave me my own key for 24-hour access, a room of my own, and use of a Xerox machine so that I could go through hundreds of thousands, if not millions, of pages of the various periodicals housed in the storage facility there. In the year that I was there—I had no teaching duties, a perk of being the institution's first Distinguished Humanities Scholar—I managed to make over 33,000 photocopies. I thank the then-chair of the history department, George McJimsey, for paying for the xeroxing. I also want to acknowledge my children, Gregory and Jocelyn, and my late father-in-law, John Wasieleski, each of whom was punished by being required to do some of the actual photocopying in the library. My father-in-law's "crime" was making his sons and sons-in-law stack wood in one place on one week and then move it all back to the original place the next, because he enjoyed being in the woods. When I discovered the ruse, he told me if I ever needed help, he'd be glad to pitch in. After I had him xerox, he never brought up moving wood again.

Iowa State's participation in the HathiTrust project helped me obtain sources I otherwise would not have been able to access. My status as an emeritus professor there has enabled me to continue to use this otherwise unavailable source, even after I relocated to Mississippi State University. The Interlibrary Loan staff at my new institution provided significant help with hard-to-find documents.

Niklas Trzaskowski, a PhD student in our history graduate program at Mississippi State, helped with the translations of German texts. My spotty knowledge of French was adequate to handle translations from that language, bolstered by an ample assist from Google Translate.

I asked Matt Lavine and Alexandra Hui, two of my colleagues at Mississippi State, and two of my PhD students here, Kasey Mosley and Katie Sullivan, to read the introduction. They provided helpful, insightful comments. I also sketched out the project to the CHASES Experiment Station, a consortium of faculty and students at Mississippi State interested in history of agriculture, science, and the environment. The discussion was spirited.

Beth Motherwell and other members of the University of Alabama Press remain a pleasure to work with. Of special note were the comments of an anonymous referee, who helped make this a better book.

I was asked some time ago why I decided to write a book on cancer.

Frankly, I do not remember. I do not have a story of a family member succumbing to the disease. I have not lost a friend prematurely that led me to this project. I think I did it simply because it seemed well nigh impossible. I have always enjoyed projects that seem to be difficult. If proof of that statement is needed, I submit the fact that I headed the history department *and* the chemistry department at Mississippi State during the two years I spent finishing this manuscript. I like being able to create a structure out of things that few today see as related or relevant, or to resurrect and explore a sense of organization from the past. My father, a World War II veteran, used to say that the army's motto during that conflict was "the difficult we do immediately. The impossible takes a little longer." I incorporated the heart of that sentiment in my latest aphorism: "The project of life is to bend reality to one's will." I hardily embrace that challenge and did so as I labored to create this book.

INTRODUCTION

On Institutions and Institutional Change

This book is not about cancer per se.[1] It is about the ideas and processes that culminated in a worldwide search for the cause of the disease known as cancer during a specific set of years. That was a search for something unknown. Its ostensive goal was to make that unknown known, to remove the mystery of cancer's cause and replace it with certainty. In the course of this cancer quest, investigators relied on tried-and-true techniques and pioneered new mechanisms to pursue the disease. The book details the repeated failure of that quest, as well as the institutional network that failure generated and helped perpetuate.

Finding cancer's cause was no small project, of course. Indeed, determining a relationship between cause and disease had been an important and defining struggle throughout the nineteenth century. Establishing a disease as a distinct, concrete malady was an essential part of that analysis. Cancer had yielded to that thrust rather early but in a limited way. Although recognized as a distinct disease before the late nineteenth century, cancer remained synonymous during this later period with but a single symptom—rapid, seemingly uncontrolled cellular growth. Beyond that, there was remarkably little agreement. Some linked the disease to established cells losing differentiation, while others fought over what kind of body cells could become cancerous. Still others questioned whether sarcoma and carcinoma were distinct diseases and debated what exactly characterized a true cancer case or tumor. In effect, medical men and investigators settled only on the most obvious symptom of cancer, not a more comprehensive definition of the malady.[2]

With that slim definition of the disease, it was not surprising that determining what caused cancer proved problematic. Earlier in the century, physicians treated the disease's obvious symptom; they tried to end the proliferation of cells, not investigate reasons for the onset of that condition. By the middle of the century, physicians, statisticians, and others sought to establish who got the disease and what activities fostered it, presuming that determining these factors would assist them in its prevention and amelioration. This etiological sense rendered cause much more important than symptom; it redefined the disease in terms of what generated it.

This nascent groping for the cause of the disease, to prohibit its inception, led to considerable speculation that can be gathered into two main camps. Proponents of the first epidemiological explanation, the Constitutionalists, considered cancer a systemic disease but with local manifestations. That dualism resolved the problem of the seeming incongruity between the disease seat and the fact that cancer often was found in several different organs. A force from outside the individual or a behavior undertaken by the individual caused the individual's system to become disrupted, unbalanced. The place where cancer surfaced—the disease seat—resulted from what taboo was violated, how it was violated, or the nature of that body part. Cancer did not so much spread from the initial manifestation as develop in a second or third site. Disorganization of the system opened potentially any site to suffer the disease.

Representatives of the second group, the Cellularists, provided a different ex post facto explanation. Advocates of Rudolph Virchow's dictum that all new cells descend from existing cells, the Cellularists included Virchow himself and many of his students, particularly Julius Cohnheim. They argued that cancer was an internal disease; its formation depended on cells already in the body. Cancer was positioned to strike even before birth. As the embryo developed, certain cells remained dormant and undifferentiated. The basic laws of fluid dynamics pushed these cells, which ultimately took refuge in what would become the body's crevices and imperfections. Only when some external mechanical or chemical agency stirred these cells did they awaken, become renegades, and spawn cancer. Metastases resulted from these animated cells coursing through the body.[3]

While both groups disagreed on how cancer emerged, both remained convinced that an external occurrence, individual behavior, or both loosed the disease on its victims. Both theories were multicausal in two distinct ways. First, both required two kinds of activities to propagate and spread the disease. One was not necessarily sufficient. But more to the point of this book and the later nineteenth century, both were multicausal in that they postulated any number of acts and behaviors that could result in the disease. Cancer remained a condition that a slew of things, actions, or conditions could spawn.[4]

The later nineteenth century cancer war was of a very different piece. Its partisans searched for *the* cause of cancer, the sole stipulation without which cancer was impossible. Philosophers of science have defined this kind of causation as "necessary." It must be found in each and every cancer case as essential to the disease's formation.[5]

This radical reorganization of cancer thought around its necessary cause paralleled a rather profound late nineteenth-century development, the rise of bacteriology and its salient epidemiological feature, the Germ Theory of Disease. To be sure, earlier in the century a few diseases had been tied causally to specific microorganisms. But the late nineteenth-century Germ Theory onslaught was massive in scale and proved tremendously alluring. Disease after disease was linked to its specific pathogen as the necessary causal agent. Numerous enigmatic diseases were rendered familiar simply by the notion of each being the consequence of a distinctive microorganism operating within a particular set of conditions. Initial successes in the germ-disease nexus quickly encouraged others to take up the mantle. Numerous investigators assumed that their diseases with theretofore unknown causes operated analogously to those that had been shown to stem from a germ, and they adopted the model of one disease, one specific causal microbe. It was in this heady era dominated by bacteriology, especially the Germ Theory of Disease, that the war on cancer was first prosecuted.[6]

Cancer gained especial attention in the later nineteenth century as demographer after demographer reported the disease increasing at a prodigious rate worldwide. The desperate situation demanded action. In this new world of bacteriological-based certainty, optimism reigned that this plague could be beaten back. While not every investigator linked cancer to a particular microbe, contemporaries felt certain that the cause of cancer would conform to an analysis consistent with the Germ Theory's most important facet. Cancer surely would have a specific cause and that cause would be found in each and every instance of the disease. It was that sentiment, coupled with the apparent threat of epidemic-like cancer, that spurred the world's first war on cancer. A massive search throughout the western world ensued to identify the nasty little culprit and implement preventive measures.

While these new seekers were cocksure of their approach, finding cancer's microbial cause proved more elusive than anticipated. As John Harley Warner and Nancy Tomes have pointed out, concrete, real-time demonstrations of the union between the Germ Theory and any particular disease have proven in each case to be complicated, more convoluted than the now common trope would imply. A single narrative for that multidimensional story has been elusive.[7] In the case of the quest for cancer's cause, the critical idea that each disease has a unique and single "necessary" cause served as a fundamental principle guiding observation, discussion, and inquiry. Operating as axiomatic, that notion eliminated or at least seriously delayed the gymnastics of ensuring that all phenomena under consideration met the Germ Theory's strictures. The heyday and apparent successes of bacteriology and its Germ Theory concomitant reified that causal combination of single causes for single diseases. One disease, one cause offered the extraordinary power of reducing mystery through establishment of an actionable, recognizable pattern even before that agent was identified.

The clarity provided by the bacteriological model—the notion that one particular microorganism necessarily produced all instances of one specific disease—cannot be overestimated.[8] During the late nineteenth century, it was the sole criterion that cancer researchers held in common. Persons who searched for cancer's cause, at least during the book's first few decades, rarely did so to the exclusion of other responsibilities. They were not oncologists in any modern sense. Nor were all necessarily conversant with laboratories and laboratory methods. Rather, they were bacteriologists, pathologists, laboratory scientists, physicians both with and without hospital privileges, specialists in the diseases of women, statisticians, apothecaries, and general practitioners. They generally dealt in their daily affairs with a wide range of patients, diseases, and subjects. Many of these people had excellent reputations in the medical and/or scientific world—and sometimes even with the public—but not for their cancer research work. Others were labeled charlatans. By and large, these late nineteenth century cancer hunters were persons certain of the idea that the cause of cancer, like that for other diseases, could be uncovered, that cancer had a single cause—likely a microbe—and that they had the skills to reveal that cause.

The actual diversity of people and types of people interested in cancer's cause itself established a powerful, persistent conundrum. How would questions surrounding cancer be adjudicated by a group of investigators who were in fact not remotely homogeneous or even truly a group? To be sure, they did not even pursue their investigations in similar sorts of facilities. Some practiced only at the bedside. Others sought cancer's cause through statistical analyses. Still others worked in hospitals. Few had first-rate bacteriological or pathological skills. Who would adjudicate questions and differences within this enquiring morass of predominantly part-time investigators? As Theodore Porter has noted, "objectivity" has been "one of the classic ideals of science." Its attributes include "truth to nature," as well as "impersonality, fairness [and] universality."[9] With so many disparate individuals, backgrounds, and competencies involved in the search, what was objectivity and how was it to be determined? No single discipline, no single type of doctor, no single type of scientist, and no single independent investigator possessed anything like the ability, authority, or power to set terms and to decide questions. In common, they had passion and a notion that the disease had a single cause, little more. At best they constituted a loosely affiliated cohort of people interested in the same thing—ridding the world of cancer.

Perhaps an example would be helpful. A report in a medical journal or newspaper might note that a physician from Louisville, Kentucky, had found certain bodies associated with cases of cancer of the esophagus. How would physicians at the Royal Medical Society of London decide the veracity of the claim? They could begin to try and collect similar data, to be sure, but medical journals often and newspapers usually did not report findings in such detail as to make them absolutely reproducible elsewhere. Temperatures might differ. Were these bodies related to any unique habits of the people in which they were found? Time of observation might be before or after death. Were the particularistic bodies associated only with esophageal cancer, digestive cancers, cancers in men, cancers in the aged? And what of attending physicians in Germany, laboratory scientists who spoke only French, or apothecaries in the English countryside? How would they and countless other discrete groupings understand these "findings"? There was an almost endless list of possible discriminants to consider and an equally numerous series of perspectives from which to evaluate them. It was truly a tower of Babel.[10]

Armed with a similar philosophy, this amorphous mass of investigators all applied a rather simple plan of attack. They took what they knew—each disease had a specific, unique cause, and microorganisms or other agents were explicitly implicated in many diseases—and applied it to what they did not know—the cause of cancer, which manifested itself in uncontrollable cell growth. Put baldly, they operated according to analogy. Just what analogies these incredibly disparate men and women chose to accentuate differed almost as greatly as did the men and women themselves, but all adopted this rigid imitative framework. They bounded themselves and circumscribed their gaze by refusing to consider that cancer did not function in a manner analogous to other bacteriological-era diseases. Cancer was a single disease with a singular cause. The events surrounding other diseases would be directly applicable to the case of cancer.[11]

For these investigators, analogies became the touchstones of verification and objectification. They provided appearance of surety during the quest for certainty, by directly comparing the known with the unknown in an effort to establish facts. Use of referents to make sense out of something ambiguous, difficult, or uncertain in the medical sciences was not restricted to cancer or the later nineteenth century. Christoph Gradmann in his essay titled,

"A Spirit of Scientific Rigour: Koch's Postulates in Twentieth-Century Medicine," has discussed how anecdotes function in a similar capacity in later twentieth-century medical science. An anecdote "presents a plausible story about an important object in a way that reduces complexity." The essentialness of anecdotes allows them to act as surrogates or proxies and makes them useful. Like analogies, anecdotes are familiar, and their familiarity and comprehensibility brings apparent clarity and comfort to an otherwise murky situation. Each anecdote gives the appearance of "not change, but stability." It suggests that things, even those not yet known, remain remarkably consistent and continuous.[12]

Late nineteenth-century analogous thinking in cancer research was ruthlessly bound by the idea that each disease had but a single necessary cause. Identification of various vitamin deficiency diseases after 1900 did not undercut the essential ideational framework.[13] True, there was no microorganism implicated in most deficiency diseases, but those illnesses retained the crucial aspect of what I am calling here bacteriological-era thinking—that each disease always had a single, unique cause—even when specific situations and conditions were required to accompany that cause.[14] That aspect of the Germ Theory remained the bedrock of reputable medical science thought in the late nineteenth and early twentieth centuries and served as the structure in and through which to consider various individual actors and agents as cancer's possible cause.

The book, then, is about matching expectations with observations and the failure and chaos that ensued. It is about confrontation in real time, the hard work of attempting to make something certain, to make something "truly" so. Contemporaries went about that task within the context of what they knew and what they did—what they deemed analogous. It was not a matter for laboratory scientists or a scientific community—let alone a profession—as we tend to employ those conceptions. Various interested parties seeking cancer's cause cleaved together as often and tenaciously as they cleaved apart. They jockeyed with each other, assisted one another, and resisted the entre of others. It was a dynamic free-for-all.[15] In the parlance of historians of science, these men and women worked within several vastly distinct and different "geographies of exploration." They were denizens of the bedside, the clinic, the dispensary, the laboratory, the field, the hospital, and elsewhere and employed methods consonant with their geographies. Nor was that all. They approached cancer from disparate viewpoints: from clinical medicine, zoology, botany, chemistry, nutrition, bacteriology, pathology, microbiology, and more. Despite their vastly different "geographic" loci and even more diffuse foci, their perspective on cancer's cause remained resolute and common in one crucial, overarching respect. Each disease had a single cause, and cancer must be analogous to something already known.[16]

Nationality mattered in this "war"[17] and not just in the sense of national medical/scientific styles. Nation-states—governments—themselves competed with each other to lead and sometimes control the cancer hunt and to fight the fight. Indeed, not all contemporaries shared the same precise perspective, but virtually all conducted their quest in a similar fashion. They did so publicly and most prominently. That was the mechanism left open to them. They wrote in medical and scientific journals, published research reports, and presented their findings to professional and medical organizations. The world's newspapers and magazines slavishly covered these efforts, reporting on the implications and potential implications of various notices. The press noted cures and discoveries, outlined arguments, interviewed investigators, highlighted points of contention, and speculated about the manifest possibilities of recent findings. They compared present efforts with those of the past and predicted what would come in the future.

History of science patterns, courses, or models of how successfully to attack the unknown—models ex post facto derived and reified as the consequence of achievement—did not come into play here. They could not. Late nineteenth- and early twentieth-century cancer investigators pursued a course that was destined to fail. They were incapable of deducing, inducing, or even stumbling upon the single cause of cancer because no such thing existed. They could not achieve what they set out to do—find cancer's cause. With evidence so difficult to confirm across geographies of inquiry, across disciplines and subdisciplines, and across national borders and oceans, it was most explicitly not a negotiation. There was nothing to negotiate. It remained an intense, publicly fought battle, ostensibly about truth, predictability, and certainty, as well as objective measures thereof. It was a battle that could be waged but never won.

Analogies as fashioned in this war often proved not helpful or irrelevant but pernicious. Analogies always constrain. They restrict inquiry to what is known and thereby indirectly label the unknown as unfathomable, outside the pale. With the unknown taboo, intolerable, or at least off the table, cancer investigators lacked the conceptual tools to resolve the epidemiological problem that had galvanized them. It was not reasoning by or use of analogies that stood as the problem. It was the unquestioned devotion to analogies derived from a theory of disease that could not be fruitful. So long as analogies based on a single cause of cancer guided cancer research, the only recourse for investigators was frustration and failure. For patients it was usually death.[18]

Historians have rarely studied situations as grotesque and convoluted as the late nineteenth and early twentieth centuries' quest for cancer's cause.[19] Participants came from many walks of life, operated in numerous localities with various spatial configurations and environments of inquiry, and possessed several types and levels of training. Not homogeneous or bound enough to suggest a community, let alone something as distinctive as a profession, they clung only to a misguided presumption that guaranteed failure. It was within that tumultuous framework that these men and women fervidly carried on their momentous pursuit. And it was within that milieu that they created several things new. Indeed, uncertainty and persistent, depressing, negative outcomes were critical to those geneses.

It strikes me that the best way to approach a complicated international public phenomenon, such as the quest for cancer's cause, is to trace it as it actually happened in its minute, dirty, gritty details. After all, the late nineteenth- and early twentieth-century publicly waged cancer battles were very much a rich tapestry of their own—contests on their own terms and for their own objectives. Looking at the matter in its gloriously morbid, often contradictory minutiae—as a series of vignettes—is not dissimilar to what the anthropologist Clifford Geertz might call "thick description" or what Michel Foucault would have called an "archaeology."[20] Exploring the situation chronologically—tracing the events as they occurred in real time—exposes in a very intimate manner the investigators' repeated lurches of promise, discoveries of hope, and the despair of reality that inevitably followed. As discoveries were trumpeted and disavowed, as institutions were built and fell, as power was seized and relinquished, and as expectations were changed and juggled, one factor undergirded the whole process: failure, dismal, abject failure, in the announced ambitions to find the singular cause of cancer.

In the course of this artful human flailing, heroes, monuments, and procedures were manufactured. The cast of characters proved remarkably fluid. Some sought cancer's cause for an instant, while others were aboard for the long slog. Roughly ten Nobel Prize winners involved themselves in this first cancer war. Two received the prize for their cancer work. Invention of cancer research laboratories was probably the most enduring legacy of what proved a quixotic quest. Funded predominantly by private bequests, these places took root in many major cities in the Western world after about 1900. They became the loci of persons engaged primarily in cancer investigation, vehicles in which people who would become known almost exclusively for cancer research practiced and trained. These laboratories were initially a work in progress. People staffing the new facilities had no singular experience as cancer investigators. Their goal and ambition was not simply to find the cancer's cause but to mold themselves into a cohort composed of members with similar skills, referents, and techniques. That process was never easy. What these new cancer scientists practiced, why they chose to practice it, who practiced there, what they practiced on, and how the institutions related to each other were perpetual sources of debate, often discord.[21] In every instance, however, self-definition preceded actual activity. These researchers declared themselves laboratory-based cancer scientists and only then did investigators in each of these often divergent institutions begin to try to define exactly what that meant.

Historians have devoted much attention to the rise of laboratories generally over the past thirty years. They have noted how they arose in different disciplines, different places, and for different purposes. They have considered their architecture, whether they were modern or premodern contrivances, and how external cultural institutions may have colored their structure and function. These findings have been so diverse that most scholars have abandoned the idea of a universal history of the laboratory per se.[22] The new cancer research laboratories reinforced that contention but take complexity and diversity to the next level. Formed for a single purpose—to find the cause of cancer—and embodying the idea that each disease had its own unique cause, you would suspect that they would exhibit a great deal of commonality. But cancer laboratories wrought large were not systematized institutions. Each emerged from the labors of a specific individual or individuals sponsored by a particular geopolitical unit. Originators were not cancer experts but doctors, surgeons, bacteriologists, pharmacists, pathological anatomists, and more. Their identities and their livelihoods reflected their diverse circumstances, talents, and interests. Each cancer laboratory was built on the back of an investigator with different expertise and skill. These investigators brought their preconceptions to the task. A final factor helped account for their remarkable differences. Cancer laboratories, even those that had secured a measure of state sanction, relied to an extraordinary degree on private funding sources—often bequests. Lab directors generally proved successful in establishing and perpetuating laboratories because they offered a vision that convinced benevolent persons—or occasionally state officials—to patronize their particularistic efforts.

The diversity in origin and emphasis of these laboratories further helped account for why researchers had such difficulty adjudicating various conflicting evidentiary reports. To be sure, these central places of cancer research communicated with each other, often sharing information. But their aforementioned differences led them to talk past one another, to investigate very different things in very different ways. Rather than constricting options, cancer laboratories together were the very embodiment of multiplicity of focus, training, competence, and assumption. They were parallel in conception and in implementation, even as they each clung to the one disease, one cause analogy.

Despite their differences, cancer research laboratories were truly the world's first oncological institutions devoted purely to research.[23] They were solemnly charged to determine cancer's causative agent and resolutely undertook that critical task. Had earlier investigators working without cancer laboratories "discovered" cancer's cause, cancer laboratories would never have been created. If the nascent structures subsequently had been successful in the cancer crusade, they might not still persist. But the laboratories' persistence did not simply acknowledge failure (or at least lack of success); it venerated that unfortunate state. Institutions proven incapable of doing what they were created to do and several times reformatted in hopes of future success came to dominate cancer research. At each stop, they secured more and more rewards—many gained their own cancer research hospitals, for instance—and more and more power.[24] Their institutionalization also institutionalized the means and methods of failure. Cancer research laboratories retained authority precisely and perversely because they failed. The work for which they were created remained to be done, and their sizable investment crowded out other forms of analysis, inquiry, and exploration. They parlayed lack of success into becoming the cancer research establishment. They claimed perennially and perpetually to be on the verge of making things so.

That apparent and continuous lack of success in determining the disease's cause did have consequences. In the years immediately before World War I, cancer laboratory directors fretted that the world war on cancer was irretrievably broken. Cancer's cause was unlikely to be uncovered in the foreseeable future. While laboratory directors lamented that depressing realization and used it as a tactic to attract further and long-term support for their institutions, many medical men and surgeons took decisive action in another direction. If cancer could not be conquered quickly, other action was mandatory. Their solution was simple but brilliant. They would seek to control cancer, not conquer it.

Controlling cancer had a practical facet. Only complete surgical removal of the tumor before it metastasized guaranteed patient survival. Therefore, they labored to identify the disease at its onset or even before it presented clinical symptoms. The key was to get the public to recognize cancer before the situation became grave and to visit a surgeon before it was too late. Surgeons, often in conjunction with physicians and using laboratory tests, could make the decision if an operation was warranted. A goodly portion of medical men thought the disease so fearsome that they recommended preventive surgery to remove suspect body parts before finding any evidence of disease invasion.

Managing cancer presented physicians and surgeons a discrete yet prominent place within the nascent cancer establishment. New institutions dedicated to public outreach—institutions analogous to those erected for tuberculosis, the "white plague of (hu)mankind"—and generally populated and guided by practitioners, not researchers, were created for the new task. They were tangible manifestations of the cancer research laboratories' inability to achieve the purpose for which they had been formed. The American Society for Cancer Control (now the American Cancer Society) was among the most prominent of these management institutions when it was established in 1913. In effect, what we now know as the modern cancer network had been firmly established by about World War I.[25]

Soon after creation of the new two-pronged cancer Leviathan, the initial assumption that had fueled the world war on cancer began to lose favor. After forty years of employing one disease, one cause as the model for the cancer quest, a few investigators cautiously questioned whether cancer did in fact conform to that exclusionary archetype. Perhaps cancer exhibited another pattern, a pattern without a simple medical analogy. The disease might be multi-causal. Several different agents might produce the nefarious disease. There could be a plethora of necessary causes.

That realization would change the character of cancer research. What it did not do was change the character of the cancer research establishment. Despite the fact that the notions upon which this establishment was predicated no longer remain viable, its institutions persisted, even thrived. Established over a century ago in the expectation of a swift, final victory over the disease, those same institutions continue their pursuit of the dread disease today.

The argument here is not to suggest that the persistence of the cancer establishment was unique. Rather, it is to indicate that there exists a fundamentally different way to look at public and private action. Rather than evaluate it solely for what its initial proponents claim it may achieve or has achieved, one also needs to acknowledge what has not been achieved in the past. Virtually every public act was undertaken in hopes of righting some wrong, removing some blight, addressing some such ill. The implication is clear. That wrong or blight had existed and was being dealt with ineffectually, or not at all, prior to the new institution being formed and implemented. The questions surrounding public acts then become what constitutes failure and when is failure no longer tolerable? When does failure generate an acknowledgement of that station—that things have failed and there remains virtually no hope for amelioration—and spawn a desperate new attempt(s) to achieve success? What then constitutes not failure per se but intolerable failure? Those questions persist, both in the case of a first institutional attempt to deal with a problem and in the persistence of those institutions once they have demonstrated failure. Is that where and when negotiation occurs? Is science or any "objective" form of reality involved in any way? Men and women by the hundreds of millions—if not billions—have died of cancer and continue to do so. Does that matter in institutional formation or persistence, or does the question devolve into one of salespersonship, power, old boy and girl networks, threats, promises? How are failed institutions enabled to remain extant, even vital, when their programs have failed to deliver year after year? Do people double down on promises, providing ever more grandiose visions of the nirvana ahead? Do they double down on threats, arguing that the situation that persists, while far from ideal, is more tolerable than what it would be without the established entities or programs? Are the old adages "prosperity is just around the corner" and "in for a dime, in for a dollar" the way public action is determined? Is institutional persistence or change simply a matter of cultural and/or social context, and exactly what do those conglomerated designations truly hide? Is designating something "context" akin to using a name as a ruse to "explain" something that is otherwise too complicated and complex to suss out? Is failure simply society chasing its tail, or is failure a potent mechanism for change and progress?

This book does not resolve those issues. What it hopes to do is to point out that they should be acknowledged to exist. Public and private action is the harbinger of failure. Institutional reorganization or change is its bellwether.

1

"Bacteriology" Is Destiny

Cancer, Certainty, and Uncertainty in the Late Nineteenth Century

"It seems more than probable that all malignant growths belong to the infectious microbic diseases, and that by to-morrow we shall have the tiny causators" identified, argued Robert T. Morris, MD, in an 1887 issue of *Popular Science Monthly*. An anonymous physician writing in the journal *Science* a year later agreed. The exact cause of cancer "is now prosecuted with more hopefulness than ever, by reason of the belief in many minds that cancer is a specific disease depending on a germ for its causation."[1] These men articulated a position common in the late nineteenth and early twentieth centuries. For about four decades after 1875, European and American investigators of different stripes, training, and reputation approached cancer from a quite similar perspective and with similar enthusiasm and optimism. They each tried to determine the single cause for the single disease of cancer. The one cause, one disease framework was the fundamental thrust of late nineteenth-century medical science and bacteriology, and the application of the Germ Theory of Disease were its most noted and visible triumphs. It was the thrill and promise of the Germ Theory of Disease that energized the quest for cancer's cause.

The Germ Theory was infectious for several reasons. Those who clung to it or even just referenced it marked themselves as knowledgeable, cutting edge. Adherence to this theory suggested that they were highly trained, up-to-date, modern. For these cancer investigators, the theory with which they prosecuted the cancer microorganism was not just a case of the ends justifying the means. The means that how the problem was aggressively broached was at least as significant as the ends—determining the cause of cancer. Put simply, these "modern" cancer investigators did not accentuate objectivity or trust in numbers in the pursuit of cancer's cause.[2] Their belief in one cause, one disease and the application of the methodology that accompanied that presumption denoted them as progressive and served as the foundation of their commonality.

Armed with a consistent, although generalized, notion of how to prosecute cancer's cause, they labored for decades to expose the microscopic culprit to no avail. These late nineteenth-century men and women never acknowledged failure of their announced mission, just lack of success so far. Despite failure after failure, they continued, steadfast in their belief that the cancer agent would soon be uncovered. The past and its successes remained the bedrock of their conceit. No matter their specific background, cancer investigators claimed a concrete, perhaps even glorious, history. The scientific/medical cohort in which these diversely located, schooled, and experienced individuals claimed historical kinship had achieved notoriety in what the cohort identified as analogous pursuits. The search for cancer's cause made members of the cohort epidemiologists, pure and simple. They followed in the metaphorical footsteps of the great names of sanitary science—Edwin Chadwick, John Snow, John Griscom, and John Simon. The sanitarians, although not necessarily ascribing to a one disease, one cause–based model of inquiry, had applied their methods to demonstrate why particular identifiable populations became liable to specific disease outbreaks, thereby vanquishing uncertainty from the equation. They too had sought the disease's cause.[3] Late nineteenth-century cancer investigators also claimed for themselves affinity to the emerging bacteriology-dependent discipline of the new epidemiologists—Rudolph Virchow, Jacob Henle, Louis Pasteur, Edwin Klebs, and most notably Robert Koch. Indeed, Koch's postulates—isolate the same pathogen in every case of the disease, grow it on sterile media, inoculate it into living things to produce the disease, and isolate it from those bodies in which it was inoculated—had persuasively and powerfully tied specific microbes to individual maladies and brooked no other cause. When viewed in light of these postulates, the Germ Theory of Disease stood as a potent force, a tangible manifestation of methodological acuity.[4]

Faced with this pantheon of proscriptions and heroes, late nineteenth-century cancer investigators took what they knew and how they knew it and applied it to what they did not know; the analogy of one disease, one cause became the essential means to pursue cancer. To be sure, contemporaries recognized that all diseases might not be so readily attributable to specific germs as had been tuberculosis, for example. The vibrio of cholera and, much later, the spirochete of syphilis proved more difficult to link to their respective diseases. Nonetheless, the heroes had positively shown those unique microbe-disease causal linkages to exist. Not surprisingly, when investigators encountered some initial difficulties in identifying the cancer bacterium, they immediately recalled tuberculosis and syphilis as diseases that at first seemed intractable and attempted to introduce techniques that had proven successful there. Some worked directly in either tuberculosis or syphilis before switching to cancer. For example, Ernst Viktor Leyden joined with Koch on tuberculosis before he immersed himself in the search for the cancer germ and became Germany's leading cancer researcher. Indeed, being able to refer firsthand to difficulties in uncovering tuberculosis and syphilis germs strengthened rather than weakened resolve and almost paradoxically seemed to guarantee success. It was just a matter of time and research.[5]

It would be hard to overstate just how critical the essential element of the Germ Theory of Disease was to the late nineteenth- and early twentieth-century cancer quest. Its fundamental kernel—that each disease had a unique single cause and that that cause was an agent that came from outside the organism—reoriented thinking about disease generally. It promised that disease as a category could be completely disaggregated into its constituent elements. Each malady would be separated and identified, and each could be tied irrevocably to a specific causative agent. That causative relationship, moreover, was universal. It would operate in every circumstance where the disease was present.[6]

That incredibly optimistic assessment extended to notions of cancer. The tenets of the Germ Theory provided a sense of concreteness and certainty that appealed to scientists and medical men, who craved definitiveness as well as objectivity. A veritable stampede ensued to find cancer's particularistic microbial cause. But even if a microbial culprit was not detected, the stricture that each disease had but a single cause provided an overpowering inducement to search further using the same template. In the twenty-five years before 1900, inability to find cancer's sole cause simply meant that science had not yet successfully located it. Digging, more digging, and thinking, especially through forming analogies to what was already known about diseases with established causes, was the prescribed path. It proved virtually irresistible, congruent with the surety necessary to label something scientific.

The one disease, one cause approach to cancer did not completely vanquish either the constitutional or cellular explanation from the medical firmament. Some senior medical men and a few scientists cleaved to the old ways. That was especially true of German pathologists, many of whom studied with and revered the great Virchow. Led by the venerable David Paul von Hansemann, they remained in the very decided minority.[7] The appeal of the Germ Theory seemed so alluring and its application in any number of diseases appeared so deterministic that it drew convert after convert. It came to dominate the war against cancer.

At the heart of this cancer quest was a series of critical, yet apparently subordinate, questions. All were similar to those posed by investigators for any number of diseases. First, why did some individuals get cancer while others did not? Liability to disease extended further back than the Germ Theory, of course. Later nineteenth-century cancer researchers focused on individual proclivities and experiences and attempted to aggregate them to expose larger patterns to account for the disease's proliferation.[8]

While inextricably joined to the one disease, one cause nexus, cancer investigators looked to the past, as well as the present and future. They sought the single necessary microbial cause of cancer but, to account for the fact that the disease did not strike everyone and that the disease's seat varied from individual to individual, researchers offered a more complicated epidemiological assessment. One disease, one cause remained necessary—essential—to cancer's production, but that cause alone might not be sufficient to generate the disease in every case. Certain circumstances, conditions, or situations also might be required aspects of the cancer constellation for the disease to occur in any single person. Put baldly, while a particular germ spawned cancer, it might operate in that fashion only when at least one representative of the appropriate auxiliary categories of phenomena accompanied that necessary microbe.

If that were not enough, the idea that cancer cases were increasing almost geometrically fortified the cancer-microbe nexus. Microorganism-borne diseases spread by contact with infected individuals and material. Physicians knew through experience that an unchecked germ would naturally filter its way through a susceptible population lacking means to defend itself. Since that situation occurred as a matter of course with diseases already linked to microbes, they naturally assumed it would be similar for cancer.[9]

Contagiousness fixed disease transmission, but explaining why cancer took root in specific organs or body parts required other metrics. Michael Worboys argued that the dominant exposition of this epidemiology model in Britain in the late nineteenth century was seed and soil. The seed—the germ—was necessary for every case of a disease, but soils—individual bodies—could be prepared in numerous different ways to enable the seed to get a foothold and sprout. Using Worboys's verbiage, then, "inflammation" gained currency in the late nineteenth century as a most prolific tiller of the soil in cancer cases. Inflammation was most frequently considered the consequence of a physical or mechanical phenomenon, akin to rubbing something raw. But inflammation was rarely rendered totally distinct from irritation, which contemporaries linked to things like smoking or making surfaces angry through heat or chemicals. Inflamed or irritated areas—damaged and therefore susceptible loci—became sites where germs of cancer invaded their victims. Both were posited as auxiliary factors for cancer, situations that acted in conjunction with the cancer microorganism to produce the disease.[10]

Inflammation and irritation justified why cancer was often found in specific sites and why some persons got the disease and others did not. Joseph Coats, pathologist at the Glasgow Western Infirmary, made the case simply when he explained how germs of cancer infiltrated organs. Believing that "a certain preparedness of the tissues must pre-exist" before cancer could occur, he accentuated inflammation—what he called "an imperfection of tissues"—as the logical place for germs to take hold. Coats postulated "that minute organisms belonging to the animal kingdom" burrowed their way into those distressed sites. There they entered "into the substance of the cells," where they underwent "their stages of evolution" and "produce[d] phenomena of a kind similar to those of cancer."[11]

G. Sims Woodhead, a member of the Royal College of Physicians, offered a more complicated position. It too relied on inflammation, but in Woodhead's analysis, the cancer bacteria caused the damage. He found that certain bacteria could act as irritants and spawn cancer if they persisted at a single locus for long periods of time. As living things, these germs underwent regular metabolic processes including "increasing in quantity and in activity." That biological activity produced constant irritation that created "proliferative changes" in cells and tissues at those very irritated sites. The result was cancer, a runaway multiplication of undifferentiated cells. Woodhead believed these special bacteria irritated cells, engendering a "proliferation of them at the expense of their functional power."[12]

More common than Woodhead's mechanical explanation was a chemical one. A specific type of microbe would, in perfectly normal cells, "induce new formations, not by a mechanical presence . . . but by the chemical changes incited by it." Cancer would be the consequence of these unidentified secretions, which yielded runaway cell growth.[13]

William Russell, fellow of the Royal College of Physicians of Edinburgh, adopted a microbial-induced chemical cancer explanation but added yet a different layer of complexity to the equation. Using the newest staining techniques, Russell identified a particle found in numerous cancers that readily accepted the fuchsine stain. These "fuchsine bodies," which he claimed were fungi closely related to yeast, were absent in roughly half the tumors he analyzed. To Russell, that did not cause a problem, even as it failed to achieve the standards set out in Koch's postulates. The answer lay in the properties of the fungi. Russell likened them to yeast, "an organism which from its very character implies the production of a fermentation product." What yeast did to sugar was analogous to what the Russell's fuchsine bodies did to healthy tissue. Yeast, he argued, produced "changes not disproportionate in magnitude to the anatomical changes present in cancer." Once those changes had occurred and cancer was running rampant, the fuchsine bodies might run out of metabolizable tissue and disappear. Researchers, therefore, would find the bodies in only some cancer cases.[14]

Russell's explanation adhered to the one necessary cause theory, but since the bacteria might die and disappear, it also made falsification extremely difficult. Those parameters were not without precedent in the realm of disease etiology. Louis Pasteur had proven that the saliva and spinal cords of rabid animals contained a "ferment" that regularly produced the disease in similar species. Physicians and others had long known that scabs from a smallpox victim could transmit the disease even though identifying the specific germ rested far outside contemporary view. These examples seemed to violate Koch's postulates that a pathogen need be repeatedly isolated, grown, and then given to a healthy individual to produce the disease in order to be identified as the true disease cause. In both instances, isolation, identification, and growth of the microorganism were not achieved. Yet scientists/physicians were not dissuaded from treating both of these diseases as being caused by specific germs. The one disease, one cause union remained such a fundamental fact of the then-contemporary disease exegesis that it could withstand almost any contrary observation.[15]

Powerful analogies—variola and rabies—rendered Russell's findings plausible by making the unusual possible and the invisible palpable. They were hardly the only mitigating factor when contemporaries evaluated Russell's claims. Cellular anatomy, morphology, and pathology seemed to offer potential corroboration. Microscopists were limited by the stains they employed. Some cells readily accepted specific stains, while other stains worked better on other types of cells. That was precisely the fuchsine body situation. But still other microbial cells, such as the tuberculosis mycobacterium with its waxy coating, proved quite difficult to stain. The upshot of this staining situation was anything but clear. Inability to find a microbe was not necessarily because it was not there. The microbe's relative invisibility could have been the product of the stains employed or the bacteria's unique properties.[16]

Or a version of the converse might be true. A. P. Ohlmacher tackled that aspect of the staining situation head on. In fact, he believed that the proliferation of cancer germ reports in Europe and America was directly attributable to the unfortunate consequences of the new micro-technical techniques—new stains and microtomy. Every day, he argued, "imperfectly digested contributions from investigators of all ranks of excellence" were published. "Almost every object which presents itself in the histological study" had been identified as the cancer germ by "over enthusiastic [*sic*] workers." This "mass of unscientific material . . . has brought the whole subject into ridicule." Rather than "increasing our knowledge . . . this worthless material" served "to burden and retard research."

Ohlmacher argued that staining itself produced distortions that misled investigators. Stains clarified and revealed extant structures, but they also produced uncountable false ones, the product of artificiality or contamination. Many of these proposed germs, he argued, were the artificial result of "a mixture of numerous reagents of unknown effect, the artificial products of the mechanical aids employed in gross and microscopic anatomy, and the artificial products of our optical appliances." To hammer his point home, Ohlmacher, professor of pathology and bacteriology at the University of Wooster, decided to stain various tumors with every stain then "in vogue among the carcinoma organism investigators." He reported on the extensive stain-dependent variation he found under the microscope. What he claimed he saw was a series of false products and bodies, simply the consequence of the new microscopy. Warning his fellow physicians of the profound dangers of the new microtomy, he proclaimed that these methods "can never, in themselves, aid us in solving the very important question of the etiology of malignant tumors."[17]

Such a diversity of perspectives and limitations of technique and ability proved an almost insurmountable obstacle to finding and then confirming cancer's etiology. H. G. Plimmer, a member of the Royal College of Surgeons and pathologist at St. Mary's Hospital, was undeterred by that criticism. He examined slides from 1,278 tumors and found among a few a proliferation of circular bodies. These bodies—soon known as Plimmer bodies—he believed to be the parasitic microorganisms that caused cancer. He carefully isolated these reputed cancer-producing organisms and injected them into rabbits and guinea pigs. In certain conditions and with certain procedures, Plimmer claimed to be able to transplant the cells that caused cancer in humans into animals and produce the disease there. He then maintained that he was able to isolate Plimmer bodies from the induced tumors and further inoculate rabbits and guinea pigs.[18]

Plimmer attributed his success to his inoculation techniques. He designed a way to introduce them into epithelial cells. Others failed to achieve Plimmer's results. While they frequently came upon the bodies he identified, they could not get these reputed microbes to induce cancer in the appropriate animals. There the matter stood. The truth remained incredibly murky. Were the bodies other investigators identified truly Plimmer bodies? Were the techniques used by other researchers absolutely identical to those employed by Plimmer? Were the animals involved in every way suitable?[19]

Ironically, Plimmer had been unable to confirm an investigator's cancer-producing microorganism experiments about five years earlier. That caused him much distress, although not because Plimmer was unsure of his methodological criticisms. The investigator in question, Alexis Korotneff, a professor at Kiev University, proposed that what became cancer actually existed in living organisms as an innocuous, commonly occurring form. Its cells turned malignant when vivified by a particular microorganism. Plimmer patiently attempted to reproduce Korotneff's experiments but found that "the staining reagents have not the reactions that Dr. Korotneff states" and that "his drawings do not correspond to the results he maintains he gets." In fact, Plimmer slammed Korotneff for his "methods of observation" as well as "interpretation," claiming that the Russian had "no true or logical basis" to make his claim.

Yet before he was willing to make these assertions in the professional, public discourse, Plimmer worried that he might be accused of being "guilty of presumption" for "criticizing . . . a worker in another branch of science." Forced to choose between his results and professional propriety, he did neither but instead sent his documented suspicions to Eli Metchnikoff, the discoverer of phagocytosis and a major figure in medical microbiology generally. Plimmer then published Metchnikoff's confirmation letter as an addendum to his study.[20]

The pains that Plimmer took to avoid directly criticizing a fellow scientist simply added yet another layer of uncertainty to the cancer quest. Strictures against professional disapproval of a fellow researcher's work, methods, and interpretations hampered falsification efforts and forced investigators to couch their disagreeable findings to seem diffident, even inconclusive. This patina of professional civility extended throughout the cancer germ search. It certainly tinged the debate of whether cancer microbes were only at the site of the infection or coursing throughout the body. The phenomenon around which this disagreement revolved was metastases, or several cancer sites in one patient. Did cancer invade the body all at once, as in the case of smallpox? Was each cancer site in an individual a unique and distinct "infection" or infestation, or did cancer germs break free from the initial site and travel through the blood or nerves to locate and work their nastiness elsewhere in the body? Why in a single individual did cancer appear in some organs and not others? Why was cancer susceptible to surgery sometimes and others not? Why did surgeons not frequently catch cancer from their patients? Could cancer be transplanted from one individual to another? In each of these instances, the Germ Theory of Disease writ large provided a model to explain the various phenomena but offered no wisdom on which of the several positions were ultimately correct.[21]

Almost nothing was objectively determined or even had a veneer of objectivity. Lack of a methodological or empirical discriminator encouraged each investigator to offer firsthand knowledge or insight on which of the possibilities appeared most likely. Indeed, that had been a primary purpose of medical societies, at least since the early nineteenth century.[22] Physicians met collectively on a regular basis to consider interesting or troubling cases. Cases were almost always brought by a single doctor, who would relate what he found curious or seminal. Discussion would go from there. This ritualized form of medical testifying often depended upon analogy. Physicians not only recounted their experience with the particular issue at hand, but also brought their observations from other diseases as a sure way to bolster their point. By using the known to suss out the unknown, analogy was often mistaken as confirmation.

Reputation, usually a concomitant of professional status, appeared to temper analogy. A researcher's prominence enhanced credibility; that person's argument appeared more persuasive and true. But a closer examination indicates that reputation was generally a product of clinical and research success.[23] And since there was no directly relevant clinical or research success—no one identified the germ of cancer—then status in that field was derived from success in a different field. For example, Koch was celebrated for his anthrax pathogen work well before he studied tuberculosis. But his identification of the tuberculosis mycobacterium catapulted his fame forward. Success in one arena seemed to increase the likelihood of success in a quite different research endeavor. Those individuals who had selected the most easily resolvable questions, either through serendipity or design, generally proved the most successful. But those who chose what proved to be more difficult or even impossible questions were no less skilled necessarily. They differed only in the blessings of Fortuna.

Again, Koch proves illustrative. His work on tuberculin as a remedy for tuberculosis drew plaudits from across the western world. The substance continued in use for an extended period simply because Koch had been "right" with his anthrax and tuberculosis mycobacterium work. It took nearly a decade for the enthusiasm that greeted tuberculin to die and for the great Koch to be identified in this case as a false prophet.[24]

Over the course of these decades, doctors and a variety of scientists identified dozens, if not hundreds, of specific bacteria, protozoa, parasites, cell vacuoles, or cell bodies as the sole germs of cancer. Europeans were most active advocates, especially in the region's leading medical centers of Vienna, Bologna, London, Berlin, and Edinburgh.[25] The sheer volume of cancer germs uncovered and the prominence of their discoverers itself became a problem. Woods Hutchinson, an English physician who taught at proprietary medical clinics in England and in medical colleges in the United States, laid the case bare. "Scores of observers have announced the discovery of 'parasites' in cancers," he noted, "but scarcely any two of them agree." Their descriptions range "all the way from the animal to the vegetable kingdom, from protozoa to bacteria." The "first work" of each "is to demolish the theories and disprove the existence of the parasites which have preceded his own." Chaos reigned. The "parasites" were declared to be "degenerated cells" or "other nuclei or cell-granules." Unlike common germs, few of these reputed cancer-causing suspects had proven "capable of cultivation outside the body." None "produce cancer in animals when injected in their tissues." To Hutchinson, "no parasite yet can be said to have survived a second or 'check' investigation by competent and entirely independent pathologists." The "germ-theory of the causation of cancer" was simply yet "not proven."[26]

Sentiments like Hutchinson's led these cancer-chasing investigators to embrace a series of other techniques to tease out various possibilities. They pondered the implications of the fact that women caught cancer far more frequently than did men. Cancer infected the breast and the uterus at a most frequent rate, far in excess of any other cancer site. They disagreed over which sex acquired cancer at a younger age. They debated whether the number of cancer cases was increasing, decreasing, or remaining the same. For all these investigations, inquisitors relied on the tried-and-true method of social statistics and statistical surveys. Statistics would generate new data that would lead to the necessary cause of cancer—the microorganism—or to an auxiliary condition, which together would be sufficient to engender the malady. These men and women demanded a sound, unambiguous conclusion; therefore, they sought refuge in numbers.

Medical staples since the early nineteenth century, these venerated, rudimentary statistical analyses promised to identify relationships and correlations hidden from casual view.[27] Researchers actively considered whether the Jewish, African, or Asian "race" caught cancer and whether certain places were rife with cancerous germs. These questions about cancer houses and the attempts to identify a group exempt from the disease harkened back to Europe's incidences of the Black Death in the fourteenth century and beyond and had become fundamental features of the anti-smallpox campaigns prior to the widespread introduction of vaccination. In that sense, these statistical categories used against cancer were less likely to reveal things unknown than to reaffirm discriminants already proven meaningful for other diseases. By drawing as they did on previous statistical work with other diseases in the search for cancer's cause, these men and women restricted themselves to the familiar. They unquestioningly assumed the situation in cancer analogous.[28]

More impressive were geographic surveys, almost topographical outlines, of land elevation, physical geography features, rainfall, and temperature used to determine where cancer most frequently resided. These repeated attempts echoed several hallowed epidemiological efforts, especially the battle to understand malaria and the attack on cholera. Both posited location as a predisposing cause—an auxiliary factor—of the disease. Both suggested that something in the locale engendered or fostered the disease. Both "proved" that moving residences from these plagued areas would prevent the disease in those able to flee the pestilential places.[29]

These cancer geographic surveys were of two types. The first focused on areas in the nation state that had markedly different cancer incidences. Epidemiologists scurried to find out what environmental factors set these places apart, what made these locales the sites and seats of cancer. But these studies were only as good as the statistics upon which they were based. Statisticians, record keepers, and residents of the areas all claimed that their data was superior and demanded that it become the basis of subsequent assessments. Each trumpeted their expertise. Statisticians examined change over time and claimed to identify arithmetically otherwise indistinguishable trends, record keepers extolled the accuracy and virtue of their recordings, and residents reported their tireless, often impressionistic observations, many of which had been accumulated over decades. Each brought their special talents to the table and demanded that these skills be employed as the basis of understanding. That itself was problematic, since the benefits of one method over any other were often not clear. These number crunchers were no more homogenous a group than the nascent cancer researchers of this period.[30]

Surveys of colonial lands seemed especially critical and constituted the second survey type. Colonies were explicitly foreign, different, a virtue in efforts to detect hidden connections. Inhabited by people visually different from Europeans, subject to climatic extremes, and populated by exotic flora and fauna, these places served turn-of the-century investigators functionally the way "sports of nature" and the New World did the seventeenth and eighteenth centuries. In both eras, exotica promised to expose through juxtaposition what was normal and what was possible. Investigators argued that, by virtue of their profound unusualness, colonial places revealed relationships that otherwise would have remained buried.[31] In effect, that presumption added another investigative dilemma to the cancer microbe quest. It privileged reports from physicians and others actually in these environs, thereby complicating questions of how to adjudicate among claims based upon different types of evidence developed by persons with different skill levels on data collected far away.

When it came to geographical surveys, correlations provided especially important clues. This was equally true both with surveys of America and Europe and of colonial and foreign lands. Even in these bows to empiricism, analogy remained central. In the 1890s, for instance, French physicians became enamored with what they determined was a crucial phenomenon—cancer rates seemed higher in woody, wet areas. Previous demographers had concentrated their attention on densely populated urban environs. An Alsace practitioner, Charles Fiessinger, was among the first to chastise his colleagues. "The topography of cancer," he argued, was "a friend of the loneliness and reveling along the course of water." The "frequency of cancer is set by its topography." Yet Fiessinger warned others about rushing to any sort of judgment. He did not want "assumed relationships" posited upon "coincidences." Men and women "too easily" make "associations" among "phenomena whose rationale eludes us."

Fiessinger recognized the one disease, one cause method ruthlessly pursued as the means to prevent folly. "Epidemiology—the science built on observation—" laid "the first stones . . . of reasoned consideration of the facts." Science had shown that both inner cities and damp rural spaces were ripe arenas for pathogenic microbes. In cities, means of possible contamination were obvious. Persons lived in intimate relations with each other. That was not the case in sparsely populated river valleys and woods. There, persons came in infrequent contact with others. Yet these men and women did share intimacy with living forms, plants and animals. He hypothesized that it was through closeness with nature that cancer microorganisms traveled to settlers. Analogy provided explanation. Researchers "had demonstrated that a microbe pathogenic for animals may become [so] for the plants." What was "more rational than to ask whether such an impact cannot be exercised in the reverse direction, if the agent harmful to the plant cell cannot become harmful for the animal cell?"[32]

Others picked up this thread and pointed to a fungus that infected plants, creating on them tumor-like projections. It was that fungus that they quickly implicated in human cancer. Subsequent investigations mimicked the essentials of Koch's postulates. Microscopists demonstrated that the fungus could be found in human tumor cells and, when injected into rabbits and dogs, soon killed them. The fungus could then be viewed as having invaded cells near insertion sites and was also recovered from the dead specimens. That proved proof enough for several physicians, and discussion persisted for years at provincial French medical societies.[33]

That theory made little headway outside of France. Demographic studies of other places provided inconclusive, even contradictory, results. Not all wet woodland areas had cancer spikes. Justifying why every damp, wooded area was not a cancer hotbed became a burden too great for the scheme ultimately to bear. But the French example was not the only statistically generated cancer explanation linking the disease to the environs. A similar sort of phenomenon occurred nearly a decade later in the United States. American investigators became quite interested in the relationship between trout and the disease. Statistical evidence indicated that cancer rates were significantly higher around fertile trout streams. Again, analogy functioned as the mechanism through which these scientists applied this understanding. Recent work in Cuba with yellow fever had confirmed that disease vectors—in that case, a particular type of mosquito—often served to spread "germs" from individual to individual. And at about the turn of the century, investigators posited rats as a critical host for the fleas that bore the bacilli of bubonic plague.[34] That trout-prolific areas also had high incidence of cancer implied a possible connection between the two seemingly disparate occurrences. Desperate epidemiologists felt compelled to follow up all leads.

Yet that was no easy matter. The vector hypothesis—the model that these investigators posited—depended on a relationship between the fish and human cancer. But just how would that relationship be consummated? How did the microbe travel from the fish to the person? Was it consumed? If so, then stream proximity may not have been as central as it initially appeared. There was no evidence that residents near trout streams ate more trout than other people or that those persons eating the greatest amount of trout were more likely to develop cancer. Did handling the fish transfer the cancer germ? Again, other studies, this time linking those who fished or prepared trout for consumption—chefs and homemakers—and incidences of cancer, needed to be undertaken. Yet this did not nearly exhaust possibilities. Perhaps both trout and people were affected by a third agent. The relationship between trout and human cancers might have stemmed from a common factor external and separate from either. In that instance, looking for a path between the two would have obscured the "true" situation.[35]

Geographic surveys carried with them a host of problems. Their chief virtue was their familiarity—they had been the basis for many of the successful sanitary measures of the mid- and late nineteenth century—and their ease of accomplishment. Those two factors were also significant vices. Surveys were a pre-microbial framework, one reliant on regular observation and categorization. These two techniques required no special abilities, just commitment. But the devil was ultimately in the details. What each of these survey results meant depended to a large degree upon context. For trout, a presumption of vectors would focus analysis in one area, while an old-fashioned reliance on predisposition would have emphasized rainfall, temperature, air pressure, type of vegetation, or other such environmental factors.

At the heart of these early statistical analyses rested the fundamental assumption that cancer was a solitary disease. A patient either had cancer or did not. There was no middle ground. The exact locus of cancer—where in the body the tumor resided—was of no particular interest; its location simply indicated what part of the body had been predisposed to the disease. Tumors of the salivary gland, lung, prostate, and breast were all cancer. In that sense, physicians and other statisticians treated cancer as analogous to other contagious diseases. Cholera was cholera, typhoid fever was typhoid fever, and tuberculosis was tuberculosis. Distinctions that might have been made among the preponderance of the site of cancer invasion and atmospheric/natural/social circumstances in that place (and any complications imposed by that view) did not figure prominently in assessments. Statisticians concentrated solely on the idea that each particular disease was caused by a specific identifiable pathogen. Where in the body the pathogen took root remained outside the microbe identification question as investigators focused directly on isolating and identifying that cancer-causing microbe.

Less popular but equally compelling for the cancer microbe search was the exciting discovery of toxin-antitoxin couplings and serum-antiserum reactions. There, the model for action was diphtheria. Physicians determined that, in the case of diphtheria, the bacteria did not cause visible illness per se. Instead, a toxin produced by the bacteria yielded the grave disease. The bacteria themselves seemed rather innocuous, but their toxin wreaked havoc on two critical body sites, the lymph glands of the throat and the nerves governing the heart. The first locus would cause a victim to smother, and the second could spark a fatal arrhythmia. Using the model of acid-base reactions, various medical men undertook a campaign to develop a substance to neutralize the poison and looked to individuals who survived the disease as potential repositories of that valuable substance. Producing that material in commercial quantities remained the last point.[36]

In cases of cancer, however, the actual germs that produced the toxin were not yet known. Investigators did the next best thing. They followed their epidemiological model. They applied to cancer cases the antitoxins and antiserums from other bacteria on the off chance that one or more would prove effective against the disease bacillus they could not yet identify. When that failed to bear fruit, they reversed the process. They gave various toxins to cancer patients, arguing that since these poisons affected healthy cells, tiny cancer germs might succumb to a lesser quantity of these venoms. Finally, they extracted various substances from cancerous tumors, chemically modified them and injected them in other tumors in expectation that they could create appropriate antitoxin substances. A similar sense of possibilities marked the work with Roentgen rays. X-rays damaged tissue. Therefore, cancer germs could be slain by non-lethal amounts of the deadly radiation, even if these invaders could not be isolated or identified.[37]

The diverse efforts to find the germ of cancer demonstrated just how creative these researchers had been. Yet that creativity was less impressive because all these men and women had been creative in precisely the same way. Their singular approach had reified, perhaps even deified, analogy as the pathway to scientific insight. To be sure, employment of a common model of pursuit—one disease, one cause—had helped foster dependence on analogy. But the method itself was more than defining; it contained some intrinsic obstacles and inherent barriers. How exactly do you disprove a hypothesis? The exact conduct of any experiment was always suspect outside of its immediate environs. What did an investigation pursued in Rome, Italy, and reported in a journal note in Cincinnati, Ohio, mean? What was done at the original research site? What questions were expressly considered and what conditions were actually involved in the experiment? How many scientists in how many different places must consider a hypothesis to falsify it? What if, as was most frequently the case, initial reports of verification attempts differed? In short, these men and women puzzled over in real time the fundamental issue of what makes something so. How is general acceptance—near unanimity—for a medico-scientific result achieved in an environment where the group to be convinced has few functional or occupational characteristics in common? What is needed for confirmation or refutation? Physicians and scientists remained definite that a cancer germ existed. Therefore, their constant pursuit of the germ led them to announce results as soon as they personally produced them. And since the quest was so broad and so encompassing, physicians and scientists in different places with many different talents and many different interests often identified different germs of cancer at the same time. There were then a number of cancer-producing microorganisms to rule out simultaneously.

These questions had no certain answers, an unacceptable situation in medical research of any kind. Methodologically pursued research demanded the luster of definitiveness. Hypotheses must be verified, confirmed, or falsified; there must be a result, a verdict. That approach was—and is—innately historical. A hypothesis needed a determination to move beyond it, to progress to the next stage or question. Questionable determinations constituted de facto bottlenecks, inhibiting further work. To overcome what was an intolerable consequence of the method they pursued, physicians and scientists involved in the cancer germ quest desperately sought mechanisms to make some things seem so and, therefore, become so.

Periodically since the 1870s, researchers had bemoaned the lack of concerted, coordinated action in cancer germ investigations. The making something so question—actually making something certain, or appear certain—loomed at the center of these laments. Without a central clearinghouse to gather, sort, and announce determinations with a single voice, uncertainty would remain rife. The discipline of conformity rather than the chaos of individual assessment appeared not simply desirable but indispensable to the cancer quest. Almost universally, these concerned researchers looked to the past. Their goal was imitation, not inspiration. They sought to create apparati that would function for cancer research questions the way that the Royal Society of London, the Academy of Sciences of Paris, the American Philosophical Society at Philadelphia, the Academy of Science at Berlin, and the Imperial Academy of Sciences at St. Petersburg did for science and invention generally.[38]

The initial thrust to enforce conformity, and therefore apparent certainty, involved adopting a method en vogue among medical societies after about 1880. These societies sought to conduct among their members what was in effect a medical plebiscite on disputed cancer questions. The profession, they reasoned, was a vast storehouse of relevant medical observations and experience. Attending physicians and their hospital counterparts served at bedsides, took medical histories, noticed the surroundings, watched the course of disease, attempted therapeutic or surgical remedies, conducted pathological examinations, and engaged in necropsies. These doctors were de facto on-site investigators. Each was intimately involved in the details of numerous cases, albeit on his own terms. These regularly occurring observations generated considerable raw, not necessarily comparable, data. What remained was to standardize, secure, and assemble these bedside observations and experiences to reveal what the profession had uncovered en passant.

Gathering experience and making these observations consistent and therefore comparable—systematizing research results—was their aim. Medical organizations had created investigative or collaborative committees to do that very thing, but generally with diseases deemed epidemic, such as diphtheria or tuberculosis. In both those and other similar cases, the committees compiled a set of questions based on disputed points or questionable events. They then publicized their queries widely in both medical and scientific periodicals. In every case, they provided a template, often as simple as a card with a series of boxes or a tabular form, for individual doctors to report in regularized, standardized fashion their narratives about the course and cause of disease. The committee would then systematically amass the information and report to the organization on a regular basis. In effect, these committees established their societies as indispensible to disease fighting, while at the same time compelling member physicians and other practitioners to adopt a similar framework to report their unique experiences. The committee then would be the repository of these systematized—through standardized accumulation—narratives, experiences, and observations. In this case, collective reportage would be used to make something so and identify possible deterministic situations or conditions.[39]

An analogous onslaught against cancer seemed promising. Collaborative committees asked practitioners if their medical histories and experience detected any discernible relationships among geography, topography, and incidence of cancer or uncovered any relationship between incidences of cancer and family members (investigations into both heredity and contagion); if the number of cancer cases and the number of cancer deaths were increasing, declining, or staying the same; and whether in their experience irritation and inflammation, such as "nervous tension," could account for the higher incidence of cancer among women, especially of the uterus and breast. Follow-up questions ensued. For example, the committee attempted to clarify the women-and-cancer question by asking if the occurrence of "female" cancers was similar in married and unmarried women.[40]

Two French medical men, Simon Duplay and Emile Henri Ozenne, launched a different but not fundamentally dissimilar effort. They established in 1896 a medical journal devoted entirely to reports about cancer. Both situated at the Hôtel-Dieu and members of the Society of Surgeons of Paris, as well as the Academy of Medicine of France, they undertook their project precisely because they were frustrated by the disorganized state of affairs. "Everywhere in France and abroad" medical men daily published numerous reports on cancer. Yet its "etiology, pathogenesis and treatment" remained in question. Their goal was not to spur new cancer studies. It was to gather information already being pursued in one place, "to provide as complete a summary as possible" of cancer papers "published in France and in other countries." This endeavor required "the goodwill" of their "colleagues in Paris and the province," and they called on their fellow medical men in France to scrutinize all reports about cancer both in French and foreign medical journals. The group would then summarize the most important and provide bibliographic information about those case studies deemed less critical. The result would be nothing less than the "centralization of all work relating to cancer." The work would reveal otherwise indistinguishable patterns, a situation that could assist in revealing the necessary cause of cancer or its auxiliary elements. It would thus replace mystery with certainty.[41]

Despite the initial promise, neither the French journal nor the collaborative committees achieved the cancer germ-determining results their partisans anticipated. The problem did not rest with participation or collaboration, however. What mattered was that the types of bedside scrutiny undertaken by attending physicians themselves lacked the definitiveness necessary to make things so in the case of cancer. It was not simply that perceptiveness among physicians varied. Rather, the kinds of things being measured were inconsistent. The medical history of any patient proved virtually unique; circumstances surrounding each case of disease were particular, and therefore any attempt to pool them collectively necessitated interpretation. Observations, experience, and narrative were all inherently subjective. Chaos remained because what was measured and how it was measured remained open to individual assessment and not collective wisdom. Increasingly, medical leaders argued that only controlled conditions and environments would provide the key evidence necessary to pinpoint the germ of cancer. Bedside observations must be formalized, standardized, and systematized.

Recognition of the necessity for standardized, precise bedside conditions and spaces dedicated expressly to the search for cancer germs ran counter to how the medical profession traditionally undertook investigations. Individual practitioners or institutional physicians reported their experiences and observations as part of their normal duties, treating the sick. Collective investigations, reporting cases to medical societies or in medical journals, and recording observations and formulating theories were ad hoc occurrences, produced in the course of the very activities that produced revenue—healing the sick and managing disease.

Communal efforts among physicians and medical societies to determine cancer's cause remained consistent with the one cause, one culprit theory of disease causation. But while the systematic assembling of the bedside data voluntarily generated by individual physicians in the course of their practices was sufficient to detect the cause of many other maladies, that same approach to cancer's etiology brought medical practitioners no closer to an explanation for the disease. Analogous practice failed to point to cancer's cause.

The French cooperative initiative among medical men established practitioners as valid and interested partners in the quest for cancer but pointed to the work yet to be done. Physicians' reporting—observations, forms, categories, and more—needed standardization and systematization for house calls to help identify cancer's necessary cause or one or more of its possible auxiliary but required factors. When that occurred throughout the medical community, it appeared inevitable to these practitioners that information essential to discovering cancer's cause would emerge.

2

Making Something So within a Nationalist Context

Cancer Laboratories, 1899–1905

Not everyone was as cocksure as practitioners of the wisdom of relying on statistical determinations derived from bedside observation to determine the cause of cancer. Part of the hesitation stemmed from the nature of medical practice. Doctors in the course of their normal activities, either at bedsides or in hospitals, could not readily develop the standardized techniques and systematized routines required to pinpoint the cancer microbe. What might be necessary was to pursue cancer systematically, in a tightly controlled space and under meticulous conditions. Laboratories were such places where conditions could be standardized. There the question would be out of the hands of physician practitioners, placed squarely in the province of laboratory researchers. Research in a precise environment, which included the creation and maintenance of disciplined space, could be mandatory to unlock cancer's secrets.

Laboratories existed, of course, but none was devoted entirely to cancer. Extant laboratories already had definitive tasks. A cancer laboratory would be a new invention, a disciplined space staffed with men and women pursuing but one task—the cause of cancer.

Such a grandiose vision required new personnel trained in the various disciplines involved in laboratory science and in what would become cancer research. It necessitated new facilities, new equipment, new administration. These new laboratories could not easily be subvened through the traditional way—patient charges or state contracts for primary or custodial care facilities. Attending physicians could not be in effect taxed to establish facilities that would replace them as central agents in the cancer quest. States were not likely to assist. Attempts to get states expressly to pay for medical research usually failed. As a member of Britain's House of Commons wrote, "the medical profession lives upon the public; the medical profession makes use of its knowledge to extract money from the public." Therefore, any state grant to create new knowledge would simply result in "money drawn from the pockets of the public to aid in the further depletion of the pockets of the public."[1]

In the late 1890s, Roswell Park overcame these obstacles. He developed a justification that the threat of cancer germs was so profound and immediate that cancer itself constituted a public health emergency. A surgeon affiliated with the Buffalo Medical School and one of two physicians who would minister to the fatally shot President William McKinley, Park galvanized state action when he produced statistics demonstrating that the Buffalo area had the highest incidence of cancer anywhere in the United States. Park, moreover, was convinced of cancer's infectiousness; citing microbial studies of syphilis, tuberculosis, and leprosy, he argued that "so many analogies between cancer" and these other diseases "known to be infectious" existed "to almost convict" cancer as an infectious malady. He therefore warned that identifying the "contagium vivum" that caused the dread disease constituted the highest public duty. Park's contention and his assertion that Buffalo led the nation in cancer cases alarmed the legislature, which followed its tradition of sponsoring extraordinary measures to battle epidemics by authorizing a state-financed cancer research laboratory within the medical college. The governor vetoed the measure, citing precedents similar to those offered by the House of Commons. In 1897, the next year, Park added another fearful statistic to the mix. He argued that if investigators did not find the cancer germ quickly, the number of cancer deaths in New York would in a decade dwarf the deaths of all other epidemic diseases combined. The legislature passed the Park bill later than year. Public pressure forced the governor to sign it.[2]

Officially named the New York State Laboratory for the Investigation of Cancer, Park's cancer laboratory became the home to well-appointed investigators, versed in the latest reports about cancer microorganisms. Researchers there would not be confined to observations at the bedside. Instead, they could attempt to produce the disease; they could initiate experiments and observe them in a controlled space. For each fresh tumor removed, the staff engaged in "a most careful study of the pathological and histological elements." They then pursued "a carefully conducted bacteriological examination with systematic endeavor to cultivate in every known culture medium whatever living parasites that may be obtained." They concluded every analysis by undertaking the "most minute investigations into physiological chemistry, including chemical and spectroscopic analysis of secretions."

These investigations were conducted in beakers, on plates or in petri dishes, or with animals, controls not subject to the vicissitudes of human life and living. They could be tracked and traced. Any circumstance investigators desired could be created. Tests could be conducted under definitive conditions and produce predictable results. Things could be made to seem so.

Or so it seemed to Park. Within six months of its opening, he proclaimed the experiment a resounding success. While noting that any "systematic report" would be "premature and unfortunate," he termed the laboratory's results "almost startling, or even dramatic." In almost every tumor, investigators found "bodies which cannot be other than parasites present in vast numbers." The "life history" of these germs was studied there "both by culture and inoculation." Outcomes proved "exceedingly satisfying . . . and exceedingly promising," so much so that Park believed anyone who observed this work would have "no doubt" that "cancer is unmistakably a parasitic, i.e., an infectious disease."[3]

Park's grandiose claims and bold gambit in securing governmental assistance for a specifically appointed cancer laboratory drew considerable interest. Often referred to as "the scientific study of cancer" to mark it as distinct from practitioner efforts, it sparked a profound spate of imitation as groups demanded analogous institutions in other localities. For example, the American Public Health Association applauded New York's effort to grant "an annual appropriation for the establishment and maintenance of a laboratory with all the modern appliances for the persistent prosecution of studies in the etiology of cancer." It then called for "state and national patronage" to "universally establish . . . special and general scientific research." Indeed, Americans recognized the originality of the Buffalo laboratory and took every opportunity to celebrate its creation and to define it as characteristically American. George H. Simmons, editor of the *Journal of the American Medical Association* in 1899, claimed that cancer laboratories now marked "the American phase of cancer investigation." J. Riddle Goffe, editor of *Medical News,* predicted that "American enterprise and inventive ingenuity" would prove successful "in the problem that so far puzzled the medical world." Harvey R. Gaylord, first science director of Park's lab, contended that up to this point "the Italian school" led the quest for cancer germs, but he felt confident that America, because of its new cancer labs, would soon assume worldwide leadership.[4]

The celebratory Americans were not alone in recognizing the virtues of their artificial creation. The Cancer Society of London sent an envoy in 1899 "to study the American methods" of the Buffalo laboratory. When he returned, the society attempted to get the British government to establish a cancer facility—"a real research commission"—to "enable skilled investigators to devote their entire attention to the investigation . . . for two or three years." The British government refused, but the Foreign Service promised to secure for British use copies of any reports authored by the Buffalo laboratory. While gaining access to these reports likely cheered some, others remained steadfast and "severely censored the refusal" to establish a British cancer lab.[5]

London's Middlesex Hospital did more than complain. It received a large bequest to establish a cancer ward and demanded that a portion of this funding go to the creation of "pathological and bacteriological laboratories" there. At this "well-equipped" site, "the carefully recorded and systematic work of highly trained investigators" would produce "work of the highest scientific character." A hospital-based "Cancer Investigative Committee" would oversee the work.[6] Even with the impressive new laboratory infrastructure, however, partisans recognized that progress would not be immediate. Thomas H. Wakely, editor of the august *Lancet*, perhaps Britain's premier medical journal, argued that the "patiently and laboriously" conducted research would take "years" for "any real or substantial advance" to occur.

Even though he appreciated that any breakthrough would take time, Wakely steadfastly championed the cancer laboratory idea. His enthusiasm for these new ventures stemmed from a certain pessimism about the status quo. For years, "men of the highest ability" had undertaken "the most exhaustive observations on the clinical aspects" of cancer and "in its various forms and geographical distribution." These had been "carefully recorded and published." But that approach was at a dead end. Little more could be gleaned from that data. Given the "very great public interest" in cancer and the weekly "imagined discovery" appearing in print, a dramatic new approach was necessary.[7]

Wakely recognized that clinical and statistical investigations had run their course. Observations and numbers could not accomplish the cancer task. They lacked the clarity and certainty that laboratory investigation promised; they could not make something so. Without a scientist-accepted certainty—a certainty based upon a perception that the non-analogous situation of a rigidly controlled laboratory environment replicated the natural world and that experiments conducted there were reproducible—the science of cancer's microbe would not progress. Researchers would continue to bicker—public disagreements hurt reputations of partisans and their kindred professionals—and to provide contradictory evidence and theories, as there existed no clear, universal means to adjudicate the disparate contentions. Determining the cause of cancer would become a pipe dream.

The editor of the *Boston Medical and Surgical Journal*, George B. Shattuck, agreed on the need for a bold new approach. "All possible methods of statistical inquiry have been employed" to determine cancer's "causation." The "association with certain geographic and geological conditions and mortality statistics have [*sic*] been tabulated." The days of physician-led demography were past. Now, a new attack was necessary. "The microscope and all the resources of the laboratory" must focus on "the problem of its origin and development." This was especially so because "pathological study" pointed "strongly toward the parasitic origin of cancer." Indeed, the laboratory "in the near future" will furnish "the remaining steps to the proof of the parasitic origin of cancer." He pointedly referred to Park's Buffalo laboratory as already producing research "of sufficient value to demonstrate the wisdom of such enlightened action by legislative bodies." Such research, he concluded, requires a laboratory "endowment and equipment." Gaylord said it even more clearly: "Scientists, as a rule, are peculiarly skeptical on the subject of statistics." In the case of cancer research, "I think it almost impossible to prove anything of importance from them."[8]

Soon after Shattuck published his plea, Harvard received a bequest from the estate of Caroline Brewer Croft, a prominent English woman, to erect its own cancer laboratory. This laboratory in 1902 became a designated section of the new Collis P. Huntington Laboratory of Pathology and Bacteriology. Beneficence as well as state sponsorship could fund cancer laboratories. The late Huntington had been a railroad and shipping magnate, notably involved in the transcontinental railroad; his friends, including industrialists J. P. Morgan and John D. Rockefeller, built the facility. Under direction of John Warren, chief of surgery, the new cancer laboratory exclusively sought the cancer germ. Columbia University in New York City opened its own cancer laboratory in 1902, when Huntington's wife established a cancer research fund in his name at the city's General Memorial Hospital. Disappointed by the failure to identify a specific causative cancer microorganism, its board left "the beaten track" and decided to attack the problem by analyzing what seemed likely products of those microbes, the "chemical constituents of tumors." Seeking "deeper insight" into "the processes involved" in the pathogenic invasion that produced cancerous lesions, the fund employed scientists from Cornell University's Loomis Laboratory to do the requisite analyses.[9]

The metastatic growth of cancer laboratories in the United States meant that more investigators had access to the latest equipment and techniques. But traditional clinical and statistical research did not go quietly into the good night. Local and national medical societies continued to debate and consider traditional cancer questions. Was the disease increasing everywhere? In the first few years of the new century, demographers in Prussia,

Saxony, Baden, Hamburg, and Augsburg in Germany; Essex, Birmingham, Dundee, North Bedfordshire, Scotland, and Ireland in the United Kingdom; Sweden, Holland, and Norway in Scandinavia; Italy, Greece, Spain, Russia, Hungary, Spain, Portugal, and Paris in Europe; Tunis, Algeria, Morocco, and Egypt in Africa; and New Zealand, India, and Australia in British Asia and Oceania all weighed in affirmatively on that question.[10] As significant, demographic cancer investigators began to break down those large discriminants in several ways. They disaggregated data by gender to show that women generally had twice the incidence of cancer as men. But the same statisticians noted that, when cancer of the breast and the female reproductive organs were ruled out, cancer rates for men and women were similar, a phenomenon reported in country after country. At what rate Jews caught cancer also focused attention. Some found cancer rates among the People of the Book low and attributed it to refusal to eat pork. Others disagreed and argued for other factors. This was especially true in London. Some there found the preponderance of Jews living in squalid conditions and contended that, since cancer was a disease of the upper classes, correlating those rates with the non-Jewish poor would demonstrate no discernible difference in cancer rates. Others suggested that the Jews of London were significantly younger than the non-Jewish population and that, since cancer rates were more pronounced in the aged, the figures for Jews were in line with others so young. Still others claimed that the rate of cancer among Jews was identical to their Gentile brethren.[11]

India also seemed rife for statistical analysis of cancer. Its massive poverty, dark peoples, relentless climate, high incidence of malaria, and non-beef– and non-pork–eating populations each seemed a way to demarcate and distinguish groups, which could then be assessed for their comparative cancer rates.[12] Indeed, statistical studies remained especially prevalent in England, where the Galton Institute and Karl Pearson had done so much to establish the utility of statistical analysis in biological issues. There, almost anything seemed possible. Alfred Wolfe, a London physician, for example, attempted a statistical correlation of cancer death rates worldwide. Relying on official records, correspondence, and just plain figuring, Wolfe tried to identify a number of discriminants as not simply meaningful but critical in the fight against cancer.[13]

Not all English statisticians took a global view. While some considered alcohol as increasing cancer mortality or recognized differential cancer rates among occupations, several posited a concrete relationship between prevalence of flooding in the Thames Valley and the region's high incidence of cancer. They concluded that this moist, damp, dark area provided a potent demonstration of the likelihood of a cancer microorganism. They reasoned that fungi and other microbes grew especially well in conditions not unlike those of the flooded valley and hypothesized that accelerated cancer rates were directly attributable to the favorable growing conditions for the hypothetical pathogen.[14]

Perhaps because of their sheer numbers, statisticians and clinicians retained public visibility even as cancer research shifted to the laboratory. Counting and parsing or recounting years of bedside experience were double-edged swords. On one hand, those attributes allowed doctors and sanitarians to continue to engage in the cancer quest, which furthered public approbation. But those very qualities that enabled them to participate also made their participation anachronistic. There were no simple methods to adjudicate among their contentions. They lacked a means to make things so. They could not defer to number use. Their involvement was invaluable to gain public support, which meant bequests and other donations. But the absence of a viable determinant among their claims rendered their studies quite insufficient.

Germany, the worldwide leader in the laboratory idea generally, planned in 1900 its first cancer laboratory. It too understood the political power of physicians and statisticians and designed its cancer effort to capitalize on these numbers. Leyden, who had studied with Johann Lukas Schonlein, an early parasitologist, and had been a colleague of Paul Ehrlich, who perfected aniline tissue staining and worked extensively with Robert Koch on tuberculosis, pioneered the effort. He called together the chairman of the National Insurance Institute, the head of the Prussian Statistical Bureau, the director of the Statistical Office of Berlin, an official of the Ministry of Culture, the Berlin city council sanitarian, the physician to the Royal Police Bureau, and a representative of the Imperial Health Office to form the Comité für Krebsforschung (Committee for Cancer Research). Operating under a 500 mark gift from the National Insurance Institute, the group coalesced because each participant represented a constituency that was appalled by the nation's apparent cancer increase. Leyden set the agenda. The group would bring together all forms of information on cancer; it would centralize and systematize each and every cancer effort. To that end, the Comité invited virtually every conceivable group to participate—medical societies and congresses, town and country doctors, police, statisticians, actuaries, governmental ministers, and many more. To the Comité, cancer was clearly a public health question, and prevention of the disease through statistical analyses and other means dominated its thinking.

The new venture did not confine its work to Germany. The group aimed to bring the world's cancer knowledge to Germany under the Comité's banner. With Leyden as president, the organization established two vice presidents—one from the advisory board to Imperial Health Office and the other from the oversight board to the Ministry of Religious, Educational, and Medical Affairs. That latter group controlled German universities, medical schools, and societies of physicians. Koch, Virchow, and five others were named honorary members. The nine so-designated foreign members included three from England, two from France, and one each from Russia, Japan, Egypt, and the United States. Plimmer, Metchnikoff, and Gaylord fell in that category. Sixty-two others were simply designated members, including Park. Without exception, persons chosen for membership received invitations due to their cancer research history.[15]

Leyden set the group's focus neatly. Certainly the insurance industry's intimate involvement in the Comité colored its mission and ambition. The group's goal was to reduce cancer risk and cancer injury at least as much as to determine cancer's cause. Leyden argued that a cancer cure was far off and that to labor in that direction squandered limited resources. Prophylaxis was more immediately possible. That goal required but two things: accurate knowledge of the disease's distribution and the means through which individuals acquired cancer. The disease's distribution cried out for collective research—the gathering of "reports" by doctors and sanitarians according to specific categories as defined on easy-to-tabulate cards. This effort would resolve "the matter of heredity, of transmission, age and professional relationships, questions of the influence of climate, employment, and of city and country."[16]

Eventually over 60 percent of German medical men participated in the cooperative data collection process. Many used Comité-designed "census forms for collective research." Extensive voluntary involvement by physicians and statisticians in this "who gets cancer" question reflected both the public interest in finding a suitable answer and the authority of insurance money.[17] But it remained the means by which persons acquire cancer that galvanized Leyden's attention. He rejected as failed any of the theories of abnormal cell formation, atypical cell proliferation, or damaged nuclei and contended that they offered no fruitful insights. The only theory consistent with the "facts, observation and today's biological theories" was the "parasitic nature of cancer." It was around that theory that Leyden called for cancer laboratories.[18]

The Comité itself engaged in no research. It existed instead to "encourage and to assist financially research work in immediate connexion [*sic*] with the causation of cancer, to collect and tabulate information bearing on the subject and to further . . . scientific knowledge" of the disease. Clearly, the organization positioned itself to lead. Its offices were in the Interior Ministry building in Berlin, and the group received a stipend to conduct its centralizing and systematizing activities.[19]

Leyden's laboratory was one of two German laboratories at which much of this Comité-approved research occurred. He explained its genesis as a consequence "of the new pathological view, which had been founded by Louis Pasteur and Robert Koch." These men had established "parasitism of diseases" as "scientific fact." The Germ Theory initially "spread slowly but with irresistible force." Its impact had been so great that "even when science was unable to find the pathogenic germ" for a particular disease, scientists now "presume the culprit will be quickly discovered." It "has become that way for cancer," a situation his new laboratory would address.[20]

Ehrlich led the other cancer laboratory, which was established at the Emperor's urging. Imperial support did not translate into money, however. Ehrlich's Frankfurt-located facility hunted the cancer microorganism entirely with funds developed through beneficence. Leyden's main source of revenue was different. He headed a special thirty-four–bed cancer ward at Berlin's Charity Hospital and received 53,000 marks per year to operate the ward and care for patients. Leyden merely diverted a significant portion of the funds to run his lab and to employ the requisite staff.[21]

Leyden then semi-clandestinely used government money to fund cancer research. He was not being hypocritical in this endeavor. He and the other Comité members generally backed direct government support for cancer laboratories as consistent with legitimate and long-standing governmental duties. Their argument was simple. Governments had the obligation to protect citizens, whether from foreign armies or foreign microbes. Determining cancer's microbial cause would enable the state to prevent the disease in many people. It was not a matter of curing or treating that they espoused; those activities rightly remained the province of medical doctors. The Comité urged only a straightforward matter of defense and called on the state to mobilize laboratories to find the cause of cancer to end the invasion of the dread disease.

Several in the Prussian House of Lords supported Leyden's contention and urged their colleagues in the chamber to fund cancer research. They never constituted a majority. The Comité's labors spawned similar institutional efforts in the Netherlands, Hungary, Russia, and Spain. Indeed, reports claimed that Russia had raised over 700,000 rubles for a cancer hospital/laboratory facility from prominent citizens even before it was built. In 1902, the

Comité published *Verhandlungen des Comité für Krebsforschung* to share the activities of its first two years with a wider audience. One year later, it created a full-fledged cancer research journal, *Zeitschrift für Krebsforschung*.[22]

The Comité's explanation for publishing the specialized journal hinted at the make something so question. A periodical devoted entirely to cancer research had become necessary because cancer investigators and their publications "were scattered over the whole world." It had become virtually impossible for any single person to keep up. In particular, the question of cancer's etiology remained to be adjudicated. Any single research effort could tip the balance. It "could highlight a new direction" and take cancer investigations "out of the prevailing darkness."[23]

To make things so and to get leverage on cancer, place after place, nation after nation created analogous institutions. Each new enterprise downplayed the bedside and attending physicians for single-purpose controlled space—cancer laboratory space—and persons adept in precision techniques—laboratory techniques. Each tackled only cancer, no other malady. Each gained impetus to a large degree because of the uncertainty surrounding the quest for the cancer microbe. Creation of similar institutions in place after place and staffed by similarly trained men and women demonstrated that the cancer germ crusade was of profound public interest. But this public interest did not always result in funding from the public purse. Benevolence, the great tradition of private giving for public purposes, provided moneys for many of these early cancer research facilities.

England's seminal effort proved among the most interesting and successful. This effort initially devolved from the Middlesex Hospital cancer laboratory, which had such a difficult time raising funds that it took out an ad in the London *Daily Mail* "earnestly solicit[ing] . . . subscriptions and donations." Henry Morris, chief of surgery at the hospital, member of the Royal College of Surgeons, and overseer to the new laboratory, was acutely concerned about the laboratory's financial plight. He also worried about the state of the cancer search in the United Kingdom. Several investigators working in non-specialized research or pathological laboratories—Russell in Edinburgh and Plimmer at St. Mary's, for instance—prosecuted cancer germ research but had presented antagonistic results.[24]

Fear that these medical men would continue to work at cross purposes—Russell and Plimmer had already had public dustups over the cancer-causing microbes they brought forth—and lack of reliable funding troubled Morris. Organization, systematization, and getting disparate laboratory results presented publicly as if with one voice were essential facets of making something so. Laboratory stability, to a great degree the consequence of consistent, dependable funding, and reduction of unnecessary research expenses generated through duplication at competing labs were Morris's keys to success in the cancer germ crusade. These several goals could be reconciled in a single, privately funded central agency in the United Kingdom assembled precisely for "systematizing and procuring endowment for research upon cancer."[25]

Opportunity presented itself in October 1901. Morris learned of a movement with potential donors to establish an experimental cancer treatment clinic in London. Always the surgeon, Morris contended that recent strides in surgery rendered the proposal obsolete; surgery to remove cancer was a patient's best option. He maintained instead that for cancer "the only immediate prospect of gaining new knowledge of any value was by laboratory research." Armed with the name of a large donor, Morris brought the matter before a special finance committee of the Royal Colleges of Surgeons and Physicians, which agreed with Morris's sentiments but deemed that the new experiments all be held at "the laboratories belonging to the Royal Colleges."[26]

That proposal resolved few if any of the issues that had mobilized Morris. The new Middlesex Hospital cancer lab would remain in financial trouble and the laboratories in the nation would persist in their frequent bickering and separate paths; the colleges' proposal would not make something so.

Death of the largest and most likely potential benefactor gave the various sides pause. The colleges now refused to assent to their original plan, for fear of being held financially responsible for all expenses. Both the king and the Prince of Wales offered their verbal support to the lab measure but declined to offer any financial backing until other benefactors could be found to establish the venture on solid footing.[27]

The Lancet's Wakely emerged as a potent force in carrying the matter forward. He surveyed other nations and found that, there, the cancer microbe "was actively pursued." Claiming that England was "behindhand," Wakely pointed explicitly to Park's lab, Germany, and Italy as laboratories already "in full activity." It is "quite time," Wakely concluded, "that this country should bestir itself."

Negotiations among the various parties continued behind the scenes. Morris pushed for a plank that the new institution would be permitted financially to "assist in the development of the Cancer Research Department of Middlesex Hospital and . . . any other . . . special cancer department," a necessary requirement in gaining a foothold over all the requisite cancer research institutions in the quest to make something so. Without coordination by a central authority, disorganization would remain the rule.[28]

With matters at a standstill, the House of Commons considered appointing a Royal Commission on Cancer. While that proposal drew some support, Alfred Balfour, First Lord of the Treasury and leader of the House of Commons, quashed the idea. He argued that, while government had a responsibility to its citizens, preventing cancer by establishing its parameters and cause was a matter best left to science. In typical droll English understatement, he urged his colleagues to "leave the matter in the hands of the medical profession" as "the number of great scientific discoveries . . . made by royal commissions has been very limited."[29]

The king himself weighed in on the subject. He sent a message to the Royal Colleges of Physicians and Surgeons declaring himself greatly interested in the prevention of cancer and pronounced himself "glad" that they were "taking up the question of cancer research." Coupled with the threat that Parliament might create its own commission, the memo galvanized the colleges, and they elected a committee "to draw up a detailed scheme" for "investigation into the causes, prevention, and treatment of cancer."[30]

Wakely offered harsh criticism of the colleges' subsequent proposition. He looked at the proposed committee membership and found it "partly composed of ex officio" members of the colleges. These people were not scientists and therefore not "in any way specifically qualified" to create a "scheme for the organized investigation of cancer." He feared that whatever money they raised "would not be wisely spent" because the committee would not choose the most "suitable men in the most perfect methods of scientific research."[31]

Wakely's objections fell on deaf ears. The English institution that finally emerged was to have a rock-solid, well-articulated footing with numerous governmental and political ties. Five trustees—members of Parliament—would solicit research funds and invest them. The presidents and censors of the Royal College of Surgeons and of the Royal College of Physicians, members of the laboratory committees of both organizations, and a representative of the nation's health officers would decide on what projects the interest would be spent. These men would also champion a central office and laboratory in London to coordinate the work nationwide and to conduct research of its own.[32]

Enabling the committee to grant funding to cancer laboratories not under direct control of the colleges, such as that at Middlesex Hospital, gave the body great latitude in what labs it supported and thus the potential to organize cancer research nationwide. Its authority to create a central office and laboratory cemented that bond. The committee established that office as the first among equals. It would stand as the arbiter of cancer research in the United Kingdom and the bully pulpit from which things could be announced as so.

Dawson Williams, editor of the well-regarded *British Medical Journal*, celebrated the new organization. To this point, Williams remembered, "research on cancer . . . has been left . . . to private enterprise." The work has been "intermittent, and sometimes misdirected, owing to ignorance." The "want of co-ordination has led to great waste of power." Now, cancer will be prosecuted "in this country by the systematic and co-ordinated efforts of a body of specially skilled investigators." This new organization can "collect the scattered rays of research, and focus them on a given point." In particular, he pointed to the new body's commitment to the "establishment of a system of intercommunication with workers in other countries." Cancer research will be greatly enhanced when "the observations made in every recognized laboratory were regularly communicated to others all over the world." Williams concluded by noting that Balfour had stated that "combination is one of the characteristics of our time." Before formation of this cancer organization, that remained "a power that had never yet been fully utilized in scientific research."[33] It was the power to make things so.

Although somewhat different that the non-English organizations in form, the new cancer fund's goal was identical. F. W. Tunnicliffe, professor of materia medica at King's College and a member of the Royal College of Surgeons, added to the case that the new institution was critical because of the making something so question. "Theories are abundant," he contended, "when facts of unmistakable significance are wanting." Explanations of cancer causation "express one enigma in terms of another." What was necessary, Tunnicliffe maintained, was not observation, "which has yielded up to the observer almost all the information it can do," but rather "pathological experiment." "New and important truths should be sought" by experiment, for there is where progress "will probably be found."[34]

The fact that Balfour, now prime minister, presided over the initial meeting of the Cancer Research Fund—Morris became its treasurer—demonstrated just how critical the English deemed the new institution. It also added de facto governmental sanction, recognition that cancer prevention constituted a legitimate public obligation. Balfour and the nation's leading physicians addressed their countrymen, pleading for contributions to find "the cause and nature of the mysterious disease which has hitherto baffled the greatest physicians." In every instance, however, medical men assured their audience that those goals would prove elusive for only a short time before physicians conquered "this terrible bane of mankind."[35]

The Prince of Wales chaired subsequent meetings, a sign that his father,

King Edward, was "greatly interested" in the work. E. F. Bashford, who had worked in Ehrlich's Frankfort cancer laboratory, became the savvy director of the new laboratory. He contacted other similar labs and attempted to divide up the scientific cancer work. "Collaboration," not redundancy or competition, was to rule the day. Each facility was called on to stake out a facet of the work and to avoid duplication. Indeed, Bashford looked at cancer research as if it were a single grand enterprise—one big laboratory—that could be cut into facets and conducted separately from the other facets.[36]

In the first few years, the various laboratories upgraded their physical plants and more neatly established their characteristic agendas. Park's lab moved in 1902 into a new building. The first floor was nothing more than laboratory space, a great central laboratory and several small private labs. The second floor contained the library, Gaylord's private lab, the chemical laboratories, and private offices. The bacteriological laboratory—which Gaylord defined to include "the study of other minute forms of life"—and an incubation room, as well as a complex for photography—dark room, a room with a skylight, and a room for photomicrography—were on floor three. Williams pronounced the lighting of all laboratories "perfect" and maintained that they were "all fitted with modern appliances." Like Bashford, Park favored coordination among cancer laboratories. He sent a staff member to tour the cancer laboratories of Europe and to exchange information. Gaylord too ventured overseas to consult with fellow investigators and to learn of European practice. Park remained proud of the system of cancer labs that had been created, maintaining that the "scientific study of cancer" had "originated" in New York and was now "followed and imitated in many other parts of the world." But he was frustrated that the cancer microbe remained elusive. More to the point, there were several investigators who were openly questioning whether there was indeed a cancer germ. Park deemed that sentiment foolhardy and pernicious, a direct repudiation of what Park believed was an "ever growing conviction" among researchers that cancer was "an infectious disease." That position, Park argued, was "both sustained and confirmed by the work" of laboratory scientists worldwide.

Park's position stressed that scientific evidence overwhelmingly pointed to a cancer parasite, even as no single microbe had been identified as the true cause of the disease. Put somewhat differently, a parasite was so. The vast majority of researchers recognized that "truth," but a handful and their misguided supporters were offering other hypotheses, which both retarded investigation and delayed identification of the pathogen. To Park, a cancer microorganism was so but required something more to make it seem so.

Park needed all cancer researchers to join together to establish as definitive and final the cancer pathogen proposition. And that is just what he tried to do; he aimed to unite individual cancer laboratories throughout the world into one great systematic enterprise. To that end, he met in Pittsburgh with leading Pennsylvania cancer researchers to "devise ways and means of raising funds for an international commission for the study of cancer." This single institution would guide and direct cancer research worldwide. There would be no waste, no false hypotheses, no sanctioned heretics. There would be no dispute. The single, sole international governing entity for cancer investigation would anoint the cancer pathogen as so.

Even as Park planned a future meeting in Buffalo to create this worldwide society and elect its officers,[37] other scientists and physicians were establishing additional cancer laboratories or expanding extant workspaces and staffs. The Middlesex Hospital's cancer laboratory got a new laboratory building in 1902, although not as grand as its American counterpart. The number of scientists supported in the new facility more than doubled. The London Hospital also opened its own cancer laboratory that year. It recruited Plimmer from Edinburgh to lead the new effort. Liverpool was not to be outdone. It opened a laboratory devoted entirely to cancer investigation in 1903 and announced creation of a cancer research fund to ensure continuous support.[38]

Liverpool's cancer laboratory was representative. T. Sutton Timmis, head of the Royal Liverpool Infirmary's board of governors, established the new facility in memory of his wife and scheduled it to close the moment cancer's cause was discovered. To facilitate work, the new laboratory was situated astride the infirmary's cancer ward. There, specimens would be readily available and possible theories tested. Noted bacteriologist Abert S. Grünbaum, a fellow of the Royal College of Physicians, was selected director. He encouraged C. S. Sherrington—later a Nobel laureate—to join him in the new effort. Together and with others, the Liverpudlians staked out a clear agenda. They would eschew any statistical musings to focus "on the cause of cancer." Until that was known, "very little can be done towards the cure, and practically nothing" towards the disease's prevention. A number of horsemen and estate owners graciously provided the investigators cancer-riddled livestock on which to experiment. Tumors were excised and meticulously scrutinized for signs of the cancer parasite.[39]

Creation of the Liverpool laboratory and the proliferation of others included significant monetary and psychic investment and commitment. That emotional and financial outlay worked against Park's international proposition; after so much hard work to secure funding and to receive approbation, it would have been extremely difficult to relinquish the primacy for the institution, its scientists, and its benefactors that the effort had created. So too did the indigenous nationalism inherent in the establishment of many cancer laboratory efforts—discovering the cause of cancer would bring incredible prestige to that nation's scientists and doctors. Coupled with an emerging agnosticism following the decades-long failure to identify cancer's causative germ, the institutional system already in place prohibited Park from establishing his unified system.[40]

Those same criteria strengthened the hand of the new laboratories over independent researchers. Clinicians increasingly seemed to lack the gravitas and resources necessary to receive a hearing in the professional literature. The quantitative precision and meticulous nature inherent in laboratory methods raised standards of evidence and even standards to achieve serious consideration in professional forums. Laboratories could not by definition make something so. That required evidence mutually agreed upon by investigators. But these new labs made some things not so, or at least less likely to be so, simply by offering what appeared more rigorous alternatives. Bedside observation, a consequence of the senses, was rendered relatively inexact and the use of verbal description a symptom of further imprecision.

Berlin's W. A. Freund's theory of senilism as "the primary etiological factor in cancer" drew little attention. Many practitioners, he argued, have observed that when a part of the body suffered a "mild and insignificant" disruption, that site may suddenly become "acutely malignant." The rapid deterioration stemmed from the forces of senilism, in this case "overwork or overworry." Cancer was the consequence of the disruption of normal activity and the subsequent rapid failure of tissues exposed to irregular stimuli. To ward off senilism necessitated a strong regime of "hygiene [and] of the regular habits of life." J. Etcheverry, writing in the Parisian medical journal *Annals of Dermatology and Syphilis*, argued differently but without much effect. Syphilis had an "active influence" on mouth cancer, he contended, "providing a soil for cancer." Syphilis generally lowered the mouth's "resisting powers," and cancer resulted.[41]

Both Etcheverry and Freund focused on cancer as opportunistic, invading when weakness occurred. Implicit was the idea that some agent availed itself of the chance to gain a foothold when available, a view totally consistent with the idea that cancer resulted directly from pathogenic activity. Yet their and many other such announcements did not receive the sort of hearing that they had only a decade earlier. Credibility of bedside- or clinical-based statements paled in wake of laboratory surety. The number of bedside or clinical reports appearing as full cancer articles in medical journals dropped markedly. These reports were relegated to letters to the editor or news notes. They no longer possessed the cachet necessary to merit more prominent exposure.

Movement to laboratory analysis also promised to hasten the date of the cancer germ's discovery. The apparent sense of exactitude in laboratory measurements seemed to guarantee quick and final determinations. Things would readily be so or not so. Ambiguity, uncertainty, and conflict would be banished. Researchers would charge ahead, and cancer's cause would be revealed in a few short years.

When these cancer laboratories were established, few believed that identifying cancer's microbe would necessitate a protracted search. Indeed, these institutions owed their creation to the idea that cancer was a microbial disease and that laboratory methods and a laboratory environment were critical to identifying the offending pathogen. A sense of mission accompanied the laboratories' formation. Investigators now possessed the tools necessary to unlock cancer's mysteries. Identity would beget certainty, and certainty would reveal truth. In less than a decade, perhaps, investigators would isolate the cancer germ and then develop "a relative simple physiological cure" to vanquish the disease.[42]

These researchers were selling immediacy, an immediacy rooted in and based upon decades of failure. Lack of success in securing the cancer germ in real-world conditions had caused physicians/scientists to abandon those conditions for situations that were truly artificial; they worked with substances and environments that did not appear in nature. The goal was to simplify a complicated matter—to divide it into constituent parts—but in doing so they needed to make it subject to absolute control and thus risked stripping their work of any authenticity and relation to reality. Such an approach assumed a mechanistic world, where organic life was little more than the sum of the various physio-mechanical and chemical processes. In the quest for the cancer microbe, investigators simply transferred an assumption made in a host of disciplines, including medicine—they specifically mentioned aniline dye-dependent staining—and applied it as if it characterized life processes generally. If a situation could be produced in the laboratory, the implication was that it must behave in a similar fashion in nature. That was an extraordinary leap of faith, but one consonant with the use of analogy. Natural situations—nature—were similar or identical to artificial situations—the laboratory. W. T. Councilman, Shattuck Professor of Pathological Anatomy at Harvard and a member of the Croft Commission, put it simply. Formerly in medical science, an hypothesis was "formed based on experience and analogy" and tested at the bedside or some other suitable natural place. Now, he continued, experiment under laboratory conditions has come to rule the day. The reason was control. "In experiment," he concluded, "it is possible to divide questions into their simpler components and make each the subject of experiment."[43]

An essential part of the new artificial laboratory environment was the equipment, and no piece of "equipment" would be more critical than laboratory animals. Despite the protestations of antivivisectionists, laboratory animals made the laboratory possible. With shorter life cycles and generations, expendable animals subjected to the minutiae of control promised the veneer of reproducibility and almost immediate progress. Discovery that mice suffered from the dread disease provided "more hope of an ultimate solution of the awful problem of cancer," maintained Smith Ely Jelliffe, editor of the *Medical News* and one of the first adherents of Freudianism in the United States. In mice and other small animals, "the history of cancer is so condensed that its study is much more fruitful and satisfactory than [it] would be even [under] the most careful clinical observations" in human beings. Because of laboratory animals, "by experimental methods cancer may be studied in its most intimate workings." Lab animals in cancer research, Jelliffe concluded, "represent an advance greater than any hitherto made in our history of cancer progress."[44]

Laboratory scientists went further than merely trumpeting their new venue. They also sold themselves and their abilities. They sought to demonstrate to the public that their efforts differed "from all previous collective researches into the natural history or pathology." Laboratories were attacking a disease "about which nothing definite is known save" that all previous attempts "have failed to cast any light on it." Only through "patient application on the part of highly trained" researchers—not observers—could cancer be conquered.[45]

The newly minted laboratories began investigations almost immediately, all the while confidently predicting that significant breakthroughs would occur quickly. Several main lines emerged, and a series of objectives predominated. Each institution took a characteristic approach, but all remained bound to investigating cancer as a pathogenic disease. The germ of cancer framed all discussion in these new labs as ruthlessly as it had for the previous quarter century. It was the parameter around which each institution measured itself.

The situation was different in one particular, however. While the decision for the institutions to divide the work among themselves significantly eliminated duplication, a bugaboo of clinical-based investigation to be sure, it also set them to work along parallel lines. Rarely if ever did research lines at different institutions intersect. Rather than serve as a grand adjudication body, the various laboratories pursued separate courses and programs. The consequence was that determinations usually did not undergo rigorous peer review through replication of experiments by the other cancer laboratories. What remained generally was for commentators to question the logic of others' assumptions, not the methodology or actual practice of their laboratory work.

3

Getting to Work, 1900–1905

In this heady atmosphere, cancer laboratories got down to business. They initiated the experiments for which they were created. Their acknowledgment of a mutual quest for the cancer germ both fueled optimism and demanded hard-headed research. They needed to articulate their research agendas, pursue the cancer microbe, and announce results. The quest seemed both heroic and mundane. To the laboratories went the glory and the toil.

Day-to-day research meant that investigators encountered challenges both unexpected and unprecedented. Sometimes courses needed correction in the midst of work. Few institutions remained more dogged in pursuing its original plan than Park's Buffalo operation. Gaylord proved even more indefatigable than his mentor in his faith in the existence of a cancer-producing microorganism. In early 1901, he found and identified a protozoon as cancer's cause. He claimed to have come across this profoundly important microbe because his laboratory techniques were fundamentally different from most of his compatriots. Unlike other laboratory researches, Gaylord worked only with fresh microbial cultures. By eschewing staining, which fixed specimens at one stage (usually postmortem), he was able to deduce that the actual protozoa of cancer was polymorphic; during its life cycle, the microorganism underwent numerous structural changes. Those several physical changes masked its ubiquity in tumors. When stained, each of its various stages was mistaken for a distinctly different organism. The sporadic reportage of different vacuoles in cancerous tumors during the past several decades—many of which were individually identified as the cancer-producing microorganism by careful investigators—merely reflected some of the various forms this organism could take. Gaylord's protozoa unified and made sense out of the reports of cancer's cause during the previous decades. The cancer protozoa was almost always there, albeit in different physical guises. His organism was difficult to plate and establish as a pure culture, in part because of the duration and specificity of its life cycle. But those facts did not dissuade Gaylord. He recognized his new agent as anatomically and physiologically similar to two other "protozoan" diseases, syphilis and variola (smallpox). Neither had had their protozoa isolated and identified, and Gaylord argued that was precisely because of how these two as yet unidentified agents morphed throughout their life cycles. Variola and syphilis were analogous organisms, and researchers had encountered analogous problems in identifying them. But in the case of the cancer microbe, Gaylord was able to overcome the difficulties by using only fresh material. And from his fresh cultures, he maintained that he could inoculate subsequent animals and transplant tumors from one to another, all the while being able to isolate his agent again and grow it in pure culture. In this way and despite its complex polymorphic masquerade, Gaylord's protozoa fulfilled all the requirements of Koch's postulates.[1]

Gaylord presented his work to scientists and medical men at every opportunity. He lectured at Johns Hopkins Hospital, went to Copenhagen to see the results of others who claimed successful inoculation, published in America's leading medical journals and relentlessly pressed his case. Newspapers showered him with praise, and some medical journalists celebrated his technical skill and novel insight. Yet investigators in news notes, editorials, and letters to the editor began to doubt Gaylord's contention. They zoomed in on two significant facts. Subsequent revelations showed Gaylord's protozoa were not truly plated but grown en masse in liquid culture, not exactly a pure culture. Nor were they precisely isolated when incubation was complete. Absence of those two stages placed them in direct contradiction to Koch's postulates. Something had to give. Either Gaylord was wrong or Gaylord's methods and plan were right and Koch's postulates were in error.[2]

Not surprisingly, Park leaped to his protégé's defense. He argued that "for these forms"—these particular polymorphic protozoa—"we do not even know that Koch's laws . . . are valid." Those rules had never been applied "to such varied conditions." Even more to the point, Park asserted that Gaylord "in practically every instance when conditions have been favorable," found "the organisms in cancer cases" and "in practically every instance" were able "by introduction of cultures made from these organisms" to produce "fatal results in animals." Park further bolstered Gaylord's contention by identifying the means by which cancer killed its host as "a terminal—a hematogenous—infection, brought about by a distinct toxemia." Cancer proved fatal in a manner analogous to other pathogens—staph, strep, and others—a realization that also suggested a microbial explanation.[3]

Park's suspicion about the validity of Koch's postulates was not unprecedented in wake of Walter Reed's work with yellow fever. That turn-of-the-century physician had proven that the disease was borne by mosquitoes (a discovery that energized those who favored environmentally based statistical surveys of cancer's incidence) and that an antiserum could be produced from its survivors, but he had not been able to identify and culture the disease-producing microorganism. Fascination with variola (smallpox) also brought Koch's theories into question. A scab from a victim could produce the disease in another, but the active agent could neither be cultured nor even identified. As one commentator noted, "no one doubted that variola . . . [was] infectious and due to the influence of micro-organisms, although no germs had, so far, been isolated." Like cancer, Park argued, variola and yellow fever were "diseases of unknown etiology." It was precisely because of these diseases that Park had favored establishing his laboratory as a multidisciplinary effort. Indeed, the key to Gaylord's identification of his new polymorphic cancer parasite was not pathology—the staining and reading of dead tissue—but rather biology, the real-time investigation of the organism in a controlled environment. Other specialties could reveal additional aspects of the disease organism and aid in its eradication or control.[4]

Such was the case with the laboratory's announcement of serum treatment for cancer in 1905. Mice first infected in Copenhagen were taken by Gaylord to Buffalo and used to inoculate mice there. Over several generations and 1,500 mice, some of the cancer-causing agents apparently became attenuated—here the analogy was to Pasteur's labors with rabies and anthrax and the concept we know as active immunity—and at least 70 animals developed tumors but recovered from the disease. The lab's chemist then prepared an antiserum from the blood of spontaneously recovered mice that caused in others "the disappearance of small tumors and the arrest of the growth of larger ones."[5]

While Gaylord certainly championed the antiserum that cured or mitigated already extant tumors, it was the instances of mice surviving cancer and then remaining free from the disease that mesmerized him. To Gaylord, this clinched the deal; cancer was behaving exactly as did smallpox. Since there was "an analogy between the agent giving rise to cancer and the agent which is responsible for smallpox," he maintained that the "infectivity" of cancer "can no longer be doubted." Cancer was caused by a microorganism. It was so.[6]

German laboratory efforts also favored a microbial explanation for cancer, although not with the exclusivity manifested in Buffalo. Leyden was in his seventies, more valuable as a publicist than as an active researcher. That did not stop him from pushing a cancer microorganism at every turn. Among his earliest projects was supporting the research of Max Schüller, who in 1901 identified a protozoon for cancer and described it in incredibly detailed form. Perhaps because of Leyden's backing or his thorough and precise description, which he claimed was now possible because of his innovative staining techniques, Schüller's discovery gained favorable comment from a wide variety of investigators.[7] But Schüller's full description ultimately led to his microbe being discredited. Several German pathological anatomists argued that his parasite was identical in structure to cork cells, a common contaminant in laboratories. Gustav Hauser, professor of pathological anatomy at Erlangen, was among the most dismissive. Upon finding that the cells Schüller claimed caused cancer were not even affixed to his specimens but merely strewn about the slides, Hauser sniffed that "any one can scrape all the parasites of cancer he desires from any ordinary cork." As significant, Hauser maintained that these cells, when transplanted to healthy individuals, did not produce cancer as Schüller argued but rather simple masses of granular tissue.[8]

The Hauser-Schüller dispute reflected a vast breach among German laboratory scientists. Chairs of pathological anatomy generally focused on the conditions and situation that they felt made it possible for a site to become cancerous, rather than on the search for the microbe that invaded that area to complete the transformation. Microbial agnostics, they maintained that tissues subjected to inflammation or irritation were potential cancer sites and used fixed slides to demonstrate their contention. Other scientists approached cancer by seeking to identify the germ culpable for the malady and generally attempted to use fresh cultures exclusively for this purpose. The consequence of this disagreement always revealed itself in public forums. Each side spent less time arguing the merits of its case than denigrating that of its opponents. Laboratory scientists were by no means monolithic, even though it was that contention that led them to receive public approbation.

These clashes between German laboratory scientists were always great spectacle. Sometimes held in venues seating over five hundred citizens, these debates featured crowds gathered outside to hear the contest reminiscent of those attending "an American football game or a horse show." Showmanship and bon mot were often as important as brute fact. Speaker after speaker picked apart the arguments of their opponents where telling phrase sometimes mattered more than cogent contention.

Leyden was an active partisan in these grand debates. To his mind, the pathogenic view was unassailable, even though no microorganism had as yet been conclusively identified. He had the apparently analogous case of variola on his side. "The unfruitful skepticism of anatomists must give way," he thundered, before the "facts which all may see who will" see. Pathological anatomists countered in several ways. First, they wondered how a pathogen could pass through healthy tissue to render an internal organ cancerous without leaving any telltale signs of the invasion. Second, they cited the seeming impossibility of trans-species infection and the exceeding difficulty of intraspecies transplantation. If cancer was truly infectious, its transmission should be clearer. Third, they used the repeated failure for decades to find a single cancer-causing pathogen as a sign that that quest was, at best, premature. The real work was to determine under exactly what conditions cancer developed. Once that was understood, there could then be a search for a causative agent or agents.[9]

At almost every opportunity where Leyden offered a public pronouncement, anatomists challenged him. That occurred even as he announced development of a dog cancer antiserum in 1902. Leyden extended his experiments to human patients using goat-based antiserum but quickly realized that the palliative effects were magnified when he added crushed tumor cells to the mix. Apparently Leyden's use of crushed cells was based on his understanding of the tuberculosis-tuberculin interaction, which Koch had mistaken as a complete cure some years earlier; he was certain that there were substances within the tumor that checked tumor growth, an essential Paracelsian principle. As a further aspect of the study, Leyden undertook an analysis of the chemical metabolites of cancer patients, hoping to see if the parasite altered essential biological functioning of infected organs.[10]

Leyden also created two new kinds of institutions based on his belief that cancer was a microbial disease. Both had the backing of the insurance industry, which hoped to reduce the amount paid out to cancer sufferers. First, he established in 1903 a cancer hospital to isolate incurable cases. Cancer hospitals to serve the indigent had long been familiar. Leyden's new establishment was different. Again, Leyden made an analogy to tuberculosis. The Imperial Health Office had mandated that advanced tuberculosis cases be separated from society and sent to sanatoria, where they were kept according to "modern principles." Since Leyden understood cancer to be infectious, he created similarly protective institutions to care for patients and to prevent them from infecting others. In this way, the alarming increase in cancer could be combated.[11]

Cancer dispensaries were his second innovation. Formed in 1904, these places mimicked tuberculosis dispensaries. There, patients learned hygienic practice "to take care of themselves and prevent contagion of others." Dispensary workers visited the "homes, families and even workshops" of those infected and established protocols to render the chances of infection nil.[12]

Leyden's new institutions reinforced, perhaps even rejuvenated, the cancer statistics movement in Germany. His establishments were based on his belief in the disease's infectiousness. Surely, if the disease was infectious, it ought to leave manifestations in areas where contact was most intense or occurred under precise circumstances. Here the goal was to identify cancer hotspots, places where cancer seemed to predominate. Its goal was simple: "to devise mechanisms which may check the spread of disease."

Resurrection of statistics, albeit it for a somewhat different end, worked to reintegrate medical practitioners into cancer research but placed them more explicitly under the auspices of laboratory workers. The key here was that practitioners were simply to identify through reporting; they were to transmit to a central body the number of cases in a household, family, street, town, trade, or some such grouping. Their experience was no longer required because it was no longer valued. Only pure numbers, now subjected to the rigor of multiple regression and other sophisticated analytic techniques, mattered to laboratory researchers.[13]

Not surprisingly, Leyden was among the earliest to take advantage of the statistical restoration. He used the contentious public forums to announce that he now had data that showed that incidences of cancer among animals—rats, cats, dogs, horses, and oxen—predominated "in the neighborhood of infirmaries and pathological institutes." These cases, he argued, must result from human to animal transmission. He further argued that few cases of cancer were found among wild animals and argued that Africans rarely developed cancer in Africa yet "American negroes suffer from the disease just as much as the white races with which they are in contact." Leyden pronounced himself ready to announce and describe a cancer microbe, but he warned his audience that, since this germ was "intracellular, it was not reasonable to suppose that it is able to survive long outside of cancer cells." This biological "fact" meant it was folly to hold it to the same criteria that researchers held the tubercule—namely, "cultivation on artificial media, and production of the specific disease by inoculation of these cultures."[14]

In contrast to Leyden's public persona, Ehrlich's cancer research was decidedly low key. He worked extensively in his laboratory on several problems—the spirochete of syphilis was en vogue at this time, and Ehrlich was hard at work on atoxyl—and devoted relatively little effort to cancer. Nonetheless, he worked to develop inoculation/transplantation techniques for mice and measured carefully the rate of success as well as the incidence of spontaneous remission.[15]

At Harvard, the Croft Commission set its initial task as determining the substantiated facts of the parasitic premise for cancer. In that endeavor, it hewed closely to the parables of Koch. Its members demanded that the germ of cancer exactly conform to his postulates and used that measure rigidly. They took exquisite care to announce every step of their analyses or experiments as they labored to provide definitive evidence. They naturally began efforts with a literature recitation and review, marshaling those experiments, observations, and conjectures that suggested a microbial cause against those that failed to uncover such activity. From there, they moved to matters that had long plagued their colleagues. In many but not all cancers, they found similar cellular structures that could be related to a microorganic invader. But experiments to cultivate these suspected culprits generally failed, as did attempts to inoculate test animals with the suspicious cellular material. Beyond that, commission researchers spent their first few years attempting to debunk the theories of others. They offered an alternative explanation for Plimmer bodies. They proved that animals in the wild could get cancer and that fish had high incidences of the disease. They failed to inoculate various laboratory and other animals with human cancers, either directly or from fresh cultures. They attempted to plate cancer cells to grow the pathogens therein. One member of the Croft Commission summed up his experiments dispassionately but directly. "Attempts to produce cancer in animals by inoculating them with bits of tissue from human cancer so far have uniformly failed. No attempt to isolate an organism from human cancer has succeeded. Inoculation of animals with the organisms" identified by others as cancer causing pathogens, he concluded, has produced "no tumor resembling cancer of human beings."[16]

By the end of 1902, the Croft group at Harvard had concluded not that there was no germ of cancer but, rather, that working exclusively along those lines had not enabled the group to make the contribution its founders had anticipated. In effect, their efforts the previous several years, wherein they served to adjudicate and refute the works of others and to stand as de facto scientific policemen, put them no closer to understanding what produced cancerous tumors. This work simply indicated what they found to be unsustainable. E. H. Nichols, who headed the Croft work, summed up the commission's frustration and sense of what could be accomplished succinctly: "[We sought] to find the cause or origin of cancer, and we have been unable to do so, although we have exploded popular theories." Cancer remained "a supreme mystery. On present lines of investigation the true cause of cancer will never be learned. Our only hope is in some new method."[17]

The Croft Commission took its words to heart, and, while it persisted in disproving the work of others, the group also initiated independent lines of inquiry. In particular, they concentrated on tumor classification, seeking to categorize these cancerous nodules by the type of cells produced and the intracellular constituents. Researchers, they maintained, had too long distinguished tumors by rapidity of growth, shape, locus, or some such determinant. None of these attributes were germane. What mattered was the type of cell that seemed to run amuck. The Croft Commission also experimented with the converse, transplanting healthy tissue from animal to animal and from tissue type to tissue type. In each instance, investigators measured to see what transplants took and then to determine the parameters upon which subsequent growth occurred.[18]

Huntington Fund researchers also deviated from the single-minded approach of uncovering the germ of cancer. They chose tumor growth as their focus and worked according to two main lines. One thread, represented by the work of Leo Loeb, the brother of the more famous Jacques Loeb, aimed at identifying the physical constraints and opportunities for tumor growth. These structural experiments—reducing osmotic pressure, placing things in intimate contact, or increasing the vascular supply—enabled Loeb to devise more dependable means to transplant or inoculate substances to transmit cancer within species and suggested some of physical situations that naturally occurred in tumor genesis.[19]

While Loeb reduced tumor growth to structure—physical principles—his laboratory compatriots went in another direction, to the chemistry of tumors. They found that tumors contained abnormally large amounts of glycogen and amino acids, possibly the precursors for their rapid, uncontrolled growth. Tumors were not more efficient than healthy cells, just more glutinous. Similarly, the chemist group found that tumors had great amounts of those enzymes required to digest various compounds and render them accessible as cellular food. The group set about to record, describe, and recount each of the reactions that they found in tumors. In their parlance, they were attempting to determine the role of various elements and compounds in tumor growth. Their explanation was necessarily chemical, reducible to the specific chemical equations and substances involved.[20]

In England, prospects of a dynamic grand cancer investigative fund centralized cancer research efforts. Other cancer labs—Middlesex, Liverpool, and a few others—depended after 1903 on at least some central fund revenue and, correspondingly, sanction. That centrality enabled Britain to avoid waste and duplication. It established the single largest cancer research agency in the world. Indeed, in 1904, the fund gained a title to fit its prowess. The Cancer Research Fund was rechristened the Imperial Cancer Fund. Receiving research from India and elsewhere, it truly had become an imperial agency. The sun never set on the Imperial Cancer Fund.[21]

Middlesex Hospital laboratory had run a vigorous cancer research program before the central fund began to constrain it. This hospital approached cancer research by attempting to work backwards to cancer's cause from the changes that occurred during cancer. For instance, researchers investigated the cytology of the blood in cancer patients and found that granular leucocytes more heavily dominated as the disease progressed. They also reported that a series of cellular bodies were found in blood films that were abnormal in cancer-free individuals. The laboratory sought to trace morbid changes in other cancerous organs, such as the pancreas and thyroid. Middlesex researchers also tried to predict the number of metastases according to the locus of the primary tumor. They compared incidences and sites of cancer between the Indian and the English populations. The laboratory board was so invested in the cancer work that it sent the lab's director, W. S. Lazarus-Barlow, who had been appointed a foreign member of the German Cancer Investigating Committee, to Germany four times yearly to attend committee meetings. In that way, the "hospital laboratories" would be kept "in touch with the best work performed" in cancer research in Germany.[22]

But perhaps the hospital laboratory's most innovative effort was to employ Karl Pearson of University College, London, and the Galton Laboratory to analyze data collected over the years. He determined that cancer rates were changing significantly in the patients served by Middlesex Hospital. The modal age of incidence had risen for women and fallen for men, cancer rates were more volatile in men than women, and male children were far more likely to suffer the malady than female children. He also determined that heredity likely played no part in cancer; incidences among family members fell within projected margins of error. He further concluded that no association existed between cancer and tuberculosis. Rates of each were independent of the other.

Of these determinations, lack of correlation between heredity and cancer drew most notice. But it did so precisely in terms of the quest for the germ of cancer. Lack of connection between kin and cancer indicated that cancer was not likely transmitted between family members; it was not overtly infectious. Observations by physicians of cancer houses where several members of a family had cancer at the same time "may be accounted for by the laws of probability." Cancer within the population was ubiquitous; it had become normal. Therefore, "there are bound to occur at times certain groups of the cases, which may at one time fall on a family, at another on a house, or a block, or a village." These cases occurred within the bounds of statistical error. They were random occurrences, predicted by statistics, not indicative of an infective agent.[23]

The Cancer Research Fund's cancer efforts proved even more novel. Cancer Research Fund director Bashford's insistence that the world's cancer investigative agencies set separate, independent courses demanded that he set out in great detail exactly what directions British cancer research would take. To this end, he turned the question of cancer on its head. Arguing that cancer research had been left to the pathological anatomists, who stained dead human tissue and then argued over what they saw therein, Bashford demanded an end to this exclusive focus on "the problem of the genesis of malignant new growths." Instead, he chose to scrutinize "the hardly touched upon" issues of the "biological, biochemical, the conditions of growth of cancerous tissue." The Ehrlich-trained Bashford wanted to establish the agenda as determining why cancer grew at the sites that it did, what parameters governed that growth, and how they did so. The "standstill to which cancer investigation" had fallen stemmed from its reliance on pathological anatomy. Bashford pushed for the "facts of cancer" to be studied "as a general and comparative biological problem" among "all races of men" and "the entire animal kingdom."

Implicit in Bashford's argument was his understanding that other diseases—he cited diphtheria and tuberculosis—cut across species and operating similarly in humans and animals. These diseases in different species were "not distinguishable" from each other "by any such characteristic differences." They showed "typical conditions" in "the frog, dog, horse, and man." He extended the analogy to cancer. That leap of faith freed him from studying humanity. Animals offered a wider diversity of living conditions, shorter life spans, and especially the ability to manipulate his subjects without facing the profound ethical issues associated with human experimentation. Animals were potential living laboratories where skilled experts could modify, arrange, and otherwise control conditions to affect or achieve a desired state or outcome. "Only with [animals]," Bashford concluded, was "it possible to perform experiments bearing on the etiology, pathology, prevention, and attempted cure."

Bashford took pains to explain that he would bring a new series of investigators into cancer research. By reorienting research and extending it, Bashford would "involve the co-operation of workers in many professions, and in many trades and fields of scientific inquiry." Their efforts would require "years of patient observation." "Cancer has hitherto been considered a subject which concerned only medical men," Bashford, a physician by training, argued. These investigators now must take a back seat to other specialists, to experts in "general biology, ethnology, zoology, and embryology."[24]

Morris, the patron saint of the Middlesex laboratory, seconded Bashford's assessment. In the prestigious Bradford Lecture delivered before the Royal

College of Surgeons, Morris examined the limitations of experiments surrounding current cancer research and pronounced them ineffective at best. “Up to the present time,” Morris, who continued to oversee the Middlesex Hospital cancer effort, was directly involved in creating the British Cancer Research Fund, and helped select Bashford as its head, noted, “the microbic theory has not advanced our knowledge of the cause of cancer one iota, in spite of all the talent and skill which have been employed upon it.” To Morris, new direction was necessary, and he proposed to explore the environment in which cancer flourished. A distant variant of the idea of predisposing causes, Morris opted for determining cancer’s local origin—its auxiliary causes. External “exciting causes”—microbes or something else outside of the body—were one thing. What went on in the body, organ, tissue, or cell that enabled cancer to develop upon introduction of an exciting agent was what he deemed the most promising investigative area.

Now workers “equally skilled” as pathological microscopists must deal with “embryological, morphological, chemical, and functional” questions. Morris had his own theory of cancer’s local cause. He harkened back to before bacteriology gained a stranglehold on cancer to adopt a version of Julius Cohnheim’s “embryonic residues.” According to Cohnheim, during development of an embryo, some cells became disconnected and mixed among the mass of the beginning-to-develop organism. There they lay until some exciting agent—a pathogen or activity, inflammation or irritation—caused these randomly placed rogues to proliferate. Morris adopted that formulation but grafted on several additions. He believed that renegade cells need not only be created during embryonic development but might also be adult, detached, migrating cells. He also posed age as an explanation for the onset of cancer. Again, it was the rogue cells that did the work. But in young healthy individuals, the body’s tissues remained strong enough physically to keep the troublemakers in check. With age came weakness—Morris called it “senility of tissue”—“impaired vitality and lessened power to resist the effects of injury.” Without that strength, the suspect cells would break free, and a tumor would result.[25]

The *British Medical Journal* understood the radical nature of Morris’s lecture and published a companion piece of similar length defending the parasitic origin of cancer. Written by Plimmer, who now was affiliated with the Liverpool laboratory, the article denigrated Morris’s theory, maintaining that “the only hopeful outlook in cancer” rested “on the ground of the parasitic theory.” Plimmer ended his essay by calling on fellow researchers to fulfill Pasteur’s dictum: “that the mind of man shall become lord over all infectious and parasitic diseases.”[26]

Both papers drew considerable notice.[27] But response was quickly swept aside by an even more compelling paper. Three researchers working under the auspices of the Cancer Research Fund presented a paper to the Royal Society on the internal workings of cancer cells. This interdisciplinary group included botanist J. Bretland Farmer, zoologist John Edmund Sharrock Moore, and cytologist Charles Edward Walker, affiliated with the new Liverpool cancer laboratory. They had noticed that all tumor cells in humans did not replicate the same way as normal cells. That was not a surprise, but their conclusion was. Chromosome numbers in the replication patterns of cancer were identical to the way that reproductive cells divided. As significant, the chromosomes in these reproductive and replicating cancer cells both exhibited a similar deviation from normal cells. The shape of these chromosomes resembled "loops, rings, aggregations of four heads."

The three authors explained why no one had discovered this phenomenon by laying blame on pathological anatomy. The objectives, methods, and staining techniques of pathological anatomists, while "admirably suited for ordinary histological investigation," proved sadly deficient "for elucidation of the finer cytological characters of individual cells." Cancer cells, not in the process of dividing, were polynucleated or non-nucleated; their nuclei were different from both normal cells and dividing cancer cells. To determine how cancer actually replicated required cells to be fixed "sometime before death supervenes." Microscopic inspection of live cultures, the province of biologists, botanists, and others, held the key to understanding cancerous neoplasms.

These investigators then set out a two-phased process. The first phase explicated how cancer grew. "The immediate cause of the development of the malignant growth" was the manner in which cells divided. This division process produced differentiation from normal tissue. But Farmer, Moore, and Walker were left to speculate about what they called "the remote cause," or why cancer originated at a particular time and site. They posited it as the consequence of "those various stimuli," such as "continuous irritation, . . . known to favour their development."[28]

That very unsatisfactory exposition was superseded by Bashford's dramatic announcement a month later. Working with a wide variety of domesticated and wild animals, he showed that these animals suffered cancer and that their tumors shared all "clinical, pathological, anatomical, and microscopical" characteristics with human tumors. Bashford's work demonstrated the "great diversity of habitat, food, and conditions of life generally" where cancer was found, a situation he maintained "relegates . . . external conditions to a subsidiary role" in disease causation. "Essential factors," the true mechanism for cancer, "must be sought in the potentialities which reside in the [organism's] cells."

Bashford next acknowledged the Farmer-Moore-Walker paper. This paper proved to him that cancer cells replicated identically to normal reproductive cells, a fact he confirmed in a series of non-human species. He used their unusual replication as a marker for the intraspecies transmission of cancer. Bashford deduced that cancer was not transmitted but rather transplanted. Tumors were carried from one animal to another in a species but these cells were "in no sense an infection." They did not invade the healthy cells but rather produced prolific growth, consistent with tumors. Tumor production occurred "without participation of the cells of the various hosts and without manifest change in structure."

Bashford took the unusual step of adding a coda to his article refusing to speculate beyond his work.[29] Others were not so circumspect. Some combined Bashford's results with the work of Farmer et al. and the theories of Morris to devise a neat cancer synthesis. These commentators boldly asserted that cancer was nothing so much as rogue germ cells, sex cells that had become dislodged when the organism was an embryo and mixed among other tissue, only to be activated years later. These unmoored germ cells then began headlong reproduction at the expense of the surrounding normal cells, preventing regular function. Others simply claimed priority for the work, citing papers written a decade earlier as precedent, while still others urged caution. The Farmer group found itself in demand, invited to talk before society after society, as the research proved especially popular in Britain.[30]

Popularity did not connote consensus. Nor did it severely weaken ideas of cancer as a parasitic disease. Wakely thought the tumor as embryo analogy a poor one and claimed that "cancerous tissue possesses the characteristics of a protozoan colony." His analogy equated tumor formation with plating a pathogen and watching a colony develop. He further warned about settling on any theory at this point, arguing that "it is a scientific mistake to theorize on insufficient data." "Adoption of premature conclusions" would "hamper greatly" the quest for cancer. Following his own dictum, he also refused to embrace the germ theory of cancer and went so far as to speculate that "parasitic etiology" was a "manifestation of" and a "reaction to" the "bacteriological epoch," which had fixated medical science. George H. Simmons, then editor of *JAMA*, appreciated the biological rather than the pathological approach but proclaimed that these papers proved little about the cause of cancer. They did not make anything so. Cancer could be produced by, according to Simmons, "a chemical change leading to cell division similar to parthenogenesis . . . or is, perhaps, even stimulated by a parasite." The true cause of cancer, he concluded, "remains to be learned."[31]

A cursory glance at the early years of cancer laboratories demonstrates a situation far different from the one laboratory proponents envisioned. Nothing was certain. Laboratories were working in different directions and often at cross purposes. Some argued for live cultures. Others championed only pathological anatomy. Chemists found solace in chemicals and biologists in cells. Some studied animals, while others remained loyal to humanity. Each gambit—and many more—had a similar thesis at its core: cancer behaved in a manner not inconsistent with what was known. It was analogous to some already understood disease. Which disease and which analogy were almost always the issues. Debates became so intense not because of actual research findings as much as actual research design. Investigators cleaved to their assumptions about cancer and often did not permit their evidence to get in the way of their conclusions.

Despite the contention, or perhaps because of it, the British centralized cancer fund received the king's blessing and his imperial designation. Bashford took pains to keep the fund newsworthy. He gathered specimens of cancer tumors from throughout the empire to determine the range, rates, and types of cancer in all areas under British dominion. He even developed his own inverse square law from this data. Although not on the order of Sir Isaac Newton's contribution, Bashford's law noted that "the extent to which cancer is recorded [by medical men and government officials] is inversely proportional to the difficulties which have to be overcome in obtaining information." That truism led him to conclude that the incidence of cancer in the British Isles was not increasing. Cancer was not spreading like an infection; it was just being more faithfully reported. Bashford also traded tumor specimens and information with most other cancer research laboratories in the world. To continue the fund's animal experiments, Bashford added a farm to study cancer in domesticated animals. There he transplanted testes and ovaries and see if cancer grew, something that might be predicted if cancer cells were merely the residue of rogue reproductive cells. When those experiments failed, Bashford tried unsuccessfully to find a correlation between the number of cancer cells undergoing reproductive division and the virulence of the disease.[32]

Bashford's research and the aggressiveness with which he pursued it had set the imperial agenda as cancer's growth, not its genesis. The Imperial Cancer Fund would more frequently work with transplanted tumors as it tried to understand the parameters of tumor growth and the relation of tumors to the functioning of neighboring healthy cells and of the organism generally.[33] The fund had established the terms of the discussion in England and galvanized comment; numerous researchers criticized or complimented the fund's investigations and conclusions.[34] The group's domineering position in British cancer research raised its visibility beyond the borders of the British empire, an important though often not stated justification for that body.

The always competitive French took particular notice of the fund's prominence. In 1904, the Crown sent a special delegation of French physicians and surgeons to England, where they visited the Imperial Laboratory and learned about its work.[35] Observing the fund in operation presented a sharp contrast to the French anti-cancer effort. Among major world powers, France remained alone in not establishing a separate cancer laboratory. The Pasteur Institute, an institution where significant research occurred, had an idiosyncratic research agenda and devoted almost no attention to cancer. Independent cancer researchers in France were left, to a large degree, to their own devices.[36]

Only the Academy of Medicine served any sort of national adjudication function. In the case of cancer, it only evaluated. The academy was composed of august practitioners, not laboratory scientists devoted to cancer or research generally. A part of central government, the academy oversaw the nation's medical policies, dealing at least as much with who could practice medicine and the ethics a physician need exhibit as anything else. Only when a situation resulted that affected the interests of the state did the organization act.[37]

The work of Eugene-Louis Doyen seemed to provide just such a challenge. Doyen had a long history with the academy. Initially offered a position at the Pasteur Institute, Doyen rejected it as too limiting and took a post in the French medical education system. The academy soon stripped him of that position for engaging in unauthorized human experimentation. Forbidden to teach, he established his own research institute to carry on his work and two medical journals to ensure its circulation among physicians. At his institute, the Parisian practiced medicine and surgery and even compounded nostrums to heal numerous ills. Doyen's modification of surgical procedures drew notice and honor, and he soon took up the personal challenge of determining the microbial origin of cancer.

In late 1901, he sent a paper to the academy claiming that, after fourteen years of painstaking research, he had isolated a specific diplococcus from many cancer tumors, was able to grow it in gelatin tubes, and could inject it into healthy animals. The cells surrounding the injection sites grew uncontrollably, developed tumors, and offered none of the markings of a bacterial infection. White blood cells did not gorge the area. Similar cultures could be obtained from the juice of these new tumors. Doyen then took the next step. He developed an antiserum. "Subcutaneous injection of the toxin of this microbe, attenuated in a special manner which Dr. Doyen has not yet made public," provided "good results in patients who have been operated upon and in whom no growth is left as far as can be ascertained. In such cases the injection appears to prevent a recurrence."

The academy offered no public assessment of Doyen's work. He provided it a further chance in early 1904. Following in a manner analogous to the great national hero Pasteur and his work with rabies and anthrax, Doyen reported that he passed his virulent cultures through several different media and species of animals and succeeded in creating "a toxin which can be given in varying degrees of virulence" that would treat cancer. The treatment took many months and needed to be done before the disease "was too far advanced." In about two thirds of all cases, Doyen reported significant improvement, with a complete recovery rate hovering at about 20 percent.

The academy's lack of urgency on the matter caused Doyen to publish a nearly six-hundred-page book outlining his work. Complete with dozens of microphotographs, he gave a copy of this work to each member of the French surgical congress that met in the fall of 1904. He also challenged its delegates to go to his institute; observe the specimens, methods, and tumors he had preserved there; and make up their own minds about the success of his techniques: "I place the verification of these facts at the disposal of my brethren. Let them come and see that is all I ask; every one will then be able to convince himself that my statements are well founded."

Several members of the congress were familiar with Doyen's work. In fact, at least two were openly skeptical, one arguing that Doyen needed to document his work as it occurred; he must "show cases before and during, as well as after, treatment." Another suggested that Doyen submit his research to a "committee of control," which Doyen rejected as ceding control of "therapeutic experiments that had been in progress for over a year." Finally, the congress decided it had no jurisdiction in the matter and urged Doyen to submit his research to a suitable investigative body.

Doyen took his case to Metchnikoff, who confirmed that Doyen's pure cultures were in fact his new microbe. In late 1904, Doyen brought the matter to the Paris Surgical Society. He exhibited two patients that had undergone complete remission due to his attenuation techniques and eight others "with advanced cancers whom he proposes to treat with his serum and to operate on later." The society chose not to offer an assessment of the demonstration. Doyen then brought his case to the Parisian Anatomical Society, which agreed to evaluate his claims. But when, in March 1905, the society had not yet offered a report, Doyen demanded that the Academy of Medicine intercede. The academy refused to do so, maintaining that the anatomical society was presently analyzing the situation.

The entire affair became increasingly bitter and was carried out in the public press. Doyen appealed directly to French citizens to help him overcome professional intransigence. His professional detractors felt compelled to use the press to "correct the erroneous impressions" produced in "the public mind by the very full reports of his work" that Doyen published.

The society also invoked the Pasteur Institute's Metchnikoff, who gave the task of further analysis to one of his assistants. The assistant confirmed the presence of the microbe in all instances, but he did not find the lesions created to be truly cancerous. He deemed them inflammatory, a fact he reported to the society. Before then, however, Doyen announced that his substance benefited cancer patients only in the early stages of cancer. Those so suffering, he contended, should seek immediate surgery if feasible. But especially in surgical cases, cancer patients needed his antiserum. It reduced "the danger of reinoculation, which so often occurs in the wound of an operation for cancer." His "anticancerous vaccination" prevented reinoculation in most cases, so he recommended no surgery until the patient had undergone "several anticancerous injections."

The society concluded its own investigation soon after Doyen's latest broadside. It agreed with Metchnikoff's assistant: Doyen's microbe did not produce true cancerous tumors. But the society also offered Doyen something. It stated that his serum ameliorated the symptoms of some cancers.[38]

This incredibly confusing situation was not immediately resolved. But that is not to say it lacked influence or precedent. Cancer had been placed at the center of a public and private debate within France. The public and government had come to the notion of what would become known as "the cancer problem." In late May 1905, the Academy of Medicine received two additional communications on development of malignant growths. Doyen or his disciples wrote neither paper. One investigator reported success on infecting a dog with human cancer, a discovery that confirmed his "earlier observation that tumour juice would set up in white rats processes giving rise to the production of neoplasms differing in form from that of the original tumour and situated far from the region of injection." The other merely discussed how a series of fungi, when grown on culture and injected into different sites, created apparently different symptoms and diseases. In fact, the author claimed to recover Plimmer bodies from some of the tumor-producing cells.[39]

With cancer research constantly before the French public, it is not surprising that the nation nominally created its first cancer league in 1906, and a laboratory thereafter.[40] That effort, however, marked the culmination of a trend that had been begun in the Western world about a decade earlier. Investigators created specialized facilities to identify the cancer microorganism and render it inert. That challenge established institutions, institutions necessary precisely because individual researchers had no means to interpret the barrage of medical information that cascaded on them. There were no readily useful mechanisms to make things so.

Cancer laboratories, monuments to the failure of more conventional approaches, also lacked the ability to achieve the ends for which they were constructed. They could not identify the cancer-causing microorganism, and they could not make things so. Johannes Orth summed up the situation neatly. Professor of pathology at the University of Berlin, Orth used his invitation to the International Congress of Arts and Sciences in St. Louis in 1904 to describe the conundrum that cancer researchers faced. "No one up to the present time has produced proof that carcinoma is of parasitic origin," he wrote. The previous few years of research had provided "no necessity to assume a parasitic etiology in carcinoma." But, he continued, "if in cancer, parasites should happen to play a part, then these parasites . . . must bear the closest relationship to the cancer cells which characterize the growth."[41] After the heady first years of these new cancer laboratories, the cancer microbe remained either so or not so. In Buffalo, in France, and with Leyden, sentiment strongly suggested it was so. Among other German investigators, the Croft group, and the Imperial Cancer Fund, the preponderance of evidence pointed to it being not so. The swift, sudden campaign to detect cancer's cause and resolve the disease quickly had proven dismally disappointing, precisely because it failed do what it was established to do. The effort had not rendered order out of chaos. Each individual cancer laboratory had made itself so with its creation, but the scientific work done in these new facilities did not make the facts so. Laboratory scientists did not present a single explanation for cancer or even a course for cancer research. The lack of a speedy resolution or even the promise of a near-term breakthrough led the usually upbeat Bashford openly to ask in 1905, "are the problems of cancer insoluble?"[42]

4

Inklings of Dis-Ease

The Cancer Problem, 1905–1910

The new turn-of-the-century cancer institutions were conceived from desperate premises. Cancer was assuming an epidemic portrait, researchers were issuing claim after unsubstantiated claim, and professional journals were filled with reports of case studies. Fear, the kind of fear that galvanized the New York State legislature to fund and establish a laboratory expressly for cancer research, gripped place after place. Far less certain than fear, however, was funding. Few governments actively supported the new cancer labs. Beneficence, contributions specified in last wills and testaments or from wealthy individuals, provided the bulk of moneys for almost every laboratory. And laboratories were expensive. Space, employees, reagents, equipment, test subjects, experimental animals, and the like proved costly.

These institutions required a continual infusion of funds. Cancer laboratories were big business, but business that promised quickly to run its course. As soon as these facilities identified the microbe of cancer, their mission would be complete. None of them except the Buffalo lab had a recurring source of funding. In theory at least, directors and others would then dismantle these structures and return to the status quo ante.

Given the desperation that engendered these institutions, it was not surprising that their staffs threw themselves into their work. They devised a wide array of experiments and investigations that they hoped would resolve the cancer question. These inquiries were marked both by ingenuity and naivety as researchers continued to reason from what they knew on the assumption that what they did not know must follow a similar track. Each laboratory, itself a highly organized entity of expertise and tasks, informally joined with the others to set out a loosely affiliated international system for pursuing cancer research. Through the medical literature, laboratory annual reports, and correspondence, these separate facilities pursued their own research agendas but paid close attention to what their compatriots did. They took the knowledge that they had learned through visits and correspondence and tried to steer a modestly different but complementary course.

The situation was not as simple as establishing discrete research programs to ward against redundancy. Quite the opposite was the case. These facilities owed their creation to the inability of researchers to adjudicate among several conflicting claims. Their methods brought matters out of nature and living bodies into confined, defined spaces. They adopted techniques contrived to be rigorous and scrupulously controlled. This was the quid pro quo of verification. It had become an essential facet of rendering something so.

The consequence of this tumultuous milieu was that making something so required many laboratories to share research protocols and engage in parallel experimentation. That requirement increased research costs, of course, but it also maximized value; when something became so, it no longer required scrutiny. Other issues then galvanized attention, and the artificially established premise or fact was applied as if axiomatic.

The very nature of how these laboratories identified the cancer question proved problematic. Since they concentrated on finding the sole cause of cancer, they viewed each experiment attempted in a rather characteristic way. Experiments that failed to achieve cancer's cause were failures—or at least not successes—rather than a sign of progress. In effect, these organizations reduced the experimental evaluation process to a binary situation: success or failure. There was no minimalism, no moving gradually toward a solution. Success would virtually end the search. Failure—in this case relentlessly recurring failure—was hugely disappointing, even depressing.

These laboratories were public in the most extraordinary sense. They had sold their publics the idea that they would find the cause of cancer. People contributed financially and emotionally to these efforts precisely because the research seemed transparent. Directors and other researchers regularly reported the conclusions of their investigations to their constituencies, the vast majority of whom were keenly invested in the laboratories' success. Expectations remained high as these institutions aggressively pursued cancer's cause.

Aggressive was not the same as successful. After about 1905, it became apparent, first to laboratory directors and scientists and then to others not affiliated with laboratories, that cancer's cause was not likely to be revealed quickly. Identifying the disease's particulars was significantly more difficult than laboratory proponents had thought. Cancer proved unwilling to give up its secrets swiftly, a situation that placed a spotlight on the laboratories and their laborers. Their proponents had promised quick resolution. That now seemed a fantasy. Like individual scientists and doctors before them, these cancer researchers had failed in exactly what they had set out to do. Cancer remained as inscrutable as it ever had been.

By 1905, it became common to refer to "the cancer problem."[1] That phrase had no precise definition. It simply meant that cancer was prevalent and that its destruction lay well in the future. Epidemic cancer was recognized as endemic and likely to remain so into the foreseeable future.

This newly named and acknowledged cancer problem was broached in many ways. Laboratory directors and other scientific employees responded to this unanticipated reality by recounting all the new knowledge generated in the pursuit of cancer's cause. This defensive yet self-congratulatory literature acknowledged the laboratories' failure to achieve the single goal for which they had been created but championed their ability to uncover new complexities and unknown facets of biological existence. Put in our terms, they celebrated spinoffs, knowledge about things for which they were not established. Despite the miserable failure of their mission, laboratory partisans declared them successful entities. These scientists argued that this alleged collateral learning and understanding—not progress towards cancer's cause—entitled them to continued, even heightened, financial support.[2]

As was often the case, Bashford took the lead. Ever philosophical, Bashford cited the noted physicist Ernst Mach's dictum that if science did not render a problem soluble, it was simply the consequence of erroneous thought. Scientists needed to reformulate the problem to make "investigation profitable." Such was the case with cancer. "The conflicting standpoints of different investigators" connoted "problems still baffling solution," an indication that they had been "wrongly formulated." Investigators persisted in their "dogmatic opinions on a subject on which we know so little" (Bashford pointedly referred to those favoring the parasitic explanation for cancer here), even as "hitherto unsuspected facts have been accumulated in recent years and are still accumulating."

Chaos had very real social costs. "Mere medical men seeking guidance" faced disappointment "in the extreme." Nothing had become so. "There were no guide-posts in the wilderness of fact and fiction," Bashford declared. Everything was characterized by "ambiguity of interpretation or [was] insufficiently supported by accurate observation." A "mass of disorderly details" lacking "obvious relation" to each other encouraged medical men and others "widely guessing at the truth" to support "solutions [that they had] advanced."

Bashford naturally proposed reconstructing "the problems" to make "their solution more helpful." He understood that any recasting would include remnants of the earlier questions—he called this bias—because all science "must be conceived in terms of a working hypothesis of some sort." The hypothesis that Bashford targeted struck directly at the situation that had emerged before the creation of laboratories and remained to a large degree in place. He saw most investigation as being pursued competitively. Competition was "the wrong spirit among those engaged in cancer research." It forced investigators "to get out some results, to claim progress when none is being made." Competition inhibited attempts to make something so. Researchers needed to justify their uniqueness—funding and the possibility of celebrity required it—something they did by holding to peculiar theories and positions. Competition also extended to scientific specialties. Experts must not "hastily conclude that one branch of science has succeeded where another has ignominiously failed." Representatives of different sciences—multidisciplinarity was critical to Bashford—must "take a modest view of their respective capacities and . . . not indulge in 'competitive research.'" They must "sacrifice themselves to 'coordinated investigation'" so that cancer research does not "lapse from one state of confusion and error into another."[3]

Bashford refined his critique two years later. Arguing that "dogmatic statements" about the nature of cancer had destroyed "more reputations than they have made," he asserted that "progress in our knowledge" of the disease had occurred "mainly by failure." Wisdom about cancer stemmed from "successive generations of investigators proving the insufficiency of knowledge and the hypotheses of their predecessors." It had been a "process of exclusion." But Bashford reminded his readers that exclusion really constituted progress. There remained "the necessity of undertaking destructive work." We must remember, he concluded, "that hypotheses and theories, like men, may rise on stepping-stones of their dead selves to higher things." Finally, to "the everlasting question, what is the cause of cancer," someday "truth is elicited."[4]

Bashford, then, acknowledged repeated failure but declared it progress. Some of the virtually infinite possibilities had been ruled out. This was grasping at straws, of course, but the demands of being a public figure and depending on moneys from the public required some optimism, some reason for individuals to provide further support.

The University of Chicago's Nicholas Senn took a more honest, less convoluted approach to the cancer problem. He certainly had a direct stake in the matter. Senn had tried to transplant a tumor from a patient to himself in 1901 to "offer strong, if not convincing proof" that cancer was not infectious. A pioneer in bringing bacteriology into military medicine, Senn pronounced the cancer quest medicine's "one dark chapter." Despite "prodigious efforts," cancer's "real cause and nature, remain unexplained." The disease's "prevalence . . . , its relentless course and obstinacy to all known methods of treatment" filled the public with "the gloom of fear and hopelessness."

Senn, too, recognized the palliative of coordination, but what he proposed dwarfed Bashford's message. He called on the 15th Annual International Medical Congress, which met in 1906 in Lisbon, to establish a mechanism to serve as a uniformity-focusing lens among researchers. It would create a structure to guide "the international study of carcinoma in all its phases." Representatives from "all nations" would participate, and a single report would be issued at the following congress. This "earnest, united work . . . representing practically the entire inhabited surface of the earth" would eventually produce "the final discovery of the essential cause of cancer."[5]

The congress neglected to take up Senn's challenge. The *BMJ*'s Williams also cast the cancer problem as a want of coordination. Scientists and physicians knew but one thing about cancer, he reported. Unless it is diagnosed "in an early stage and then promptly excised, it is . . . inevitably fatal." It was "there that our substantial knowledge ends." The most immediate challenge, he continued, was to "recognize, clearly and unmistakably, that cancer research has not yet grasped the key to its problem." The "causation of cancer is unknown," and the "science of all vital processes" remained "in its infancy."

Williams explained his proposal in military metaphors. "Attacking the cancer problem is like fighting a mysterious and evasive enemy in an unknown country. We have not learnt the secret of his strength, and our attempts to pursue him are hampered at every turn by our imperfect knowledge" of the terrain "we have to travel," Williams maintained. He called for scientists to mobilize to plan the "campaign" and suggested that they "adopt a wide encircling movement." "All available forces of scientific knowledge" would move "over this wide field of operations" to converge "gradually and very laboriously" on "our still imperfectly located objective." The result would be glorious. The "army . . . at work and steadily pursuing a concerted plan of campaign" would "inevitably continue until it has attained its object." Each soldier needed to dispense with his or her "theory," for until that occurred, "we acquire little enlightenment but much confusion." There were not "true theories about cancer," Williams reminded prospective recruits. Only "working hypotheses" existed, good only because of "their efficacy as incentives to good scientific work." The "real value of a piece of cancer research" is "its addition to the store of accumulated facts."

Williams's admission about cancer research's real value was startling. No longer was the goal to find the cause of cancer immediately. It was not even the ultimate conquest of the disease. Rather, it was the production of new scientific knowledge. This knowledge was not directed. This knowledge was not exactly knowledge for knowledge's sake, but it was close. It was knowledge that researchers could employ to form hypotheses about anything that the knowledge exposed. A warehouse of data would enable investigators in any field to frame informed hypotheses and to fight whatever campaigns they chose. Williams found no result insignificant in this data accumulation quest. He proved particularly adept at justifying, even praising results of experiments that were unsuccessful. "A negative result, in accurate scientific work, does not mean failure," he reasoned. It was essential "to the process of induction by exclusion and elimination." That, he argued, stood as "one of the requirements on which the validity of positive construction depends."[6]

Williams was not the first to redefine the purpose of cancer labs, changing their mission from deciding the cause of the disease to producing knowledge that could be used in any endeavor. Indeed, the concept of original or basic research, or pure science, emerged forcefully at about this time, precisely to explain either lack of success in the project for which the research initially was sought or to free investigators from any accountability except to their like-minded peers. Pure science became a commonplace validation for results that failed to produce what had been promised. In this intellectual nexus, investigators often suggested that what was produced was far more useful than what had been promised, even as it bore almost no bearing on the initial question. Success, then, was declared in a battle other than that which researchers claimed to have fought.[7]

The other facet of Williams's argument also proved popular. Like Senn and Bashford, and Park years before them, Williams wanted scientists to mobilize for a war on cancer. That sentiment provided the motivation for the French to establish their first cancer league in 1906. In the first few months of that year, two broadsides by different authors appeared. Both were titled "The War Against Cancer," and each one was presumably written without knowledge of the other. Etienne Burnet's, in the *Revue de Paris*, was published first. Formerly an assistant in Amédée Borrel's microbiology laboratory at the Pasteur Institute, the bacteriologist Burnet recently had become director of immunization for the city of Paris. He used this bully pulpit to call for a war against cancer. Burnet wanted this war to mimic the war against tuberculosis, because "cancer is as worthy" as that disease. Laboratory research during the past decade placed cancer "almost at the point of tuberculosis" when Koch "demonstrated its infectiousness and inoculability." The key discovery so far had been the realization that cancer attacked virtually every animal species. Because of this fact, Burnet predicted that the laboratory mouse in the hands of scientists will "be the liberator of man." The situation was primed for action. "Cancer waits its discoverer of its microbe; it awaits its Robert Koch." These germs—Burnet called them "microbes not yet seen"—remained hidden because no one has yet found "the staining process" for these creatures, or because "they are very small."

Concerted action would win this war, but "in France there is nothing." There were no institutions, just "goodwill and isolated talents." "Observations [and] experiments, the material of science" were "scattered, largely lost." Mobilizing to create a full range of cancer research institutions was essential for "the country of Pasteur."

René Ledoux-Lebard's doctoral thesis at the University of Paris hammered on similar themes. He too undertook a historical analysis of efforts to determine the cause of cancer, likened the disease to tuberculosis as well as syphilis, and called on his countrymen to act. But Ledoux-Lebard also stressed what had been done outside of France, especially collective efforts. He identified Gaylord's Buffalo lab as "one of the most important" efforts and celebrated its full-ranged research laboratory as "appropriate," with expertise in "pathological anatomy, chemistry, bacteriology, experimental pathology, etc." The Germans sought to battle cancer through "science," attacking it with "number and mass" of investigators. Their assault was organizational, "their method and customary discipline." The British naturally gravitated to plotting out a comprehensive grand strategy, for "they know how to treat the big issues." France stood "woefully behind all other major nations." It did not "have a single institution truly devoted to the study of cancer."

That travesty need not occur. Ledoux-Lebard thought French prospects promising. The warriors existed, "a phalanx of scientists significant by their number." This army could tackle cancer "with enthusiasm and without truce, [with] a diversity of research approaches, varying experiences and trying all techniques." The scientific corps would "put to the service of laboratory science all the resources the imagination of an inventive nation of men" could muster.

Mobilizing scientists to fight cancer "rationally, vigorously and collectively" should be "a French imperative." Everywhere governments began the onslaught "by encouraging timidly private efforts, scientific research and laboratory work." But the "large states of Europe and North America" had taken the next critical step. Each had "grouped its medical men and scientists under the same flag for public defense."

Ledoux-Lebard saw combination within nations as the way to wage the cancer war. The prominent Borrel agreed but offered a more straightforward argument. All civilized countries but France had founded committees and associations and devoted significant resources "to maintain special laboratories to gather all experience" about cancer. France "regrettably has no similar association. Researchers remain isolated, left to their own resources." One investigator's findings were not shared with another. Borrel concluded his plea by calling for France to establish its own cancer research organization.[8]

The French took no action at that time. But while Williams's call to arms bore little tangible fruit in France, it resonated clearly with others. In particular, German investigators shared Williams's assessment and had worked to establish an organization to wage just such a campaign. Creating the Committee for Cancer Research in 1900, electing foreign members, and establishing a journal devoted entirely to cancer research a few years later proved to be preliminary steps in forming an aspiring worldwide cancer research entity. In 1906, Vincenz Czerny, professor of surgery at Heidelberg, took the next step. He knew of a call in 1905 by Buffalo's Gaylord—he had visited the New York facility in 1901 and learned of its operation—for a special international cancer congress to discuss the cancer problem. He then followed the express direction of the German cancer committee and used the occasion of the opening of a grand new cancer laboratory/cancer hospital complex—the Institute for Experimental Cancer Research—at the university to call an international cancer research conference. Ehrlich lent his stature to the project, promising to have the assemblage visit his new cancer facility in Frankfurt on the Main as a further inducement to attend.[9]

Czerny's conference initiative fit nicely within the established German cancer research paradigm. From the start, a single entity—the Committee for Cancer Research—tried to guide the German effort. This committee fostered the creation of cancer laboratories, to be sure. But it also used its authority over German cancer research to try to rationalize clinical observation, a means to gain some semblance of control over practitioners (and to mollify the nation's pathological anatomists, who generally looked askance at biological and microbial cancer explanations) and their predominantly idiosyncratic reports. Perhaps because of its organic affiliation with German insurance interests and public health officials, the committee gathered statistics at a time when other countries were beginning to dismiss that approach as unrewarding. The Germans relied on the country's practitioners to report data as well as cases they encountered. These statistical and clinical reports lacked consistency, a factor that rendered them almost useless in the effort to make something so.[10]

The Germans moved decisively to resolve both issues. The committee established specific forms for practitioners to complete to make statistical efforts conform to a single template and worked diligently to formalize reporting. Systematizing cancer observation and later trials required something greater. Municipality after municipality, university after university, decided to erect clinical institutions in intimate relation to the new cancer laboratories. Cancer research hospitals became a staple of the German cancer effort.

It was just that sort of new systematic approach that Czerny celebrated when he issued his invitation to the world's cancer researchers. Leyden, the patriarch of German cancer investigation, and his associate, George Meyer, handled the invitations. And it was those invitations that galvanized Parisian medical men finally to form their collective, L'Association Française Pour L'Étude du Cancer.

All was not as it seemed. The new French organization proved a total sham, simply a face-saving gesture. France hypothetically had an organized cancer research entity like other European, North American, and South American countries; it had seemingly joined the league of cancer-fighting nations. The L'Association Française, however, never met before the Heidelberg meeting; had no facilities, budget, or periodical; and sponsored no activities. It would remain dormant for years.

The French and almost all the other investigators who received invitations to the international conclave pledged to attend. Representatives from most European and North American countries graced the meeting and various countries in Asia and Africa also sent delegations. Directors of all the major cancer laboratories came. Only about fifty of the eight hundred invitations were declined. Despite the enthusiastic response, many attendees were taken aback by the Meyer-established meeting protocol. He permitted no comment on conference papers. That stipulation prevented arguments, such as those over cancer's cause, but it also eliminated in-depth, public examinations of a paper's merits. Another meeting-related situation also raised concern. Most prominent German pathological anatomists had declined invitations and were absent from the assemblage. Their objection was intellectual and long-standing. It had manifested itself in vituperative meetings that had rocked German medical societies when discussing cancer. The anatomists refused to be party to any organization that stressed non-pathological measurements as more vital than their techniques. In particular, they seriously disputed whether animal cancers were comparable to human cancers and dismissed animal research almost out of hand. They had concluded that much of the conference was likely to be wrongheaded and a waste of time.[11]

In his introduction to the conference, Leyden laid out as an explicit goal of the conference to "consider whether it is now appropriate to establish an international association to combat" cancer, patterned after "the international organization to combat tuberculosis." Such an international effort seemed prudent because science and medicine "knows [*sic*] no distinction of nations." All must "join hands for common work." Several other dignitaries celebrated the gathering, taking their turn at lionizing the German effort. To these men, the German committee initiated organized cancer research. Czerny placed his new institute within that context. Its focus on "etiological researches" to determine cause placed the new entity "shoulder to shoulder with its sister institutes home and abroad," especially Leyden's Institute for Cancer Research/Charity Hospital and Ehrlich's Frankfurt Institute. The inspiration for this facility, Czerny noted, came from his trip in 1901 to the "institute for cancer research in Buffalo." This visit fixed in his mind what beneficence, tempered with official sanction, could accomplish.[12]

In his congratulatory address, Bashford took a swipe at the absent pathological anatomists. He was pleased to be at a facility structured according to an "enlightened spirit"; this structure recognized that "our knowledge of cancer is only to be expected from the experimental and comparative biological study of the disease," which included "ample provision made for the study of the disease in animals." He then presented his idea of what constituted organized research: the cooperation and "collaboration between the workers in different laboratories and free exchange of ideas." That was and would continue to be the British model, Bashford continued. He championed an international organization but only if it adhered to several fundamental principles. Progress in the cancer fight would occur most expeditiously when numerous approaches were broached. There, "freedom of intercourse and discussion between the workers in different institutions engaged in similar work," including "a free exchange of the material" delivered "value far above" any rigidly directed, centralized system.[13]

Bashford staked out a position contrary to the German organizational model and at odds with the anatomical pathologists. George Meyer, second in command at the Comite Für Krebsforschung, issued an opposing view. He claimed that, since on cancer "the views of experts, are naturally still widely divergent," prohibiting discussion at the conference seemed sensible. The committee mandated that there would be no freedom of discussion.[14]

Perhaps Meyer's history with the German pathological anatomists colored his perspective. Certainly their attendance would have poisoned the conference.

The anatomists' assumption that animal experiments, which they saw as suspect and unnecessary, would comprise the bulk of the conference proved correct. The Jensen mouse, the first mouse strain that most investigators agreed had undergone successful cancer transplants, served as the focus of numerous papers. Identified by a Copenhagen investigator shortly after the turn of the century, the strain had been delivered to laboratories throughout the world soon after its discovery. Within short order it had emerged as the de facto cancer laboratory animal. It gave researchers a common referent as they subjected the mice to a variety of experiments. Francis Carter Wood, later a major figure in Columbia University's cancer laboratory, put the significance of the Jensen mouse in bold relief. Because of his work creating the Jensen mouse, Wood claimed that Jensen should be "considered the Pasteur of cancer research."[15]

Investigators had worked to increase transplant success, considered whether transplantation was akin to infection, failed to transplant mouse cancer to other animals or breeds of mice, and tried to explain and take advantage of spontaneous cures. Ehrlich's lab had been especially aggressive in pursuing mouse experiments. He had excised 280 mouse tumors by the time of the conference and had over 1,200 mice in his facility. As one conference participant noted, among the meeting's most important facets was the profound acknowledgement and the near universal assessment that "cancer in mice is comparable to cancer in man."[16]

Leyden was even more direct. He acknowledged as "fruitful" the then-present state of cancer research but demanded that the group "recognize" that the mechanism for "progress in cancer research is the introduction of experiments on animals." "These little creatures," he continued, "have taught us a lot." They stood as "the classic subject of scientific research" for cancer. Animal experimentation had become the source of "significant advance in the study of cancer."[17]

Among the other phenomena emerging from the conference was a reexamination of the relationship between cancer and parasitism. Initially proposed in full by Henry Butlin, chair of the surgical section of the Royal College of Physicians in his 1905 Bradshaw lecture, this new theory took the radical approach of considering the cancer cell itself a parasite. Leyden pushed hard for this understanding at the conference because he felt it reconciled the long-standing debate among scientists looking for the cancer-causing parasite and those arguing that the disease resulted from somehow abhorrent cells or tissues. He offered his own experiments as corroboration. Leyden claimed that cancer cells had a different chemistry than normal cells and that they produced an enzyme that weakened the resisting power of nearby cells.[18]

Cancer research framed the meeting. But in wake of the realization that discovery of the germ of cancer likely remained years in the future, researchers at the convention did not limit themselves to the cause or biology of cancer. They broadened their gaze so much that it constituted almost an entirely new debate. The group discussed treatment experiments and called for adoption of methods to prevent cancer. Proponents reasoned that a firm understanding of causation was not necessary to investigate treatment. Successfully mitigated diseases of unknown etiology provided a potent model. Treatment or prophylaxis could be deduced by other means, as Pasteur had done for rabies and Jenner had done for smallpox. The experimental mouse offered a reasonably convenient means on which to test their speculation.[19]

The gathering replaced the straightforward question of the cause of cancer with issues of origin and genesis of the disease. Discovery of the scourge's cause remained a distant goal, of course, but questions that had seemed moot when cause was thought imminent emerged as vital. As a consequence, the meeting sanctioned the transformation of cancer research. Research now seemed appropriate into cancer's cause, its cure, its prevention, and its genesis.[20]

Ledoux-Lebard issued this call to battle. He urged his colleagues from many nations to join together "powerfully and effectively to intervene" in all facets of the cancer question. Even "the smallest victory over cancer" was "more than enough to justify a long struggle" against the disease. With each new fact, he continued, closer comes the day "where we can confront cancer with better weapons." Perhaps stirred by Ledoux-Lebard's rhetoric and remembering Leyden's opening plea, the conference resolved to become a permanent body. Details were left in abeyance, but the assembled appointed the officers of the German committee to hash out the particulars of the new organization.

The committee wasted little time after the convention adjourned. Its initial plans for the new union planned for the group to meet biennially. The committee even tentatively proposed a London meeting. Their suggestion of London was no accident. It was an olive branch to Bashford. If the organization was truly to become a guiding body for cancer research worldwide, English researchers needed to fall in line.[21]

The Germans clearly recognized the importance of the British, but not as equals. They would be subordinate to the German-dominated central organization. Soon after the conference, the German committee sent Bashford letters proposing a Berlin-located international cancer organization and asked him to organize all British cancer facilities—there were about ten places receiving ICRF moneys in 1906—as a single affiliate to the new entity.

Bashford declined the imperial overture as offensive. It spit in the face of his insistence that freedom of inquiry and voluntary cooperation stand as the cornerstone of any international cancer effort. Bashford also thought the German proposal premature, an attempt to make something so that was definitely not so. The organization would be structured to speak with a single German-dominated voice at a time when the note or even octave was unknown. Citing the lack of "exact knowledge of the etiology of cancer" as his reason to resist combination, he favored research that sought to answer that question; he claimed that cancer research could make most efficient progress if researchers worldwide focused their efforts there and shared information and experiments voluntarily. Defining cancer research to include statisticians and practitioners—the way that the Germans long had and the new organization now proposed—had severe limitations.[22] It opened the group to the vicissitudes of practitioners and unqualified nostrum vendors. The former group lacked the perspicacity to do systematic research, while the latter would trumpet false cancer cures and slow the entire investigative effort. Bashford also feared that the German actuarial/public health connection—political hacks and glory seekers—would dominate the new organization. He therefore argued that the greater good would come from "encouraging active individual intercourse and exchange . . . between those investigators who were *actually* [italics mine] studying cancer in the laboratories of different countries."

The ICRF board agreed with Bashford, and England declined the German offer.[23] The case in the United States was different. Americans had been conspicuous by their 1906 cancer conference absence. Gaylord, the nation's sole invitee, did not attend. Concerned about becoming peripheral to the worldwide cancer effort, eleven cancer researchers based in Buffalo, New York City, and Boston greeted the post-convention entrée to affiliate most favorably. Among their number were several researchers affiliated with the new Rockefeller Institute for Medical Research. Endowed by John D. Rockefeller in 1901, the New York City–based institute's resources dwarfed all others in the United States. Its director, Simon Flexner, chose in the middle of the decade to move investigation decidedly into a new area, cancer research. Flexner implemented that decision simply by reorienting the institute's standing organization. Unlike the specially constructed cancer research facilities in the United States, the Rockefeller Institute approached the cancer question as a matter of biology. It aimed to understand the biology of cancer rather than simply to detect cancer's cause. In that sense, it was much closer to the Huntington model than the Buffalo lab.

With this powerful new entity at its side, investigators from the other American cancer research laboratories met in May 1907 during the Washington, DC, meeting of the American Association of Pathologists and Bacteriologists. There, they formed the American Association for Cancer Research (AACR). Citing "the growing need for understanding the causes of cancer and for improvement in cancer research," the new national organization planned to meet twice yearly at the national meeting of the pathologists and bacteriologists and at one of their members' laboratories.

The new American organization approached its mandate passionately and reflected the Huntington and new Rockefeller influences. Earliest papers considered the types of animal tumors generated by transplantation, the biological consequences of those tumors, and possible cancer causes. The organization stood ready to join the international effort, which it did in May 1908 when Germany formally established the International Association for Cancer Investigation (IACI).[24]

The French, under the guise of L'Association Française Pour L'Étude du Cancer, also participated. In the month after the IACI's creation, the French group finally held its first meeting. This gathering followed another plea from Burnet, again in the *Revue de Paris*. Great hope accompanied the renewed venture. The association wrote a detailed constitution, laying out specific types of memberships. Now active, the French association agreed to convene monthly at the college of medicine in Paris to offer the individual work of one or more of its members. Discussion was to ensue. The secretary was to collect the papers and issue them for distribution.[25]

The association also anticipated becoming a critically important organization. Its first meeting was filled with consideration of any number of legal issues as it set who could speak for the French society and who would represent it in court and civil society. Its constitution and by-laws specified the types of facilities it hoped to erect and own—laboratory, dispensary, and hospital—how they would be funded and how the organization's reserve funding would be invested to best advantage to ensure an active cancer research enterprise.

This new cancer investigating corporation expected to flourish because it hoped to be labeled a public utility by the state. It applied for that status right after its initial meeting. Being a public utility reflected governmental sanction. Public utilities received the blessing of the appropriate branch of government, gained funding and the ability to dispense funds to constituent efforts, and stood as an indication that the institution so designated served a compelling state interest. Being labeled a public utility encouraged people to donate significant sums for a high noble purpose.[26]

Even without an immediate public utility designation, the French organization was finally up and running. It persevered as its members reported on work ongoing in the facilities where they earned their livelihoods. That gave the new international organization thirteen affiliates. Twelve were European—but not the British—and the thirteenth was the AACR. Its charter set its mission as "the promotion of arrangements for cancer investigation, the care of cancer patients and the combating of cancerous disease." The group also pledged to establish "uniform, international cancer statistics," an "international information office for all questions pertaining to cancer investigation," a cancer journal, and annual cancer conferences. Each affiliate was permitted to appoint a certain number of members according to population, but the new organization required affiliated societies to send Berlin the equivalent of 100 marks annually for each member. Put more simply, the organization took as its mandate research into all things conceivably related to cancer, creation of a standardized statistical bureau, a board to coordinate and direct cancer research worldwide, a means to fund its efforts, and a journal through which to communicate with members. The journal itself began in 1909 and was published in German, French, and English.[27]

On paper, the international association seized for itself powers necessary to rationalize the cancer quest in its myriad aspects and to get researchers to speak with one voice. Russia and Japan both quickly joined the internationalist movement. By 1908, Russia had its own cancer research journal and had established chairs of cancer research at major universities. Japan established its cancer research journal in 1907.[28] But these new converts to the cancer cause did not enable the international association to exert control over cancer research. Without authority over the British effort, the organization could never establish any sort of hegemony. That was not the only problem the new association faced. Its leaders soon recognized that the cause of cancer was not likely to be uncovered soon, so organization looked to expand its utility. Leyden and others who had avidly sought research coordination now extended their gaze to cancer cures and insisted upon a grand central entity to undertake those experiments. But others in Germany demanded that the association support existing facilities and allow them to pursue whatever courses of research their boards and directors favored. The situation never became a true impasse. The association resolved conflict by offering continued support to the institutions the German committee had traditionally backed and creating a small Berlin-based facility to experiment with cures. With that situation papered over, the IACI again tried to entice Bashford to join, but he responded verbatim as he had to the earlier request. The IACI also renewed its inducement to hold the next meeting in England, but that too was rebuffed.[29]

Paris provided the venue for the 1910 meeting, the first for the new international association. Again, an IACI declaration provided a spur to French association action. The group had engaged in no collective or concerted research or outreach since its initial 1908 meeting. It had failed in its attempts to be designated a public utility, a sine qua non for large-scale fundraising. As the 1910 Paris meeting approached, the French cancer collective avoided international embarrassment by taking the paltry sum its fund-raising efforts had netted and prevailing upon one of its members to open his laboratory for l'Association use.

Despite l'Association's failure to be designated a public utility—a de facto rebuff by the French government—Pierre Delbet, the society's secretary, argued that the French association had "become one of the foremost centers in the world for research into the terrible scourge of cancer."[30] That claim was highly suspect, of course, but it would befit an organization chosen to host the IACI's first international meeting. For that gathering to have real substance, the English needed to actively participate. The German-dominated organization recognized this and, as the date of the meeting neared, took the unprecedented action of appealing for Britain to join through petition directly to the English king. He turned the overture down. The ICRF reaffirmed its decision to remain independent. It claimed that its research results were open to all, both within the Empire and without, and provided a list of laboratories in British cities that it funded. That list included laboratories in London, Manchester, Liverpool, Dundee, Aberdeen, and Edinburgh. The group also claimed to offer material support to twenty-three cancer researchers in Germany, three in Austria, two each in Italy and the United States, and one each in Belgium, Norway, Hungary, Romania, Denmark, France, Russia, Holland, Spain, Japan, and New Zealand. At the same time that the ICRF was puffing its international research prowess, the IACI was entertaining the idea of establishing a regular network of cancer diagnosis stations. Concerned individuals could be examined there for cancer; early detection meant early surgery, the sole cancer "cure." The IACI also considered establishing cancer museums to acquaint the public with the cancer menace, which would foster early detection and revenues for cancer research.[31]

Those sorts of activities were an anathema to Bashford, who had argued that cancer research was a distinct activity, separate from treatment or prophylaxis. Bashford understood their importance, of course, but he recognized the biology of cancer as the essential issue. Nothing should stop that quest to understand the disease's biological parameters. Nothing should draw money away from the fundamental issue of learning the biology of the cancer cell. Without that basic scientific knowledge, any attempt to move against cancer was simply speculative, anti-scientific, and a likely waste of resources.

As the international association prepared for its Paris meeting, the group adopted a new set of rules to define more narrowly the parameters for presentations. Each paper giver was taxed 25 francs for the honor of presenting, and all had to be association members. That latter provision excluded British investigators. Papers were limited to a strict fifteen minutes, but the five-minute comment period could be extended if the moderator deemed it appropriate. Given the quasi-governmental aims of this new organization, it was no surprise that it authorized the French government to invite an official observer from each nation to watch sessions.[32]

That made things especially interesting, because the ICRF board recommended and the crown agreed to send Bashford as Britain's official non-member designee.[33] Bashford's appearance as official observer and the IACI's attempt to lure Britain into the fold became a highlight of the Paris sessions. Pierre Doumergue, the French minister of public instruction, welcomed the group of over 150 with a gentle plea for Britain to join the association, arguing that spontaneous congresses for the good of humanity were a "characteristic of our generation." Without these combinations, men and women of good faith faced the "futility of isolation." Bashford's opening address laid out his position. He championed collaboration and cited the ICRF's record there. But he adamantly argued that Britain remained opposed to the organization "upon purely scientific grounds only." Reminding the gathering that he was not there as a scientist but rather as a representative of the Crown, he maintained that now was "the time for work—much work—in the hope of advancing knowledge of a disease of which [we know] practically nothing about." Holding a conference and forming an international group was "premature, since [we have] nothing to discuss or to agree upon." What cancer investigators lacked was knowledge, and the conference put them no closer to that goal. "What is wanted at present is rather an army of independent active workers, for," Bashford concluded, "advances in knowledge are expected from individual investigation rather than from the deliberations of national committees or international conferences."[34]

Much of the actual meeting concerned itself with cancer nomenclature and cancer statistics. Emphasis on statistics both reflected the broadening of what constituted appropriate cancer research, a development clearly manifested at the 1906 meeting, but also a French-led and German-supported retreat to past and, in this case, discredited practice. Czerny emerged as the spokesman for the renewed movement. Citing the French investigators, who were "in direct communication with practitioners," he claimed that tabulating cancer statistics by site of infection and correlating those figures with "neighborhoods, houses and families" proved "most promising for determining etiology." These localized analyses, compiled by the very practitioners that denizens of the new laboratories had forcefully dismissed, seemed to Czerny to make it "possible . . . [for] more rapid progress than by general and universal statistics." That shocking acknowledgment of the cancer laboratory's limitations, an acknowledgement that Bashford found unconscionable, was followed by another similar pronouncement. Czerny conceded that high incidences of cancer "in certain localities and certain houses" indicated "a parasitical cause" for cancer even though "innumerable investigators" have as yet failed to isolate the culprit. David Paul von Hansemann, professor of pathological anatomy at the University of Berlin, demurred. He threw cold water on any attempt to use physician-generated statistics. Hansemann asserted that various practitioners (and some investigators) each used their own terminology to describe cancer cells as well as the relation of those outlaw cells to healthy tissue. This tower of Babel situation produced confusion and, since "the same lesions received different names and the same words were employed in different senses," any sort of statistical comparison would be fatally hampered.

Delbet, one of the organizers of the conference, proposed an extensive cancer nomenclature to set the matter straight. This nomenclature rested heavily on description and divided cancers by cell type, cell shape, cell depth, and organ type. It made a clear distinction between cancers of the epithelium and those of what it called the conjunctive-vascular. It established yet another category for cancers that had invaded multiple tissue types.

Delbet's scheme generated much heat but little light. The group argued over the nomenclature/classification question without resolution. It finally decided to empanel a special committee to seek "common ground" and, when that ground was uncovered, to establish that nomenclature as the IACI's official verbiage.[35] That resolved nothing, of course. If common ground had existed, the various convention partisans would have seized it.

Statistics fared nominally better. The IACI knew that it had access to three distinct types of statistical data. The first was morality reports. But the group complained that these official documents were subject to "unreliable diagnosis and dissimilar treatment . . . in statistical offices." The second type stemmed from collective investigations. Collective investigations usually started when a national or local medical society constructed cards through which individual members recorded their individual experience with a certain disease. These cards almost always had a series of yes/no questions, questions that could easily be tabulated. Investigations of this type proved notoriously unreliable for a variety of reasons. In the case of cancer, the assembled investigators complained about "irregular cooperation" by the very physicians undertaking the survey, as well as "uncertain diagnosis" due to a lack of a consistent nomenclature for disease and due to inconsistent training by attending physicians, "considerations of comfort, [and] indolence of patients." The third kind of data came from a single person—usually a physician but perhaps an actuary—pursuing his own statistical survey. These results remained the most garbled. They included some of the most precise, articulated data, while other investigators measured different factors and recorded an entirely different set of incidences. These statistics were not "of equal value." The convention agreed that the various statistics that had been so far produced "cannot be generally utilised [*sic*] for the purpose of drawing comparisons."

Despite the inconsistent, unreliable, and incomparable data, statisticians at the meeting put together a series of issues that they maintained could be resolved by a keen, dependable, rationalized set of statistics. These included number of cancer patients by country, whether the disease was increasing, the sex of cancer patients, proportional sites of the disease, and the efficacy of surgery as a curative. Statistics could show correlations between age and onset of the disease and between age and site of the disease. They could prove if any vocation or social position was disproportionally affected or if the disease struck more frequently in towns or in the countryside. A role for race and for heredity in the disease could be established or falsified, as could the possibility of infection. Finally, statistics could determine if alcohol, tobacco, syphilis, ulcerations, trauma, childbirth, nursing, and tuberculosis made individuals more liable to cancer.

Ledoux-Lebard, the other co-sponsor of the conference and, like his colleague, a professor at the University of Paris, was every bit as invested in a proper cancer statistics as Delbet was in a common nomenclature. Noting that unified cancer statistics was an issue of such "importance and complexity" that it could not be resolved at the conference, he urged his fellow attendees to devise a coherent set of agreed upon questions and metrics that would make statistics "really profitable." But even a rational statistical system was not enough. Cancer statistics were "really scientific research," he contended, and required practitioners to adopt the same "extreme rigor" in their method as prevailed in all other facets of the scientific enterprise. In short, he demanded that statisticians employ the same deductive techniques with their numbers that laboratory scientists did in their investigations.[36]

After several days and various and sundry papers on statistics and nomenclature, the organization held its closing session. Czerny, speaking in German, directly appealed to Bashford to use his influence to bring Great Britain into the union. He contended that he had always admired Bashford's research and that of the ICRF and stated that the new international body needed Bashford to get in line; it required his "support, experience and assistance." Czerny hoped that whatever objections Bashford held could be resolved before the executive board's meeting in Dresden the next year and that he would attend the session as a member. Bashford defended his institution's independence in English, arguing that the ICRF's research sponsorships demonstrated "international collaboration of a practical and useful kind," an implicit condemnation of the new group's efforts. He then addressed the German contingent in German and told them how much he admired their research. He said absolutely nothing of the international association's affairs.

Bashford's and the Czerny's speeches were pro-forma and masked the heated dispute that rested at the heart of the matter. Earlier at the conference, Czerny, Meyer, and Hansemann had come to the table where Bashford was eating. There, the Germans strenuously demanded that the British join the international association. Bashford demurred and asked pointedly why Britain should join. Was it so the Germans could "claim to lead and monopolize research on cancer?" "What have you done in Berlin," he continued, "only statistical nonsense." The verbal affront elicited a strong physical reaction by the Germans. Hansemann, "large, big, blond, short-sighted in the dyed pink, became scarlet with the eyes protruding and bloodshot." Meyer, "a small man wide and stocky, big square head, was purple. His fists were clenched and, he was grinding his teeth so forcefully that the skin of his cheeks rippled in waves because of the contraction of his jaw muscles." The two advanced threateningly toward Bashford. At that point, the French intervened, and while they had "a lot of trouble restoring calm," the dinner ended without further incident.

Even without the confrontation, everyone recognized tension between the two sides. Delbet and Ledoux-Lebard, both officers in the French association, were directly responsible for the meeting's success. Overseeing a gathering where the assembled "agreed on one point only—the pressing need for the solution of problems which almost each delegate stated in a different formulary," was no simple task. It required "bringing together, in intimate intercourse, strong men of varied nationality, holding strong and conflicting opinions."[37]

Despite Bashford's protestations and his nation's refusal to kowtow to the German monolith, ICRF had incorporated something similar to what the Germans were advocating from the Comité's beginnings; the fund was in part an offshoot of a scheme to fund a cancer lab for Middlesex Hospital. By 1905, the hospital's laboratory had explicitly moved in the clinical direction when it pledged trials for "any new remedy which [*sic*] even remotely promises success."[38] Philosophical differences—pursuing different avenues through which to locate cancer's cause—graphically separated England from Germany, but nationalism also stood as a major factor. England refused to cede any authority to the German juggernaut. British medicine and science demanded a leading role in the cancer struggle and would not acknowledge German preeminence.

The French had more nearly adopted the German model than the English. The entire history of the French laboratory effort emphasized clinical investigation more than its European neighbors. The way the cancer laboratory idea gained acceptance—through the strikingly public assertions of Doyen about the cause and cure of human cancer—guaranteed that a clinical component would rest at the center of the French anticancer fight.[39]

Although clinical investigation held an important place in the French effort, the Pasteur Institute's Amédée Borrel explained in the new organization's first paper that "physical experimentation" stood at the core of the new unit. Experimentation had banished "speculation," and for the mouse, researchers should "rejoice." Mice were liable to cancers similar to humans, had a short life span, and produced generations quickly. They were inexpensive, easy to care for, and kept in small spaces. Since they were found in every hamlet, village, and city, investigators could even perform statistical surveys on incidences of natural mouse cancers. In short, they had proven exquisite experimental creatures. "Mouse experimentation," Borrel concluded, has "taught us more than twenty centuries of sterile observations." These tiny animals promised to speed resolution of the cancer problem.

Borrel's ode to the mouse placed the French investigative effort in opposition to the German pathologists. The French investigator even recommended that the new international cancer union adopt the mouse as its "emblem!"[40] Americans generally remained aloof from European organizational squabbles, but the main cancer laboratories in the United States soon gravitated toward adding clinical work. Cause now made way for treatment, cure, and genesis in cancer research. In the case of the Rockefeller effort, John D. Rockefeller gave an additional endowment in 1908 to build a state-of-the-art hospital as an arm of the institute. There, investigators would engage in clinical observation and human trials, techniques likely to produce immediately applicable results.[41] Human testing might provide a direct answer to the question examined—it could become so—but it almost certainly produced headlines. Publicity was an important factor in the anti-cancer effort. Then as now, beneficence followed success. People proved more willing to give or even offer tacit backing to an endeavor when an immediate resolution rested at hand. Repeated indecision was synonymous to failure and jeopardized continued public support. It imperiled the future.

Antivivisectionists also menaced cancer laboratories. This was especially critical in New York. Antivivisectionists labored to force the state legislature to outlaw animal experiments as unethical and inhumane. Tales of needlessly sacrificed, even tortured, laboratory animals called into question not only the methods of investigators but also their character. Persons engaged in these barbaric practices hardly deserved public support and approbation.

Flexner was especially wary of the antivivisectionists' political power and became an avid crusader in explaining the necessity of animal experimentation to the public. He maintained that medicine demanded statistical certainty; only by enumerable, impeccably controlled trials could a fact be considered so. "In medical research," Flexner wrote, "reliable results can be obtained by comparisons and averages, requiring months, even years, of experiment." With humans, "there is no opportunity to observe many cases at a time." More to the point, each individual gave a slightly different cancer portrait. "Disease is like a personality," he continued, "a thing distinct and different in each." Investigators could overcome these hurdles by using mice and other small animals. "Experiments may be continued indefinitely," Flexner explained, "The subjects are easy to obtain and observe. Symptoms of cancer" could "be followed in many mice. The variations may be noted and eliminated." That approach brought tangible results: "From the symptoms [that] are common to all it is possible to arrive at conclusions that are universal so far as that phase of the disease is concerned." It ceased to be, according to Flexner, "a condition peculiar to a single mouse or even a group of them. It is the basis of truth." Knowledge of cancer was extended "point by point."

James Ewing, an AACR founder and in 1909 its president, seconded Flexner's assessment. Our "entire knowledge" about cancer had come "almost solely from vivisection of animals." Further progress toward defeating the disease could "be gained in no other way." Ewing, also the director of the Cornell-controlled Huntington Cancer Laboratory in New York City, dramatized his contention. Before animal experimentation, cancer research "was barren ground." Now, if animal vivisection was allowed to persist unabated,

Ewing felt confident enough to predict "that these experiments will ultimately result in the cure of the disease."[42]

Ewing and Flexner demanded that animal experimentation remain the basis of cancer research. They responded to the antivivisectionist campaign with such vituperation and passion because they recognized it for what it truly was, a direct threat to their enterprise. To Ewing, Flexner, and others, science itself was under assault. Their method of investigation was undergoing a fundamental challenge. Getting the public to understand that their essential manner of philosophic inquiry was indistinguishable from the results that they would produce remained paramount.

That recognition led them to broaden their defense of the necessity of animal testing to embrace a defense of science itself. Repeatedly they extolled science's virtues, pronouncing efforts an unqualified success. Ewing acknowledged that "some uninformed persons" had labeled "modern cancer research . . . wholly fruitless." He vehemently disagreed. Ewing asserted that "genuine progress has been made into the dark domain of cancer pathology by means of the experimental method." He urged skeptics to compare the progress of the "new era of experimental research," introduced only recently, with the results of the preceding "thousand years." "It was only thorough the repetition of experiments that we have learned all we know," he contended; our contemporary knowledge of cancer "could be acquired in no other way." In "study of cancer, more than any other disease," Ewing affirmed, "it has been proved that the investigator should be permitted absolute freedom in animal experimentation." Ewing believed it "the duty of every layman toward animal experimentation and cancer" to provide enthusiastic support. He claimed that history would be most unkind to whomever "may dare to lay obstacles in the way of this progress." Cancer researchers demanded and confidently expected "the moral support of every intelligent person." Ewing was so sure of his case that he "anticipate[d] that men of large minds and large means will come forward and adorn the land with one thoroughly organized and fully equipped institution for cancer research."[43]

Ewing predicted one grand cancer research effort. Funded entirely by beneficence, the facility would rationalize and systematize all the nation's cancer research work. It would stand as a greater version of the ICRF. The *New York Times* offered a contrary vision, but like Ewing's formulation, it too depended on philanthropy. In a feature piece titled "Wealth and Science Joining Hands for the Conquest of Cancer," the newspaper likened science to a "giant searchlight of world-illuminating power." At "a thousand laboratories," in "countless clinics," and "at the bedsides of hosts of patients," scientists search for a "flash from the heavens," a "gleam of knowledge," a "ray of hope." In "back of all this work" was "the power of gold." But all was not right. "Vast wealth to prosecute the study of cancer is still needed."

The *Times* identified cancer hospitals as the next logical stage in the cancer battle. "Devoted to the exclusive care and study of cancer," these institutions were "'clearing houses' of the 'cures'" for cancer. Here were "the exploited cures, the evanescent remedial agents which prove . . . failures when subjected to prolonged scientific tests." Already science had rejected "theories and 'cures' by the score." Laboratories as initially conceived had proven wanting. This "study and experimentation necessary to learn the truth" took place because of "the generosity of wealthy humanitarians." Coupled with the "devotion and heroism of an army of surgeons, laboratory workers, and nurses," these cancer research hospitals would offer "hope of the solution of the cancer problem."[44]

The often hyperbolic Flexner personalized the heroic element. At the same time, he elevated animal testing by recognizing the need for human clinical trials and observations. "If I could be assured" that cancer would be cured as a result, "I would gladly be one of thirty men to sacrifice my life" in an experiment. Many others would volunteer; it was the nature of the species. "Men risk their lives in war and deeds of daring, . . . ends less momentous than this cure for disease," he concluded.[45]

Alluding to human trials and animal experimentation in the same breath not only sanctified the latter, but also made new cancer hospitals a natural step in the cancer fight. Investigators needed to confirm that insights gained from experiments conducted on animals translated to people. This clinical complement to the cancer laboratory had another benison. Testing cures, treatments, or diagnostic agents in a world where cancer's cause seemed distant had become a new, legitimate research form. Clinical trials provided the public the appearance of success and more important motion. Cancer investigators seemed responsive to public concerns, not an insignificant factor in raising private donations. Loeb even thought that manifestations of progress were critical to the investigators themselves; lack of such benchmarks had "a paralyzing effect" on investigators.[46]

For these varied reasons, clinical cancer research facilities, a profound repudiation of the impetus to establishing laboratories some five years earlier, became the next institutions to join the American cancer fight. As early as 1908, Harvard's Croft Fund faculty began to call for a special cancer hospital to engage in cancer research "from a clinical standpoint." J. Collins Warren, the group's head, argued that cancer research "has now reached a point where it is possible to take a new departure" into clinical investigation. A new cancer hospital "would place the clinical and the laboratory work in close juxtaposition in such a way as to produce results which it is not possible" if they remained separate. As significant, a cancer hospital would provide cases enough to develop statistical inferences, something "the material of private practice" could not accomplish. Warren closed by noting that tuberculosis hospitals already existed and that the effort to cure that disease siphoned off money necessary to pay for new cancer hospitals. What he sought was a reallocation of "a moderate portion of the vast sums of money" now going to tuberculosis research to fund his vision. Indeed, he reminded his audience that cancer stood as the "next most dreaded disease of modern times."

In 1910, Warren and the commission refined their cancer hospital plans and justifications. They highlighted that the proposed Cambridge hospital would be presided "over by laboratory men," investigators steeped in the methods of the laboratory. Replacing practitioners and other clinicians with scientists had never "hitherto been attempted." Trained investigators "in a more intimate relation with living cancer" would "study the natural history of disease and observe the efficacy of new methods of treatment." More to the point, their special knowledge, training, and techniques would cause them to see things in a new way. A laboratory scientist–staffed and controlled cancer hospital would "lead to new observations and new interpretations of some of the phenomena attending the generalization of cancer." Cancer scientists possessed the ability to recognize phenomena that others not so highly tuned had surely missed.

This attempt to routinize and control clinical cancer observation rendered these new hospitals pseudo laboratories. Experiments there would take place. Cases of particular types would be so numerous that meaningful statistics could be gathered and then correlated. Variation would be eliminated or at least greatly diminished. Clinical science would achieve the same rigor that had marked the laboratory. The reason for this was clear. Laboratory scientists would run the hospitals. No place existed in this scheme for practitioners and other conventional medical men.

Part of this thrust stemmed in America from the very obvious decision to mimic facilities created to battle tuberculosis. These institutions gave tuberculosis a profound public presence, a permanent part of the civic experience. These landmarks to the disease were also landmarks to those who sought to conquer the disease; they established these researchers as central to the public weal and deserving of public approbation. In the case of the new cancer research hospitals, however, an additional inducement existed. They promised to channel public sentiment in a precise direction. Studies at these institutions would adjudicate whatever claims were made about a purported cure's efficacy. Laboratory rigor and clarity would reign. Cancer research hospitals would root out the various claims of nostrum vendors and others, activities that would both lessen the credibility of those offering them and raise that of researchers than put them asunder.

The Harvard Commission acquired funding for the hospital in 1910 and began construction a year later.[47] By that time, the Buffalo group also had secured funding for a cancer hospital. Gaylord had led that campaign. He testified to the legislature that the work at his laboratory had "progressed to the point" to "justify treatment to human beings in a hospital." The proposed institution needed to be under laboratory auspices. Without particular, meticulous investigation, results in the Buffalo cancer hospital could not be correlated with those elsewhere. Comparability was essential. Gaylord shamelessly asserted that researchers were on the verge of "revolutionising [*sic*] treatment of malignant disease" and worried that incomparable results would delay acceptance of an "epoch-making" breakthrough.

When, in early 1911, the legislature authorized and funded the New York State Institute for the Study of Malignant Disease, William Warren Potter, editor of the *Buffalo Medical Journal*, hailed its creation as the "consummation of a fifteen year campaign" to erect appropriate institutions to battle cancer. That statement was absolutely incorrect. The hospital became desirable only after the nature of cancer research had changed. The original thrust had failed. Clinical study by laboratory scientists emerged as a viable research agenda when hope of a quick discovery of the cause of cancer disappeared. Gaylord proudly noted that Buffalo had now joined Heidelberg, the Rockefeller Institute, and the anticipated Croft facility as cancer laboratories to which a cancer research hospital had been affixed. Like the others, the new Buffalo hospital "will be conducted exclusively in the interests of science." There will be no visiting physicians, only laboratory personnel. The only patients admitted will be those who "through investigation [or] experimental treatment, . . . prove of benefit to medical research." Procedures would be instituted to ensure that each patient, upon admission, received the same battery of standardized tests. These tests set base lines for patients. They established normality and thus created a place from which to evaluate experimental therapies.[48]

Not to be outdone, Ewing agitated for a similar new structure in New York City, affiliated with the Loomis laboratory. In 1912, Cornell received a donation large enough to purchase control over one-half of the already extant New York General Memorial Hospital. The Cornell-run part was divided further. Half would be used to train medical students in clinical medicine. The rest became a cancer research hospital under the Loomis Laboratory's authority. Two years later, Ewing had convinced Dr. James Douglas, then principal of both the Copper Queen Mine and the El Paso & Southwestern

Railroad, to donate over a million dollars to create a separate cancer research facility, "the largest cancer hospital in the country and next in size only to the London (Middlesex) and Heidelberg Hospitals." In addition, Douglas pledged the first 7 grams of radium salt—worth an estimated $500,000—produced by his newest Colorado mine to treat cancer.[49]

Columbia University also joined the cancer quest, albeit in a slightly different way. In 1908, George Crocker gave the university money enough to fund a cancer laboratory, which opened almost immediately. He bequeathed a multimillion-dollar estate to Columbia upon his death the next year. Crocker had a long relationship with cancer research, but as a litigant. In 1906, he filed suit in Paris against Doyen for fraud, for exercising "'verifiable moral violence' in making [Crocker] believe it was possible to cure his wife," who had perished after suffering the disease.

The university quickly decided to use the bequest exclusively for "cancer research," promised to pursue it "experimentally" in laboratories and hospitals, and pledged that "close co-operation" among "scientists engaged in cancer research" would mark the two facilities. It did not rush to erect a new edifice. Instead, its president, Nicholas Murray Butler, toured the laboratories of Europe to view research facilities there. The university also involved the city's medical men in its early experiments. It urged them to identify incipient cancer cases. "Every patient of middle age," when suffering "hemorrhages and catarrhs," should be checked for the disease." The university would examine "samples of suspected tissues" and, if they were found to be cancerous, would propose an experimental method of treatment.

A lawsuit by the Crocker heirs delayed introduction of a revamped research program for nearly two years. When the matter was finally adjudicated, Francis Carter Wood, the school's professor of pathology, was appointed to lead the effort. Among his earliest initiatives was to contemplate establishing a separate facility to breed mice and rats. This rodent farm would guarantee that the laboratory would receive animals of uniform breed and age. It would permit investigators to control an additional animal research variable. For various reasons, including the possibility of fire or epizootic to wipe out the entire supply, Wood chose to enter into long-term contracts with several breeders to reduce that catastrophic risk. Also among Wood's first acts at the Crocker was to inoculate a reported five thousand mice with cancer. Whenever a new curative method was proposed that seemed "worthy of consideration," tumors were transplanted into one hundred mice on which to test the new substance's efficacy.

Perhaps the most important decision Wood made for the institution's future was inducing William H. Woglom to leave his post as Bashford's assistant at the ICRF. Bringing Woglom to Columbia ensured that the new facility would more nearly mimic the English model than the German. Columbia did not create a distinct cancer hospital from the Crocker estate. Rather, it negotiated an agreement with the neighboring St. Luke's Hospital to undertake clinical cancer research experiments there, an approach reminiscent of the ICRF's relationship with Middlesex Hospital. More than any of its prominent American contemporaries, Columbia's Crocker Fund complex placed some distance between laboratory and clinical cancer research efforts.[50]

In effect, laboratories attempted to resolve the cancer problem by erecting new artifices. The reason for that was straightforward. As it was conceived, the cancer problem was a problem of misdiagnosis; researchers misunderstood the difficulties that they would face in their laboratories as they searched from cancer's cause. They anticipated a consistent, relatively quick resolution to the question, as laboratories throughout the Western world labored on the same course and in the same way. Nothing could have been further from the truth. There was precious little commonality in the process and no meaningful mechanisms to make things so. Even as international efforts were under way, spats emerged among nations, among medical specialties, among laboratory scientists and statisticians, among animal experimenters, and more. Partisans employed analogy after analogy in support of their contentions, but these analogies failed to persuade. They frequently referenced different, often contradictory things.

Each of these disagreements among people and places remained powerful, but failure to find cancer's cause was most threatening. This failure disheartened researchers and promised to end funding. As a consequence, laboratory directors began to champion a new consequence of their laboratories. They maintained that the laboratory's real purpose was knowledge creation, knowledge that ultimately came to bear on human health. The quest for cancer's culprit took a backseat. Laboratory survival and survival of the persons engaged there became tantamount.

It is from that impetus that cancer hospitals emerged. The laboratory opened a second front on the war for cancer. This new kind of bedside and hospital observation regained some currency at the continued expense of traditional medical men and other practitioners. These new cancer hospitals were the province of the laboratory. In effect, laboratories offered a kind of resolution to the scientific problem they could not overcome through a more intense and extensive organization. The laboratory-inspired cancer hospitals were subjected to the same scrutiny, the same standards, as laboratories themselves. But unlike laboratories, cancer hospitals offered the public an additional blessing. They would also test remedies and rule on the effectiveness of cancer treatments. Ironically, their utility was inversely proportional to that of the laboratory. The longer laboratory scientists failed to find cancer's cause, the more necessary cancer hospitals seemed. Practitioners and others would propose more treatments and offer more elixirs, each of which had to be scrutinized according to the newest laboratory methods in the guise of attempting to protect a defenseless public. Revenue to run the laboratory and laboratory hospital could well follow each of these hospital successes . . . and continued laboratory failures.

5

Return to Babel, 1905–1910

Creating cancer hospitals in conjunction with cancer laboratories nominally integrated clinical research into the cancer quest. Human patients and human cancers were now to become the subject of rigorous controlled experiments. The individuals undertaking those experiments possessed the credentials and skills necessary for success in the laboratory. They would passionately seek to control variables. They would strive to detect deviations from normality. They would describe, classify, and interpret with abandon.

Cancer hospitals would be venues in which laboratory scientists plied their characteristic trades. But that belies the issue of why these new institutions seemed necessary. Why in a few short years after agitating for and receiving cancer laboratories did these same investigators return to their benefactors and ask for new, different institutions? To be sure, the new requests were for scientific institutions, institutions designed and created to be operated by scientists and for the pursuit of scientific research. Yet these new entities seemed to contemporaries essential precisely because their proponents determined and argued that they lacked the facilities at hand to resolve the questions that those previous bodies were established to resolve. Simply put, laboratories did not seem capable of securing the cause of cancer in anything approaching an acceptable period of time. Mountains of deaths would accrue as they prosecuted the search.

That was the genesis after about 1905 of what researchers repeatedly called the "cancer problem." Their ardent pursuit of the resolution of that problem continued for the rest of the decade and beyond. They had institutions that they initially believed to be suited for that pursuit. Increasingly, however, the "cancer problem" too seemed irredeemable, at least in the immediate future. Cancer research towards the "cancer problem" as it had been defined in 1905—a lack of coordinated action—had been corrected with the various formalized institutions and networks beyond the laboratory. And with this web of knowledge and interaction in place, surely the lack of comparability of research and results that had marked the previous decades would be resolved. It was a matter of organization, and that is what the national and international associations were established for and attempted to accomplish.

While they might contribute to the quest for cancer's cause, cancer hospitals were primarily a public diversion. Their purpose was to provide laboratories time, time to continue research already apace. Laboratories rarely revamped or scrapped their preexisting research lines. Buffalo remained passionately committed to finding the cancer parasite. The ICRF continued its research into and research support of cancer's biology. Questions of the transplantation of cancer continued to be vital, and immunity from the disease gained special currency.

As the decade neared its end, laboratories—and organization itself—seemed to move the various investigators no closer to resolving conflicting interpretations, evidence, and theories. With respect to cancer, laboratories, professional societies, and other bodies could not make things so. They could not speak with one or at least a dominant voice; they failed to produce unambiguous experimental results or theoretical assertions that could be championed by their memberships and beyond. Affiliates only had what they started with, a storehouse of analogies and a method, technique, and training to pursue their problem in a specific manner. Investigators in the new century's first decade had little more than a single grand synthesis or shared overarching vision: cancer had a single cause. Outside of that, their training, and their predilection to resort to analogies, they had precious little to agree upon.

Their method was their madness. The premises upon which they operated made it virtually impossible to move beyond what they already knew and remain respected within their disciplines. Indeed, theories of cancer remained as diverse and as murky as ever. George H. Simmons approached the matter backwards. Knowing that parasites—germs—must produce cancer, he used "past experience" (analogy) to reason "why we can not see these micro-organisms." Editor of *JAMA* in 1906, Simmons concluded that the cancer "parasite may be ultramicroscopic, . . . unstainable by methods at present known, or . . . so closely resemble the cells of the host as to be indistinguishable." After further deliberations, he singled out studies by the German pathologist Otto Schmidt, who posited that amoebae, often found in tumor cultures, were cancer vectors; they hosted a cancer-producing parasite.[1]

Simmons's reasoning proved illustrative because it demonstrated the depths to which medical men had plummeted as they tenaciously clung to a microbial cancer explanation. Here was a leading member of the American medical community so certain that a pathogenic agent was responsible for the disease that he was willing to suspend reliance on any sort of sensory evidence. He knew what he knew—he knew the present state of the art—and refused to brook any other hypothesis.

Nor was Simmons unique. Amédée Borrel also offered a similarly deterministic perspective. Working with Metchnikoff at the Pasteur Institute, Borrel noted what he called epidemics of cancer among caged mice. This he knew to be analogous to cancer houses or localities, situations where an unanticipated number of closely situated residents suffered the disease. With that assumption in hand, Borrel debated how such an occurrence might happen. First, he concluded that the causes must be local. Only an emphasis on the locality explained why one cage of mice had high incidences of the disease while others might have none. He then checked the cancer cage surroundings and the bodies of diseased mice. There he discovered a rather tiny nematode in a surprising number of incidences. Borrel's ultimate conclusion was that the nematode was a cancer vector; some as yet unidentified cancer-causing agent went from mouse to mouse through the nematode, causing in each case a separate infection. But Borrel continued his circular reasoning to show just how his cancer house/caged mice analogy now produced new information about human cancer. To Borrel, his findings proved "why cancer is common in damp countries, in places where manure heaps are so badly kept close to human habitations, and in places where irrigation of sewage is carried on."[2]

The problem with Borrel's environmental assumption, of course, was that it was based solely on impressionistic evidence. In the last years of the nineteenth century and the first years of the twentieth, there had been numerous studies of cancer and environmental suitability. They proved remarkably inconclusive. Investigators had reported so much contradictory information as to discredit statistical utility for the cancer problem. Environmental statistics and cancer distribution had yielded to the hypothetical certainty of laboratories.

Borrel was neither the only investigator to detect localized cancer outbreaks among laboratory animals nor the only one to interpret them as he did. Still others offered alternative explanations. For example, Gaylord focused on a similar phenomenon but did not consider environmental quality. "Spontaneous" cancer outbreaks had arisen among mice in certain cages in his Buffalo laboratory. Searching through the recent medico-scientific literature, Gaylord uncovered several incidences throughout the world of these localized laboratory epidemics. But his purpose in exposing this recurring phenomenon was somewhat different from Borrel's. A longtime enthusiast of a microbial explanation for cancer, Gaylord seized upon these epizootics occurring among laboratory animals as demonstrable evidence that cancer was infectious. In these studies, Gaylord was not attempting to identify the cancer-causing agent; he was simply trying to unsully his reputation after several of his previous pronouncements proved grossly premature. The data that Gaylord had compiled, he argued, "should tend to combat the belief among pathologists" that cancer was not contagious. He argued it "probable" that infection of the surroundings accounted for "cancer houses" and called on physicians to sterilize dressings of cancer patients as well as "the rooms which they have occupied."[3]

Gaylord's renewed contention that cancer was of microbial origin got a boost from Gary N. Calkins, professor of zoology at Columbia University and a colleague of Gaylord's at the Buffalo lab. Calkins reported that he and others had isolated spirochetes from virtually every mouse tumor and suspected that these miniscule microorganisms might produce cancer. Calkins named the strain of these microbes *Spirocheata gaylordi* to celebrate his lab director. He also contended that similar, although not necessarily identical, spirochetes were found in human tumors.[4]

These microbes seemed to fulfill the various prophecies that Simmons and others had predicted for cancer's ultimate cause. They were small, almost infinitesimal, barely at the edge of what could be seen under a conventional microscope. They did not respond to the common aniline stains but required radically different staining reagents and techniques. In fact, staining these particular spirochetes only became possible a few months earlier, when the Buffalo group adapted a new stain created at the Pasteur Institute explicitly for staining the newly identified spirochete of syphilis, a disease almost as fearsome as cancer. Gaylord even argued that the cancer-associated spirochetes went through an incredible number of morphological changes as they entered the body and became engaged with tumors, an occurrence that rendered them difficult to detect as a single consistent microbial entity.[5]

Gaylord quickly went to otherwise "uncontaminated" mice—mice not housed in the infectious cages—and inoculated them with both parts of a Jensen mouse tumor and the suspicious spirochetes. He reported that these mice developed cancer of the breast in unprecedented numbers. Yet he remained cautious. "It is obviously too early to draw far-reaching conclusions from the presence of these organisms in our mouse tumors," he noted. "Our observations do not as yet establish an etiologic relationship between this organism and cancer." But the "presence of the organism in primary mouse cancer," greatly "increasing in number as the tumors increase in virulence," coupled with the fact that it enhances transplantation—something that bacterial colonies inhibited—"is suggestive," reported Gaylord.[6] Gaylord had taken care not to claim that these entities caused cancer. He merely argued that, in all the mouse tumors he had observed, these entities were present. He also asserted that these spirochetes were correlated both with enhanced tumor transplantation and virulence.

Such reticence to claim more for the work was striking, and Calkins explained why he and Gaylord took such a conservative approach. They did so because they were scientists. "From such men the public hears little or nothing, for familiarity with the subject breeds with them only the deeper sense of its subtlety," Calkins noted, "and with it a keen appreciation of the false hopes aroused and the disappointments that will surely follow the premature publication of hasty and unproved conclusions." Matters of science must be resolved among scientists before they were related to the public. To do otherwise would be the mark of a charlatan, bilking the public and undercutting its appreciation of the virtue of science. "Fed only on the popularized conceptions which science exploiters furnish," Calkins continued, "it is small wonder that the general reader grows to accept ill-timed and unbalanced theories of cause or cure, which, being afterward refuted, awaken in him a distrust of any theory whatsoever." The public's only salvation rested in the methods of science. "If rigorously followed," he concluded, those methods "are bound to produce accurate and reliable results which are sure of an ultimate acceptance that will dispel the crude theories by which the popular mind has been more or less misled."[7]

Calkins's statements were realpolitik in action. They came from a profound understanding of the limitations of the laboratories in which he and other like-minded researchers labored. Victory over cancer had been promised to be swift. That it had not proven so posed a huge problem for those whose research and livelihoods depended primarily on beneficence. Anything that questioned their centrality, anything that challenged their preeminence, threatened both the project and their person. Anything that increased public patience would prove a benison.

Calkins issued his apologia with a precise situation in mind. That event had been roiling in the public press for nearly a year, garnering considerable attention and proving a potent threat to laboratory labors. Ironically, the turmoil-causing work stemmed not from a huckster but rather a researcher far more respected that Calkins.[8]

James Beard, a lecturer in embryology at the University of Edinburgh, was the scientist around whose work controversy had surfaced. His full, nuanced explanation for cancer had resulted in Beard receiving a Nobel Prize for Medicine nomination. Beard's theory did not depend initially on an outside infectious agent but rather on what occurred within the body. Beard combined the insights of Butlin, who saw the cancer cell itself to be a parasite, and conclusions of the first Farmer, Moore, and Walker paper, especially their contention that cancer cells replicated in a manner similar to sex cells. He then added his own investigations into embryology, as well as wild flights of analogy, to fashion in 1906 a compelling theory of cancer and its cure.[9]

Under a grant from the Carnegie Trust for Scotland, Beard had spent much of his early career studying fish embryos. He noted among his discoveries that germ cells in embryonic fishes regularly moved through the entire organism as they made their way to what would become incipient gonads. Often these mobile cells never reached their destination; they migrated to various nooks and crannies within the emergent creature.

To Beard, these lost germ cells in fish seemed analogous to cancer in the same species. They divided asexually and took root in random places. Therefore, he concluded that cancer must not be the consequence of an outside agency but rather a natural phenomenon; cancer in fishes was the manifestation of a natural process that others mistakenly identified as an invasive disease. But Beard also recognized and wrote about how analogous much of fish embryology was to mammalian embryology and ultimately to human embryology. He found himself fascinated with the mechanism by which a barely differentiated mammalian embryo managed to attach itself to the placenta to receive nutrients from its mother. These trophoblastic cells, among the first to become discernible in a mammalian embryo, seemed to invade the mothers' tissues as they attached the incipient dependent organism to the placenta.

Embryonic trophoblasts worked according to biological rules. They behaved predictably. Cancer did not. To denote the similarity between cancer and trophoblastic cells and to show the analogy there, Beard argued that cancer cells acted like "irresponsible trophoblasts," attaching themselves to otherwise normal cells and multiplying out of control. Their deployment and rapid proliferation overwhelmed regular tissue and prevented normal functioning.

An enzyme provided the mammalian embryo the mechanism that enabled the trophoblasts to attach themselves to the placenta. Therefore, Beard postulated that an enzyme—he often called it a ferment—might also work to insinuate cancer cells among healthy ones, which produced tumor growth. This predicted substance Beard called malignin.

But Beard went further. He wondered why the embryonic mammalian trophoblasts did not continue to invade tissue after affixing the embryo to the placenta. His studies led him to conclude that those wandering, unattached trophoblasts declined and disappeared at precisely the time that the pancreas became differentiated and began functioning. Further analysis led him to detect a series of pancreatic enzymes in the fetus, and he postulated that the production of these enzymes terminated unfixed trophoblastic activity.

What Beard had supposed in effect was something analogous to a serum-antiserum reaction but that naturally occurred with enzymes in mammalian embryos. One substance caused invasion, another, unleashed later, prohibited it. To Beard, the whole process was nothing more than a matter of dosage (although Beard referred to this as power). Whichever enzyme was the most prolific—the most "powerful"—dictated the progress or regress of cancer.[10]

Since he reasoned that cancer was analogous to trophoblastic action and he believed that embryonic pancreatic enzymes destroyed these "irresponsible" actors, it did not require a great leap for Beard to test pancreatic enzymes on human cancer. In a matter of months, he announced that one enzyme, trypsin, demonstrated considerable cancer-inhibiting properties.

Leyden and his supporters were among the first to put this chemotherapeutic agent—this purified natural abstract—to the test. They found it quite active in lysing cancer cells.[11] Beard himself turned to the Jensen mouse. There a series of unfortunate occurrences—mice getting stuck between bars in cages and suffocating, for instance—a dearth of mice upon which to experiment, and results described verbally and subjectively rather than by physical measurement contributed to a less-than-compelling paper. Nonetheless, Beard pronounced himself elated with the results. "In advance I know," he contended, "that no matter how often we repeat this experiment, even with much smaller doses [of trypsin], the like results will invariably be obtained. In the nature of things it must be so." This was because "in the cancer ferment, malignin, and in trypsin, we have an antithesis of ferments, of which the latter is more powerful."[12]

Beard's analogy-based, highly unscientific statements mattered little. His prestige within the scientific community gave his research force. The medical press and medical societies greeted his work cautiously but optimistically. For example, a London practitioner, A. Howard Pirie, who would later be elected a fellow of the faculty of radiology of the Royal College of Surgeons in Ireland, decided to try trypsin on a uterine cancer patient. Although she died some weeks into the treatment, Pirie still declared the experiment successful. His patient did not die of the tumor per se, he recounted. As trypsin digested the tumor, there was a "setting free of the products of the tumour, and these products in the weak condition of the patient proved too much for her and caused her death." Pirie did not conduct a necropsy to confirm his speculation—he knew it to be true—but nonetheless warned fellow physicians to treat with trypsin "early before the patient has lost much strength."[13]

W. A. Pusey, a Chicago-based practitioner and pioneer roentgenologist, offered a different assessment. His human experiments on seven hopeless cases led him to conclude that trypsin directly injected into a tumor could indeed decrease the mass. But he also noted that injection sites often became quite angry and painful. This he attributed to the trypsin itself. In some patients, trypsin injections produced "chills" and "cachexia" with patients failing "more rapidly than they were failing before." He was forced to conclude that trypsin did "appreciable harm" to those patients. "I should try trypsin again," he agreed, but only in instances where "a few injections [could] destroy a localized mass."[14]

Cautious optimism of practitioners gave way to unbridled enthusiasm in the public press. Caleb W. Saleeby, a British physician who had studied with Beard and a prominent eugenicist whose 1904 book *The Cycle of Life*, an exposition on the glory of social Spencerianism, converted him into a prominent literary figure, was the culprit. He wrote a series of articles in American periodicals touting Beard's work as signaling the imminent victory over cancer. Capitalizing on the new ten cent magazines and their muckraking approach, Saleeby proclaimed first "the coming conquest of cancer" and then "the conquest of cancer," even writing an entire volume in 1907 with that title to mark this seminal moment. Saleeby justified his brazenness by arguing that "this is no time for hiding such a light under a bushel." It "would be cruel and cowardly to refrain" from "giving . . . the widest and most immediate publicity to these facts." A "series of miraculous interventions with the course of nature . . . promises to put an end forever to what is perhaps the most appalling of all the ills that flesh is heir to." As he sang the praises of Beard and trypsin, Saleeby called on his fellow physicians throughout the world to begin immediate human trials.[15]

Newspapers quickly picked up this story, hailing Beard and trypsin as potential saviors and urging physicians to get on board. Most curious was the self congratulatory tone to the articles. Writers viewed trypsin as a success in "the war against cancer." Everyday "special laboratories are springing up in all countries and they have staffs obligated to investigate cancer and to devote their whole time to this duty."[16] But that conceit about the sanguinity of these special cancer labs was misplaced. In the case of trypsin and many other remedies and questions, the facilities could not do what they promised. They could not make trypsin so.

Saleeby's public pronouncements marked a watershed, and a negative one at that. Medical journals and physicians railed against an unsanctioned person bringing what they deemed a professional matter to the public and soon came to identify trypsin with "other" forms of quackery. Saleeby had committed the unpardonable sin. He had taken what was to be a medical, scientific matter—a matter for the new cancer laboratories, not for litterateurs—and converted it to a public debate where any practitioner could offer evidence and research. Wakely summed up the case succinctly, explaining how Saleeby's comments undercut the ambitions of the preeminence of organized medicine. Trypsin "has been much extolled by the lay press" and the public has "forced the use of trypsin on the profession." We "deprecate any attempt to bring before the [public] questions which are *sub judice* in the profession. Only evil will result" from bringing such matters "to such an incompetent tribunal."[17]

Despite opposition from medical organizations in Britain, America, and Germany, trypsin would remain for years a staple of the medical and public cancer discourses. Beard continued to back the drug, and his scientific stature gave investigators pause. But the real explanation for its persistence rested on the appalling lack of standardization for human and animal experimentation, the very sort of thing cancer laboratories had expected to resolve. Coupled with opening the debate to individual medical practitioners—not just institutions that purportedly would speak with one voice—the matter began to resemble the tower of Babel. Dozens of medical men tested the drug on patients. Several scientists looked at the drug in mice. None of these experiments proved deterministic to their contemporaries. And that was the case even as a significant portion of medical institutions stood predisposed to disbelieve positive results because of Saleeby's heresy. Results of experiments varied and whenever they did, a member of the opposing camp offered a plausible explanation. For example, many, perhaps most, practitioners noted that the cancers of some subjects—persons or animals—treated with trypsin seemed to respond to the drug. But what did that mean? How did that compare with a normal, trypsin-less course? Was there something peculiar about the location of the tumor, the regimen, the synthesis or preparation of this not quite common chemical? Why did it not seem to work in other cases? Was it introduced in too great or too small quantities to neutralize the cancer? Was it given to subjects too early or too late in the disease's course? Should it have been administered orally, subcutaneously, intramuscularly, intravenously, or directly into the tumor? What exactly did "respond to the drug" mean? Was it freedom from all vestiges of the disease, shrinkage of the tumor, prolonged life span, or something else?

What time span should testing protocols use? How comparable were mice and human testing in the case of trypsin? Did trypsin need another agent to assist its anti-cancer properties? Leyden, his laboratories, and the new IACI certainly thought so. They postulated that a certain abstract of the liver magnified the power of trypsin and converted it into a potent, active anti-cancer drug. Given that, in almost every one of these varied, contradictory studies, the number of subjects upon which each idiosyncratic report was issued was extremely small—usually significantly less than a dozen—no generalizations were truly possible from this chaotic, incomparable data.[18]

The British medical press, Middlesex Hospital, and the ICRF worked hard to quell the trypsin wave. Their critique of the drug came quickly. After Saleeby's first essays, the *BMJ* refused to publish articles or letters by Beard. It also denigrated the German studies supporting the drug.[19] As part of its new expansion of research to include consideration of reputed cancer cures, Middlesex Hospital seized on trypsin rather quickly. The hospital worked with Beard in an attempt to translate his experiments into practical clinical trials but refused to follow critical parts of his protocol. ICRF did not even feign objectivity. It summarily announced in its 1907 and 1908 annual reports that it had tested the drug and found it not useful but offered no evidence to support its claim. The group's separate 1908 edition of scientific work, which supposedly detailed ICRF research during the preceding year, included not a single mention of any trypsin research. This break with past practice made it impossible for Beard to offer an experiment-by-experiment refutation or explanation. He was not privy to any ICRF trypsin research. While response proved considerably more varied in America and ultimately Germany, the trypsin boom had ended in the first years of the next decade.[20]

The quest for a cure did not rest at trypsin. Roentgen rays were frequently tested on existing tumors. They were found somewhat useful in burning off surface lesions but little else. Fulguration also had its adherents.[21] But the most consistent approaches toward a cure during the last years of the century's first decade were to develop an antitoxin, create a vaccine to prevent the disease, find a chemical toxic to cancer cells but reasonably safe to the host, or produce antibodies to fight the malady. These techniques had been long established by Pasteur, Ehrlich, and Von Behring and adopted by Doyen and a host of more-well-regarded researchers. They were standard techniques for diseases consistent with the germ theory of disease. They were known. The simple process of analogy allowed them for this instance to mimic what was already established protocol.[22]

An important caveat needs to be mentioned here. Each of the aforementioned therapies was based upon the idea that each of those diseases had a specific pathogen and that those pathogens were infectious or contagious. Neither was necessarily true in the case of cancer. Investigators need not accept cancer as the product of an invasive agent. They needed only to believe in the power of analogy, that already extant therapies might be adapted to a disease with a single cause that did not meet the criteria from which the procedure was created.

A necessary first step in preparation of any of the above therapies was to identify true cases of human cancer that had undergone complete, permanent remission. Gaylord led that charge. To be sure, there had been sporadic reports in the literature of individuals with desperate cases of the disease that became cancer-free, but those instances always were suspect; they depended on the word and skill of the practitioners in charge and were not verifiable. Gaylord's contribution was to begin the process with Jensen mice and then to use statistics to determine what percentage of these animals underwent spontaneous cure. His 101 cases where the tumor totally disappeared constituted about 23 percent of these artificially induced cancers. But Gaylord did not stop there. He recognized that mouse cancer and the human disease were quite different—you could not transplant human cancer to mice—but he believed they were analogous and supposed that there might be analogous instances of spontaneous remission in humans. He therefore pored through case reports in medical journals compiling all incidences of spontaneous human remission. Gaylord's initial conclusion was that, due to "the frequency of the occurrence and its distribution in animals," spontaneous cures "may be more frequent in human beings than is generally supposed." He followed that up with a bolder statement. He argued that these cures reflected "the existence of immune forces capable of terminating the disease" and urged his laboratory colleagues to accelerate "research directed toward the discovery of a serum-therapeutic treatment."[23]

This presumption was not taken at face value. In fact, W. Roger Williams took the significant occurrence of cancer-ridden Jensen mice becoming cancer-free to question whether the Jensen tumor was indeed cancer. No unaffiliated doctor, Williams was a fellow of the Royal College of Surgeons and a frequent contributor to the medical literature. He was especially suspicious at the relative ease by which the Jensen tumor was transmitted and posited that that itself was a sign of misdiagnosis. He did not doubt that the Jensen tumor caused a proliferation of cells, but he did not believe that all cellular proliferations were cancer. He cited precedent. There were several earlier misdiagnoses in which diseases seemed to imitate some aspects of cancerous tumors but were later proven to be unrelated. This was another such case, "a mere bogey, the lineal descendant of other such bogeys." That such misidentification could occur testified to what Williams considered the state of the art of "experimental cancer research." It was "a medley of 'chaos, clouds and tongues,' in which there is neither light nor leading."[24]

Such a harsh pronouncement did not persuade laboratories generally to eschew the Jensen mouse. But attempting to create other strains of tumors in other families of mice proved a common occurrence. Several investigators voiced concern that standardizing techniques and approaches around one type of tumor in one rodent strain limited investigators too much. Years of study on the Jensen tumor had led investigators to plot out its virulence and basic metabolism. In the years after 1905, Gaylord's Buffalo group developed the Brooklyn tumor and Springfield tumors in mice and then tried to measure such things as spontaneous recoveries, ease of incubation, response to different chemicals, and the ability to convey immunity through the blood serum of recovered mice, as well as the recovered mice's own resistance to a subsequent bout of the disease. Among their most significant findings were that recovered mice were immune to reinoculation and that their blood carried some immunizing properties to as yet healthy mice but virtually none for mice with early cases of cancer.[25]

It should be noted that attempts to develop new strains of cancer in certain closely related laboratory mice ran contrary to earlier assessments of cancer and heredity. Indeed, the noted Pearson, so instrumental in the eugenics movement in Great Britain, had disavowed any meaningful statistical relationship between cancer and human relations. Yet, in the case of laboratory animals, researchers took as gospel that, with respect to cancer, closely related animals would breed true; they would develop the same tendency toward a specific type of tumor. They believed that you could standardize laboratory animals by tumors and so have the control of variables so dear to laboratory work.[26]

Some groups, including Flexner's Rockefeller contingent, worked with species other than mice. They, too, retained the fundamental assumptions about the hereditability of tumors. Rats, the choice of the institute, and dogs proved the most common. Experimenting on a species different from the one on which most investigation occurred promised to remove species-specific phenomena from the equation. But the work undertaken by Flexner and his associates was not fundamentally different in character or in results from the work of those researchers who continued with various mice strains. Their most important observation was reporting that a cancerous tumor of one tissue type could, over generations of transplanting, "learn" to become a tumor of a different tissue. In then-contemporary parlance, a carcinoma could become a sarcoma, a factor that brought into question the whole concept of tumor taxonomies and typing. Rather than clarifying the cancer problem, the Rockefeller effort complicated it.[27]

Explanations offered to account for this phenomenon made the situation even more tenuous. Two basic positions for the tumor conversion over time presented themselves. Some investigators suggested that frequent transplantation weakened the affinity of the cancer parasite for one type of tissue—a sort of tissue-specific antibiosis resulted—and, in either a Darwinian or Lamarckian fashion, the tumor cells established themselves firmly in tissues that had previously seemed resistant, even antagonistic. The other group offered a simple mechanical explanation. Repeated transplants and inoculations unleashed a substance that caused the tissues of the initial inoculation to become the source of an "irritating influence." That influence proved, over generations, to be potent enough to manufacture a suitable locus—a weakness or injury—in other tissue where the tumor cells could take root.[28]

A disease of dogs aroused special concern. Usually reported as a lymphosarcoma, it was characterized by genital tumors, but histological reports varied considerably as to the nature of these tumors. Some researchers identified them as carcinoma, others as sarcoma, and yet others as canine syphilis. This last group, and others still who did not think the disease syphilitic, objected to the nodes being designated tumors. This final group attributed the tumor-like nodules to an irritation, such as the type that followed a bacterial infection. The disease's manner of transmission proved particularly controversial. It was almost always associated with copulation.

Two main investigative camps emerged. Led by Bashford, an English group asserted that the disease's transmission by intercourse demonstrated it was not cancer but, rather, a disease that mimicked cancer. They further bolstered their case by arguing that tuberculosis mycobacterium was frequently associated with the disease and that the disease was comparatively rare in older dogs. The former suggested a specific microbial origin, while the latter was inconsistent with the normal age distribution for cancer.

Gaylord and others rabidly disagreed. Long denizens of a microbial explanation for cancer, they seized on the histology and argued that it proved the disease to be cancer. That it appeared infectious led them to conclude that this particular malady demonstrated that cancer generally was parasitic and contagious.[29]

This debate continued for much of the century's first decade. Two Loomis Lab investigators, George C. Crile and S. P. Beebe, offered a plausible third position. Starting from the assumption that the disease exhibited many of the signposts of cancer, such as metastases, lack of an identifiable microorganism found in all cases, and the fact that the tumor tissue could be transplanted over a wide temperature range and still yield the disease, they then set their minds to how it was transmitted. They began with the act of coitus itself. Examining numerous animals after intercourse, they almost always found "some abrasions of the mucous membranes." That led them to conclude that the method of transmission was not infection but, rather, transplantation. The "tumor cell" of one animal was transplanted to "the abraded surface" of the other.[30]

This explanation did not end debate, but it certainly reduced its intensity. That lack of resolution demonstrated just how difficult it was to correlate studies over various species and breeds and to arrive at something approaching consensus. As the histological determinations revealed, it was not always possible even to compare a single, straightforward scientific assessment between laboratories an ocean apart. Despite these technical and philosophical difficulties, animal studies remained an essential facet of the laboratory arsenal.

Ehrlich was especially active in animal studies. He chose mice as his laboratory subject and devised his own tumor strain, Stamm II. He offered the most transparent of reasons for taking up the cancer chase in this manner. "Transmissible tumors" in animals has made ending cancer "through vaccination or specific serum" seem possible. Acknowledging that in cancer "no parasitic etiological factor has as yet been demonstrated," he argued none was necessary to devise a means to terminate the scourge. The reason was rabies and smallpox, "two diseases that may be successfully prevented . . . despite the fact that we possess little or no exact knowledge as to the etiological agent in either of these maladies."[31] Ehrlich's medical and scientific colleagues took notice of Ehrlich's analogy-based optimism. Walter M. Brickner, editor of the *American Journal of Surgery* in 1907, made the case simply: "It is assuring . . . that such a man as Ehrlich is devoting all the resources of his mind, his energy, and his laboratory to the problem." He had never undertaken a project "in which he has not added something fundamental."[32]

Ehrlich's cellular staining work, toxin-antitoxin studies, theory of immunology, and attempt to fashion precise chemotherapeutic agents for specific diseases had placed him in the first rank of microbiologists. His skill and accomplishments marked him as special, but like his contemporaries, he recognized biology as essentially structural and mechanical. Processes of life could be explained and understood in chemical and geometric, or more properly perhaps, physical terms. Health to Ehrlich was static. Each body part performed its specific operation without outside interference. Disease was the manifestation of an invasion that caused the malfunctioning of a single part. Cure resulted from the restoration of that part through chemical or physical means.

This thinking pervaded Ehrlich's research. One example from his earlier work demonstrates Ehrlich's structure-based thinking. His theory of immunology presumed that pathogens or pathogenic substances were chemically configured in such a way that they (or portions of them) attached to specific groups of cells within the body and impaired the bound cells' normal function. The body responded to this pathogenic invasion by producing massive numbers of antibodies. Each of these new, identical antibodies possessed a similar configuration or site—a chemical side chain—and these sites were identical to those of the cells under attack. The rest was simply a matter of statistics. The preponderance of antibodies enhanced chances for maintenance of regular function among menaced but still healthy cells. Instead of uniting with the invaders' original targets, pathogens encountered the antibodies' structurally similar side chains and, due to the far greater numbers of these antibodies, generally linked with them. This situation rendered the bound pathogens harmless to vital cells. The intruders fit with the antibodies, noted Ehrlich, remembering the phrases of Louis Pasteur and Emil Fischer, "as male and female screw or as lock and key."[33]

Ehrlich and his laboratory published at least forty papers on immunity prior to 1906.[34] In cancer, then, Ehrlich supposed the cancer cell behaved like an invading pathogen. Its structure enabled it to compete with host cells for nutrients or bond with them, ultimately blocking them from receiving sustenance. His work with his Stamm II mice produced cancer of unprecedented virulence. It was one of eleven distinct primary tumors that his laboratory produced as he sought alternatives to the Jensen mouse. Nearly 100 percent of his Stamm II mice that developed cancer from transplantation died of the disease. He then set about to imitate Pasteur's work with rabies but, rather than chemically attenuate the pathogenic substance, Ehrlich attempted to transplant the various new mouse tumors he had created in order of virulence. His least aggressive transplant produced the disease in about 1 percent of the mice. In those who remained free of the disease—theoretically, mouse-created antibodies had prohibited it from gaining a foothold in the transplanted vermin—he progressively stepped up the regimen, attempting to transplant the next most virulent material in the series.

That constituted one research strain. Ehrlich's laboratory also worked with mice that developed cancer spontaneously. Ehrlich and his assistants found it difficult to transplant that "natural" cancer into healthy mice. Ehrlich also noted that this inoculation conveyed a measure of immunity. Those mice treated with the spontaneous tumor substance and who did not develop cancer from this inoculation proved in significant numbers to be protected from the disease, even if the most virulent material was later injected. This immunity, which appeared in at least two-thirds of the mice treated, proved temporary, persisting for several weeks or months. Ehrlich found that vaccinating mice a second time with virulent material enhanced the immunity and extended to all possible inoculation sites.[35]

Bashford and several other investigators shunned the tumor material per se and focused instead on the blood of recovered, cancer-free mice. They found that this substance provided immunity to healthy animals of the same species but that the immunity was only temporary. Its duration was related to the quantity of blood injected and the number of times the injections occurred.[36]

Ehrlich had dealt with naturally occurring cancer and cancer transplanted from a standardized, consistent tumor family. In both cases, his specific conclusions were similar. Ehrlich argued since tumors were species specific, they must be composed of two parts. The first was the tumor, of course, but the second was a "substance 'x' transplanted along with the tumour [*sic*]." This substance was "necessary for continued growth and found only in the mouse." He indicated that tumor receptors—structures—took up "growth material." Ehrlich postulated that these receptors made cancer cells "more avid" than non-cancerous cells and therefore enabled them to dominate. Ehrlich equated avidness with virulence, thus explaining why some tumors were more tenacious than others. This as of yet undefined growth material enabled the cancer cells to engorge themselves through creation "of more numerous and more rapacious 'nourishment receptors.'" To Ehrlich, this was important. It suggested that researchers should regard and proceed as if the "cancer cell" were "in itself, a colony-forming parasite."

Ehrlich carried the "substance x" experiments to the next level. He found that if he made a trans-species tumor transplantation, the tumor would persist for about eight days before it disappeared. He explained this short persistence by suggesting that the transplant brought the tumor and the "x substance," which provided a brief period of nourishment. But if the dying tumor was implanted in another individual from the original species, it would rebound, even flourish. He then went a bit further. Ehrlich claimed that different sites in the animal body had greater or lesser amounts of "x substance," which accounted for why they grew differentially. Yet he also hypothesized that a second transplanted tumor would rarely grow in an animal; the first tumor monopolized the "x substance." Initial research seemed to confirm Ehrlich's position, but other investigators quickly found that tumors transplanted simultaneously grew equally well. Still others would develop protocols to grow a second tumor in a single animal. Ehrlich countered these arguments by claiming that these investigators employed shoddy laboratory practice. The first tumor was too slow growing or the second tumor was transplanted too quickly. In either cases, the primary tumor had not yet monopolized the "x substance" when the second tumor was prematurely introduced.[37]

Ehrlich issued his "x substance" hypothesis at the same time that the Rockefeller Institute's Alexis Carrel announced that he was able to grow and maintain living tissue on a plasma-based media. Growing animal tissue indefinitely or at least for long periods of time in vitro provided researchers another experimental means by which to investigate tumors. In fact, tumors, perhaps because of their profusion of cells, became among the first tissues Carrel plated. Carrel's work seriously challenged Ehrlich's "x substance" hypothesis. Not only could tissues grow in culture for considerable lengths of time without using up the transplanted "x substance," but they could be transplanted into another living being of that species. If the tissue were cancerous, the transplant recipient would develop the disease. To Carrel and others, something within the plated tumor or healthy tissue animated and sustained the integrity of life and did not dissipate over time.[38]

Carrel's work complicated the immunity question, but the work of two Columbia investigators funded by the Crocker bequest proved even more befuddling. Robert A. Lambert and Frederic M. Hanes plated tissue from one species on the plasma-based media of another. Cells of one species could grow outside the body nourished by the blood of a second species. The Columbia men found that the length of time the growth could be sustained differed depending on the two species involved. In some cases, such as mouse tissue and goat blood, the culture could not be maintained at all. Nonetheless, they had more completely disproved Ehrlich's contention that a "x substance" necessarily sustained transplanted tumors.

Lambert and Hanes did not stop there. They sought to manipulate living tumor cultures to test immunity. Their results disappointed. Tumors could be grown on plasma cultures from immune animals; immunity was not transmitted in the blood's plasma portion.[39] This study provided little clarity. A summary provided by Harvard's Frederick Gay, a leading American immunologist, showed just how complicated immunity remained. Ehrlich's influence stood strong. His work persisted as the measure against which others posed their theories. Gay cited literature specifying that young animals were more susceptible to transplants than older ones but that older tumors transplanted more readily than younger ones, that susceptibility differed markedly "between races of the same animal species," and that "a change of environment would lead to a different resistance in a given race." To make the last point clear, Gay pointed to studies that indicated that "Berlin mice in Norway . . . failed to take the Ehrlich tumor, whereas, in Berlin, they were very susceptible to it." Gay also claimed that variation among mice led to "probable differences in individual resistance" to tumors. Gay mentioned that Jensen maintained that animals of a race and species known to be transplantable but who failed to acquire cancer when implanted demonstrated natural immunity.

Gay further argued from the literature that "individual parts of a given tumor [may] vary in their virulence." He also contended that studies had shown that the locus upon which an animal was implanted made a difference in the success rate of the transplant. Gay maintained that the quantity of material inoculated made a difference in the rate of success; the greater the implantation, the greater the chances cancer would develop. But metastatic tumors offered an additional profile. They seemed to grow quicker and more virulently than the primary and metastasize sooner. Any attempt to undertake a taxonomy of tumors had to deal with a fact often reported in the literature. Successive transplants sometimes led malignancies to change cellular types. Cancers might become sarcomas and vice versa.[40]

This was the maze than engulfed cancer immunity studies. It occurred in real time. Investigators were bombarded with all this data and multiple theories almost simultaneously. Two questions galvanized most practical attention: could a serum be developed from healthy or treated individuals that would fight cancer already established in another individual; and could a serum agglutination test similar to that devised by Wassermann and others for syphilis be created for cancer? Of the two, the former was more questionable. Several investigators published reports documenting cases of amelioration, but most research seemed to indicate that any serum had at best a transitory effect. What constituted success was always problematic. Did the animal in question truly have the disease? Was the serum introduced too early or in insufficient dose? Where did spontaneous cure come in?[41]

Agglutination studies had their own application. Early diagnosis and radical surgery was the sole dependable weapon against cancer. With most pathologists convinced that cancer cells remained physically discrete from normal cells, the key was to remove the entire tumor. If the surgeon encapsulated the tumor site with the scalpel and excised normal tissue surrounding the tumor, the long-term prognosis for recovery stood much higher. The quicker an individual was identified as harboring the disease, the more likely it was that an invasive procedure could be undertaken that would enable surgeons to remove the cancerous mass.

Unfortunately, serum reaction research was beset by the same uncertainty and lack of concreteness that hampered immunity and other studies. Investigators disputed techniques, methods, and outcomes.[42] The relatively simple dichotomy between those seeking a microbial origin and those who favored a mechanical or developmental explanation for cancer had been replaced by a more complicated schematic. The notion of a contagium vivum, a very old idea to account for the supposition that some animated principle produced pestilence and disease, became a relatively common way of discussing cancer's cause. Like smallpox, rabies, and until just a few years earlier spirochetes and trypanosomes, advocates argued that cancer could be transmitted but that the agents through which it was transmitted were unknown and unseen. Genuflecting to the Germ Theory required there to be an understanding that some single living or active principle produced the disease. But this hypothetical principle did not act as bacteria, protozoa, fungi, or other identified pathogens. It could not be grown in pure culture. Inoculation required cellular material from previous tumors. And these introduced cells multiplied; they did not invade adjacent tissue, although they might lyse it.

Bashford was having none of this. "Cancer has no analogy with any form of infective disease," he plainly stated. No evidence existed that laboratory mice "caught" cancer from other laboratory mice and no "laboratory workers" have "ever been shown to take it" from the diseased laboratory animals. Wakely objected to Bashford's stridency and argued for more laboratory work. "If a microbial origin of cancer" was ultimately proven, it would be disastrous if the present generation of researchers refused to consider that possibility. Ignorance, the flailing around of uncertainty and confusion, was part of science, he maintained. The unknown lay just over the next horizon. Cancer laboratory researchers should not be too hard on themselves, he claimed. It was not "a reproach to physics that the nature of positive or negative electricity is not yet known."[43]

Lines were clearly drawn, but the British group—J. E. Salvin Moore, J. O. Wakelin Barratt, and Charles Walker—muddled the situation further. In separate experiments, this Liverpool cancer laboratory group took two distinct mice tumors—a Jensen mouse tumor in one experiment and a Stamm II tumor in the other—froze them with liquid air (-195 degrees), and then ground them in that environment. After a period of from twenty minutes to a half hour, they inoculated healthy mice with the frozen material. In a significant portion of population, cancer developed. Gaylord extended these experiments and showed that the ground material could withstand the frigid temperature for nearly an hour and a half and still produce cancer.

These findings led the Liverpudlians to deduce that cancer was not produced by the cancer cell, which had been obliterated by grinding and cold. Indeed, Gaylord's comparative experiments showed that normal mouse tissue was destroyed within twenty minutes when subjected to liquid air. If the cell was not the parasite per se, or acting like a parasite, the Liverpool contingent hypothesized that an ultramicroscopic organism, even smaller than the recently identified spirochetes, must produce the disease.[44] That too soon seemed untenable. Various investigators who worked with the Jensen, Stamm II, and other tumors, though not at low temperatures, found that if they ground up the tumor and filtered the emulsion through ordinary filter paper, the filtrate would not produce the disease in otherwise susceptible animals. Apparently, the ultramicroscopic organism did not produce a toxic-like, cancer-causing substance and was larger than the pores of the filter paper, a commonsensical improbability since it should therefore been large enough to have been identified or at least detected. Furthermore, several of these researchers found that ground cellular material kept at room or body temperature upon its removal from a laboratory animal quickly lost the power to produce the disease when inoculated. This latter observation implied two things difficult to reconcile. Either the material contained a contagium vivum that perished quickly outside the animal body, which meant it was not truly alive in the sense that it could be plated and therefore failed to adhere to the tenets of the Germ Theory, or the cell was indeed the parasite and grinding it at room or body temperature damaged it irretrievably and led to its speedy demise. That latter explanation conflicted with the liquid air experiments.[45]

The Rockefeller Institute's Peyton Rous provided a more interesting dilemma soon after. Heading the institute's cancer work after Flexner moved to the study of polio, Rous tried to set the parameters for immunity and then for tumors. He grew interested in a cancer experiment undertaken by Crile and Beebe in which blood from a spontaneously cured animal was used to replace the blood of a vigorously healthy animal to see if it could acquire passive immunity to the disease. The two researchers found that, if nearly 50 percent of the blood in excess of the amount drained from the healthy animal was substituted, then immunity was conveyed and an implanted tumor would shrivel. Rous extended the study in a slightly different way. Rather than use transfusions, he affixed two separate animals together as if they were conjoined twins. One animal had a large cancerous tumor while its much larger partner possessed natural immunity to the particular cancer. Much to Rous's chagrin, he found that when conjoined, the healthy animal had no effect on the diseased animal's tumor.[46]

Rous next turned to Beard's discredited work and tested some of its fundamental assumptions. Implicit in its derivation was the notion that embryos behaved in some ways like tumor cells. To that end, he took "embryonic tissue and a method which has proven effective for the production of immunity to implanted tumor" and produced in the mouse immunity to the embryo. This immunity, noted Rous, behaved exactly like immunity to cancer. There was no biological connection established between the embryo and the host that transferred the blood and nutrients "necessary to life of the engrafted tissue."[47]

This led Rous to conceive "of the tumor problem as a tissue problem," and his next experiment drew on two well-known phenomena. Rous drew together studies that cancers could change tissue types—from carcinoma, for example, into sarcoma—with often cited reports that irritation or inflammation could make healthy tissue cancerous. Rather than use normal healthy tissue for his experiments, Rous employed the exquisitely sensitive embryonic tissue. While normal embryos seemed analogous in some ways to tumors, embryos, unlike tumors, differentiated by cell function and type.

What Rous did next was illustrative. He ground up tumors and embryos to make a relatively homogeneous solution and then injected the mix into healthy susceptible mice. In most instances, one or the other tissue types predominated and wiped out the other. But in a few, the two tissues appeared "in direct union." They remained identifiably discrete in that the cells of each were easily discernible, but they existed through symbiotic interaction. That led Rous to question the established notion that normal cells and tumors must remain distinct in the animal body. Indeed, investigators employed that trope as one method to detect true cancer. Cancer could not enter a union with normal cells but, rather, overwhelmed them.

Rous then returned to the immunity question and once again selected embryos as an important factor. This time he chose to test the observation that pregnancy inhibited tumor growth. Some attributed that to competition for nutrients, but Rous argued that pregnancy was actually "a stimulus" to growth. His earlier experiments had shown tumor and embryo immunity. He now hoped to demonstrate that pregnancy was just "another special instance of a more general [immunological] phenomena." He had some suggestive possibilities that such was the case. Leo Loeb argued that a specific chemical substance—what he called a "hormon" [*sic*]—controlled uterine growth, and Rous argued that "it was not beyond possibility" that the growth of embryos was governed in the same way. The implications of such an occurrence were profound. The hypothetical substance could be isolated and used to diminish tumor growth.

Mice again provided the medium on which Rous experimented. Two specific findings proved deterministic. First, if embryo cells from a pregnant mouse were planted elsewhere on the mouse, the cells would not grow or differentiate. But they did not die either. They simply survived. But if that mouse's pregnancy was terminated, the transplanted tissue would then develop. This indicated that a pregnancy-related substance might be refined to halt tumor growth, but Rous's subsequent experiment undercut that notion. He took two pregnant mice, gave them hysterectomies, and implanted two embryos—one from each mouse—on each. In the mother mouse, the embryo grew profusely. On the alien mouse, the embryo withered and died. Rous attributed this to "auto-transplantation." Pregnancy may well have conveyed a substance inhibiting growth but that substance was individual-specific. It could produce no general class of chemotherapeutic substance.[48]

Rous ended his Beard-inspired phase with that experiment and returned to the work that initially had animated him. He studied immunity by looking at anomalies, such as canine lymphosarcoma. His search of the literature had turned up a fish cancer epidemic and a species of hare that apparently could develop cancer normally associated with rabbits, an interspecies transmission. These "transmittable new growths of unusual behavior" caused Rous to determine that "our conception of tumor-behavior, based as it is on observation of a few species, is too narrow." Rous decided to look outside of mammalian species and quickly gravitated to birds. Others had considered tumors of birds, but no investigator had successfully found a transplantable tumor. Rous quickly found the first. It was a sarcoma in a particular breed of common chicken.[49]

That expanded knowledge of animal species through which cancer could be transferred, but what Rous did next truly transformed the situation. He found that the chicken sarcoma was not transferred by tumor cells but rather from a filtrate. This agent that produced his special chicken sarcoma passed through the standard filter Rous used in his laboratory to separate germs from the filtrate.[50]

Investigators long had used the filtration process as an essential facet of the disease organism search. It enabled them to gather the residue from the filters to plate the suspected pathogens. At about the turn of the century, however, some bacteriologists found that the filtrate, not the filter, contained the infectious material. By the time of Rous's work, about thirty such agents had been identified by their sole similar attribute. They could pass through the filter and regularly produce a specific disease.

Investigators characteristically called these pathogenic substances "ultramicroscopic" or "filterable viruses." Yellow fever, hog cholera, typhus fever, and a slew of other recognizable diseases were thought to be of their number. Despite the two dissimilar names, researchers generally agreed that what separated them from other pathogens was simply size. Some of these wee microbes were deemed to be bacteria, others protozoa, and still others subject to dispute. In fact, one researcher reported that he had found types of trypanosomes and spirochetes so tiny that they too could transverse the filter barrier. The idea that these filterable microbes might belong to the same or similar biological taxa offered yet another possibility to Harvard's S. B. Wolbach. He reasoned that any remedy effective against one of these ultramicroscopic germs might well be effective against them all. A single discovery could wipe out the entire class of ultramicroscopic-caused disease.[51]

Although Rous never called his agent a microbe, others interpreted it that way. That act of definition brought up several issues. If it were a microscopic germ, then cancer might well be contagious. Physicians and relatives needed to be as aware of people with cancer as they were with those infected with tuberculosis. Its infectivity would account for what most recognized as a persistent cancer increase. Rous's agent affected only one breed of chickens. If there were a cancer germ, might it strike just one race of humanity? Finding the cancer germ in chickens resurrected the question posed years earlier, namely how representative—how useful—was animal experimentation? Did humans get cancer by germ or did only one breed of chicken get the disease that way?

That last question proved critical to a large number of cancer investigators. Bashford and several others had worked for much of the decade to prove that cancer did not stem from introduction of an outside pathogen. Were they now confronted with evidence that their work rested on an erroneous foundation? Rous's agent passed through the standard laboratory filter. But a second filter somewhat smaller apparently stopped the pathogen; this filtrate did not produce the disease. That suggested an agent larger than the tiniest ultramicroscopic microorganisms, another factor in favor of a microbial explanation.

What Rous's discovery also accomplished was to help reintroduce the question, exactly what was cancer? Was the chicken sarcoma truly cancer? To be sure, it was marked by the rapid proliferation of cells. But was that what cancer was? Was chicken biology unique?

As had long been the case in cancer research, challenging assumptions rarely went unchallenged. Without extensive experiments attempting to confirm the new finding, its validity remained in question. These subsequent experiments rarely could provide actual unambiguous confirmation, but the course of action was clear. Each new "fact" must be tested experimentally. More often than not, however, researchers also embarked on a congruent project. They took the hypothetical new insight and proposed to test what they considered an analogous situation. More than new insights, facts, or discoveries, analogy became the mechanism to extend knowledge. Gaylord said it succinctly. Faced with Rous's startling results, he "suppose[d] that everyone again repeated the old experiments in attempting to filter out a specific agent for mouse carcinoma and rat sarcoma." The logic behind that approach was problematic. Researchers took a questionable phenomenon and applied that "truth." What they did, in effect, was create a second variable. The initial insight, the insight that had spawned interest, may have been false or the instance in which researchers sought to apply it may not have been truly analogous. In either situation, the actual application rarely elucidated matters. In the case of the recreated rat and mice experiments, several investigators announced that they had achieved a modicum of success in detecting filtrate-produced cancer and posited an ultramicroscopic being as the cause. Others examining the same data suggested a different possibility: cancer cells found their way into the filtrate either because of investigator careless or because the filter itself was defective. They therefore rejected microbes as causative agents.[52] The matter remained even less settled than before.

All of the discoveries, theories, incidences, and discussions in this chapter took place during a few short years. They were all the product of the last years of the first decade of the twentieth century. That brief span of time exacerbated the situation tremendously. Investigators worldwide were bombarded in a few years with a great number of dramatic theories and contentions, many of which demanded their serious attention. All necessitated confirmation and most explication. But that was not possible. Researchers had to grasp this tumultuous quantity of material undigested. Simultaneity bred immediacy as answers—decisions, intellectual determinations, and procedures—were required in real time. Such an onslaught of experimental results proved truly overwhelming. Cancer laboratory scientists usually took what was presented to them at face value. There was no time for anything else. And since much of the new investigations were contradictory and otherwise incomplete, laboratory men and women turned to the tried and true; they cleaved to established precepts, tempering what had become tropes with popular analogies. They evaluated new research according to the reputation of the scientist espousing the position—the reason Beard and Ehrlich received such sustained attention—or its utility in confirming their own research positions. Rather than change minds, the various scientific machinations of the years just before 1910 generally hardened them. The discoveries were so broad, the meanings were so vague, and the procedures were so particularistic and unspecific that laboratories incorporated the data that fit their a priori assumptions comfortably and dismissed much of the rest. Since these investigators long had been at sixes and sevens with each other over the question of cancer's cause, little changed. Each and every group seemed to gain more arrows in its quiver. And with this new material, they were even more certain that their competitors' perspectives were dead wrong. Disagreements flared as researchers moved further afield than ever. Each group dug its heels in the wake of the massive influx of rich, simultaneously produced information and misinformation. Which was not a matter for scientific scrutiny or even calm reflection. There was none of that. Idiosyncrasy determined the relevance of investigations. Each rested in the eye of the beholder.

6

Imitation Is the Sincerest Form of Science, 1910–1915

Rous's discovery of a particular agent that passed through one standard filter but not another, and produced a characteristic type of cancer in chickens, did not produce a raft of experiments seeking to corroborate or falsify his determinations. It had little traction in Europe. Journals there tended to ignore such an unexpected research development. Few if any European laboratory workers commented on the studies. In America, however, the case was mentioned prominently in numerous publications. Here, too, there were few attempts to verify Rous's work, but various researchers pointedly employed it as an analogy to "confirm" other, quite diverse cancer investigations. That was especially true for scientists wedded to a microbial cancer explanation. Beyond its use in that endeavor, the clearest consequence of Rous's work was pleas to integrate chickens into the laboratory. Chickens would provide a new front from which to investigate cancer. To Rous, Bashford, and others, especially the Rockefeller researchers, the more diverse and unusual specimens and types of cancer encountered, the better. Examining the grand panoply of biological experience seemed to circumscribe options. The more data available the stricter the limitations placed upon cancer's cause. New facts constituted new constraints, boundaries within which discussions about the cause of cancer needed to operate. Implicit in this formulation was the idea that cancer was a single, discrete disease produced from a precise cause, even if that necessary cause required one or more auxiliary factors.

In that sense, the quest for cancer had not changed. The call to add chickens to the experimental arsenal merely reinforced established practice. But it would be wrong to think the situation in the five years after 1910 was identical to the preceding years. The chaos of the first years of the new century and the profoundly contradictory experiments of that earlier period frustrated investigators and threatened public support. By no means immune to these intensifying pressures, researchers extended their gazes and brought the authority of analogy to a new level. They proved willing to embrace new possibilities and incorporate discoveries in collateral fields. Their seemingly desperate position encouraged new kinds of experimentation, even flights of analogy.

Leopards do not change their spots and neither did cancer laboratories. They remained true to the fundamental thrusts that inspired them. Researchers seeking the germ of cancer continued that quest. Those who had been seeking solace and answers within the realm of biology followed that path. What had changed was that investigators removed the shackles that had constrained their imaginations. They sought answers in places they had heretofore been wary to look. New species susceptible to the disease, new models of transmission, and new cancer clues from unusual places were all countenanced.

In the years around 1910, thyroid cancer epidemics among trout and other fish assumed center stage. Investigations into this type of cancer promised to expose new facts that would help delimit theories of cancer's cause. As early as 1902, Marianne Plehn, a member of the faculty of the Royal Veterinary College in Munich, noted significant occurrence of cancer among fish. Bashford reported on the phenomenon two years later. Plehn published much more detailed studies of the distribution and type of cancer in fishes soon after. Berlin pathologist Anton Sticker confirmed her discovery of a particularistic tumor in trout and salmon—in up to 10 percent of the fish population in some places—in 1906. An expert on thyroid tumors, Sticker claimed that a cancer-causing parasite lived in the soil of streams and ponds where epidemic outbreaks occurred and infected resident trout. He also wondered about a possible relationship between this suspected cancer parasite and unexpected incidences of human cancer near these contaminated trout ponds. Americans also investigated a trout-cancer linkage. Early in1907, Cornell's Ewing received several fish from a Pennsylvania hatchery with large, rapidly growing tumors. He reported his findings to the American Association for Cancer Research in 1908.[1]

All that was relatively ordinary. Cancer had been reported in various marine species for years. Because they were found in wet marshy places or in streams, fish cancer stories had been periodically recounted in the literature. When the peripatetic Gaylord took up the trout tumor mantle in 1909, he brought the whole situation to a new level. For the next two years, he conducted field experiments at a Pennsylvania hatchery. He found the disease extensive in an upper tank there. As part of his experiments, Gaylord sought to demonstrate that cancer was contagious, and so he ordered the lower tanks emptied, scrubbed, and stocked with trout from a place "where the disease is not known to exist." The trout in the test vats quickly developed cancer, leading Gaylord to suppose that the infectious agent from the upper tank corrupted the cleansed lower tanks. His experiment pointed, Gaylord contended, "very strongly to the infectious nature of this form of cancer and that the contagion is water-borne." Gaylord did more than talk. He undertook a further series of investigations at a number of hatcheries to see if he could deduce the exact conditions under which these epidemics occurred.[2]

Gaylord also embarked upon another set of investigations with ominous human implications. He wanted "to discover whether or not cancer is communicated to human beings by the fish they eat or whether the water of streams is infected by the cancer germ of fish." Quite simply, Gaylord wanted to see if there was a trans-species relationship between fish cancer and human incidences of the disease. His inquiries aimed to determine if "the fish infect the water in which they live" and if "cancer germs are entirely destroyed by the heat of cooking." The New York Forest, Fish and Game Commission gathered trout from the various state hatcheries and participated in the experiments.[3]

The United States commissioner of fisheries, George M. Bowers, brought his agency into the trout cancer program. Explicitly working with Gaylord, the Bureau of Fisheries promised to "devote every energy and facility at its disposal for the prompt and thorough elucidation" of cancer's cause. The bureau initially focused on comparing two localities where cancer among trout was epidemic in "young and old fish in government, state, and private hatcheries" as well as "wild fish in open waters." The bureau also created a special fish laboratory in Buffalo to work with the cancer laboratory there. Apparatus included "two aquaria on the closed-circulation plan, with full provision for refrigeration and aeration of water."[4]

Gaylord reported back to the AACR at the end of 1909. In both of his suspect hatcheries, Gaylord found that infected fish received water from ponds with cancerous fish and that infection rates were consistently elevated in the hatcheries. Gaylord also found that a considerable number of fish naturally possessed immunity. And he learned that not every kind of trout fell victim to thyroid cancer, no matter how extensively they had been exposed. Scotch sea trout and hybrid salmon never bought the disease. Brook and rainbow trout became lousy with it.

Much to Gaylord's surprise, very young trout developed epidemic cancer most easily. That fact ran counter to most of what was known about the disease; researchers considered cancer a disease of older age. He also found that the tumors grew exceedingly quickly and seemed to infiltrate areas outside the thyroid quite readily. To Gaylord, the ease with which fish thyroid cancer left that gland demonstrated a potent metastatic effect—a critical cancer characteristic—and confirmed the disease's presence. He summed up his conclusions neatly. "Evidence of infectivity and contagion appear . . . conclusive, . . . the greatest support to the parasitic theory we have yet encountered." He reasoned further that "the environment and the conditions under which fish are artificially propagated" made the causal link apparent.[5]

Finding an infective fish cancer that attacked a particular locus on a specific type of trout was consonant with Rous's chicken sarcoma. In effect, the two situations reinforced each other and offered de facto corroboration. Events deemed analogous functioned as proof for otherwise indeterminate contentions.

Not everyone recognized the two occurrences as analogous. A few argued that the thyroid of trout was not encapsulated and that a hyperactive thyroid would send tissue migrating throughout the upper body. This migrated tissue could have accounted for what appeared as the proliferation of tumors beyond a discrete area. Gaylord was having none of that, however. He interpreted the phenomenon within the context of what he knew. It was the similarity to what he anticipated—cancer metastasizes—that galvanized Gaylord.

Gaylord did not let the matter rest there. Indeed, his interest in trout stemmed from an earlier understanding of human cancer demography. As were several German investigators, Gaylord remained convinced that the disease was much more prevalent in "well wooded, well watered and mountainous regions." He found it "a remarkable coincidence" that the area "with the great number of human cancer cases is almost identical with the area" where trout thrived. He maintained that some investigators thought "cancer might be distributed through the medium of water," while others contended cancer might be spread "by fish." Several took Gaylord's sentiments to the next level, claiming that cancer was most extensive "where the consumption of trout was most general." These people worried that cancer rates were likely to increase as beef and pork became more expensive and more Americans turned to eating more fish.[6]

A recapitulation is necessary here. Early investigators demonstrated that fish got cancer. Gaylord discovered epidemics of the disease among the nation's trout hatcheries. Statisticians relying on the sporadic reporting of physicians and others claimed from these ad hoc, uncontrolled studies that cancer struck particular regions at rates proportionally greater than others, and Gaylord maintained that these peak cancer areas correlated quite closely to the distribution of trout streams and ponds. A causal link was posited as a result of these two statistical claims when weighted in light of the earlier evidence.

Nowhere was it demonstrated that cancer struck trout in considerable number outside of hatcheries. There were no other special associations among trout and cancer. Yet Gaylord's theories fit neatly within the contemporary epidemiological nexus. Yellow fever, Rous's chicken sarcoma, the discovery of the spirochete of syphilis, and other epidemiological models proved so overpowering—and seemingly analogous—as to lead Gaylord down an extremely questionable road. That was the romance and method of the science; that was how science was prosecuted. He was striking down a well trod, deterministic path. That it might yield inappropriate results mattered less than the conviction by which it was pursued.

The trout-cancer nexus entered the political arena during the last months of 1909 and the first months of 1910. President William Howard Taft had proposed a national public health agency, and the AACR designated Gaylord, then the organization's president, to request creation of a cancer research department within the new unit. Taft was sympathetic to the initiative but wanted the group to submit its proposition to the new agency's director once Congress authorized the new organization. Gaylord visited Taft about the AACR's petition but also discussed with the president his trout and human cancer theory.[7]

Gaylord proved quite persuasive on the latter issue. Taft would even venture to Buffalo, tour Gaylord's laboratories, and discuss the trout question further. But Gaylord's real success was getting the president to consult with the secretaries of commerce and labor and the head of the Bureau of Fisheries, and on April 9, 1910, to memorialize Congress. He asked for an extraordinary appropriation of $50,000 to create a special laboratory and to hire personnel explicitly to investigate the suspected trout-human cancer linkage. This new laboratory would work in conjunction with Gaylord's Buffalo effort. Taft put the case succinctly. "We have every reason to believe," he wrote, "that a close investigation into the subject of cancer in fishes, which are frequently swept away by an epidemic of it, may give us light upon this dreadful human scourge."

A note from Gaylord accompanied Taft's congressional request. The scientist repeated his contention that the distribution of trout thyroid cancer was virtually identical to the "concentrations" of cancer in the United States. "A map of one might as well be taken as a map of the other," he asserted. Gaylord indicated "that careful study" would "eliminate the disease from among fish" and be "of an invaluable character for humanity."[8]

Congress mulled over Taft's request as the *Washington Post* urged swift congressional action. The *New York Times* concurred. It provided Gaylord a bully pulpit to press his point. Gaylord argued that the trout-human cancer connection "should not necessarily be taken to mean that fish causes cancer in human beings." It could be that "both men and fish develop cancer from the same cause." The special initiative was necessary because the Bureau of Fisheries lacked the staff and facilities to undertake a full-scale experimental investigation of the connection. Paraphrasing Gaylord's letter to Taft, the *Times* noted the established public campaign against tuberculosis and argued that cancer demanded no less. The tuberculosis campaign had exceeded "the hopes of those who started it. It is now assured that tuberculosis can be cured," the paper maintained. That was just the latest success in modern medicine. "Various 'incurable' diseases have been taken up as cancer is now being attacked," the paper declared "and the cure has been found and applied." The *Times* confidently predicted that in the case of cancer, "there can be little doubt" that "the cause will presently be discovered and the cure effected." The mechanism that led to victory of "incurable disease" was laboratory experimentation, and "in all such campaigns the lower animals have been the medium of discovery." Indeed, the paper noted, Taft made that exact point in his congressional memorial.[9]

JAMA's Simmons also supported the presidential initiative. He cited experiments in a disease-free hatchery where the introduction of ova "from elsewhere" was "followed by the appearance of the peculiar tumors in many of the fish raised from the imported ova" *and* in "the indigenous stock." No doubt aware of Rous's work, Simmons declared fish thyroid cancer both "hereditary as well as contagious," a quite unusual duality. Trout, he concluded, may be the most "favorable animal . . . for the experimental study of cancer."[10]

Trout epidemics provided the focus of the American anti-cancer campaign. Overseas, there was less support. Gaylord did present his thesis to the 1910 IACI meeting but received a lukewarm response. When apprised of Taft's congressional request, Bashford vehemently disagreed with its premise. He acknowledged that cancer attacked fish but contended that the trout at hatcheries often "are swept away by goiter, not by cancer." This was a subject that the "Imperial Cancer Fund has been engaged for a long time past," and Bashford was sure that Gaylord had erred.[11]

Two Western Reserve University researchers, working in conjunction with the Pennsylvania State Fish Commission, reinforced Bashford's conclusions. David Marine and C. H. Lenhart undertook a number of experiments demonstrating that the "cancer" disappeared when the fish were given iodine or released into an open brook. The reputed "epidemic cancer" only occurred among young fish in dense, crowded environments with limited water supplies, such as those at a hatchery. The two investigators asserted that reported metastases, an important characteristic of true cancer, were not relevant when discussing fish thyroid tissue. The "widely and loosely distributed nonencapsulated gland" gave "the histological appearance of invasion of the surrounding tissue."[12]

The Marine/Lenhart paper did little to quell the trout cancer excitement. In fact, Park thought the study, coupled with Gaylord's work, opened a compelling new front in the cancer war. He considered Gaylord's experiments as demonstrating trout thyroid cancer's pathogenic infectivity and therefore recognized iodine as a curative substance, a true chemotherapeutic agent.[13] The *Washington Post* optimistically predicted that the germ of cancer would soon be uncovered. The paper surmised that such a varmint would be ultramicroscopic and assured its readers that its virtual invisibility would not hamper efforts to contain it. After all, the article reasoned, "science is able to deal with yellow fever by preventing the breeding of the mosquitoes that carry its germs." Once the germ was revealed, researchers would quickly determine if it was air- or waterborne and what kind of animal harbored it. Once those factors were known, the disease could be prevented.

The *Post* also offered the possibility of an eventual cure. A vaccine, produced "by breeding microbes in beef soup, killing them with heat and putting up the fluid thus obtained in fire-sealed tubes," would be the first step in overcoming cancer. "Hypodermic syringes" would introduce the vaccine "into the circulation" and, "according to scientific theory, quickly put a stop to the ravages of the devouring malady."

The *Post* took care to discuss some of the various experiments already under way. In Gaylord's laboratory in Buffalo, for example, the newspaper reported on how groups of three trout were kept in aerated jars and fed fish tumors from other fish. Another similarly situated group was fed cancerous human livers, "obtained at autopsies, which they ate greedily." Bureau of Fisheries investigators at a trout hatchery in Maine undertook grander experiments. Trout were injected in the thyroid gland with a solution of fish cancer. Results were pending, but none of the first trout inoculated had developed the disease. Also at Maine, the bureau secured a number of dogs, taught them to eat fish, and then fed them an exclusive diet of cancerous trout. According to the *Post*, "the scientists decided that if the dogs could catch the disease from fish it would be practically proved that the same rule would apply to men and women." The staff kept active while waiting for infection to commence, creating a kind of morbid anatomy exhibit in which they preserved specimens of trout suffering cancer in virtually every organ.

The *Post* closed its discussion by noting that some scientists claimed "that cancer is the agency by which the human race is being changed into a higher type of creation;" cancer was the evolutionary mechanism, a factor bolstered by the fact that cancer appeared throughout the animal kingdom.[14]

Each of these speculations and all of these experiments were undertaken without the provision of Taft's special appropriation. Congress failed to act, and Bowers expressed great consternation. It was difficult to secure fish from hatcheries certified as cancer-free and "above suspicion of infection," so the bureau needed to trap them from wild streams. Such care and meticulousness was imperative to a scientific investigation. "Progress is made only by slow painstaking steps and by the use of the most approved appliances and methods," Bowers maintained. The cancer situation in the nation's trout hatcheries was critical. Cancer epidemics raged at hatcheries in Pennsylvania, Vermont, Ohio, and West Virginia. Things were so bad that the bureau was considering abandoning its trout propagation work. Such a move would be tragic, he argued, because the "annually increasing mortality from cancer in man and certain remarkable coincidences in the geographical distribution of the disease in man and fish render it imperative that it should be made the subject of minute inquiry." The bureau continued its investigations, Bowers stated, but he "emphatically" argued that without special research facilities "it can make little progress."[15]

Marine and Lenhart published more extensive experiments early in 1911. The thrust of this research was to "follow step by step the development of thyroid hyperplasia" in trout and thus demonstrate once and for all that Gaylord's cancer epidemic was merely epidemic goiter caused by unique fish hatchery conditions. "A limited water supply, overcrowding, and overfeeding with a highly artificial and incomplete food" contributed to the disease, which the investigators supposed derived from a "metabolic and nutritional disturbance." They set a time line for thyroid overgrowth, which predicted when the tissue would fill the aortic cavity and begin to infiltrate muscle and bone. They also developed an elaborate protocol to determine the rate and locus at which iodine reduced the tumor, taking care to establish separate age-dependent portraits. Their contention was that goiter was endemic to all trout hatcheries but became epidemic when overcrowded conditions persisted.[16]

JAMA's Simmons weighed the work of the Western Reserve researchers against that of Gaylord and declared the Buffalo doctor likely mistaken. He even went so far as to describe just how thyroid tissue invaded healthy structures by first expanding into hollow areas and then through "pressure atrophy" causing nearby structures to wither and be replaced with thyroid material. That process was what Gaylord falsely "described as carcinoma of the thyroid."[17]

Neither Gaylord nor the Bureau of Fisheries was convinced by *JAMA*'s rebuke or the Western Reserve investigators' evidence. The bureau returned to the fish cancer as "of the same nature as human cancer" argument to plead for additional resources, the need for which was "self-evident in its humanitarian aspects."[18] With Gaylord, investigations continued and resulted in a nearly 175-page Bureau Bulletin. Dated 1912, the bulletin was published in 1914.

Evidence marshaled in the massive report was of several major types. Much was anatomical as the investigators recounted how normal trout anatomy was differentiated from that of those suffering the apparent cancer epidemic. They also did numerous tissue sections and other pathological anatomical investigations to bolster their contention that the disease was truly cancer.

The actual conditions under which trout lived also drew their gaze. They discussed trout in the wild and in confinement, taking care to design a disease portrait for each. They noted differences in breeds, discussed the various geological formations in which wild trout lived, and undertook chemical analyses of the water supplies, even taking care to measure the quantity of dissolved oxygen. Gaylord and the bureau's researchers described the disease's course and its seats at the several hatcheries, estimated morbidity and mortality rates, considered the relationship between the disease and blood hemoglobin, and took particular note of spontaneous recoveries. They also collected accounts of trout cancer epidemics from around the country and world as they sought to parse out those factors that bound them together.

Their attempts to create the disease experimentally were nearly as extensive. They ran experiments wherein they dumped tumor material into standing water and then introduced trout fry. These fry ate trout thyroid tumor, as well as other parts of afflicted fish. Investigators fed trout human liver cancer in meticulously created experimental tanks, as well as other vessels, and undertook any number of transplantation and inoculation experiments. Interspecies experiments were also pursued. Gaylord tried to give the fish disease to over two dozen dogs and twenty rats

Their section entitled "Chemotherapy" proved most interesting. Such a section was nearly essential in the wake of Ehrlich's atoxyl and then salvarsan work. For the first time, a dread disease—syphilis—had a cure artificially and specifically designed for it. That syphilis was caused by a pathogen formerly considered ultramicroscopic resonated with Rous's chicken sarcoma discovery. It also reflected Park's assertion that iodine "cured" thyroid cancer in fish. Indeed, the whole idea that a chemotherapeutic agent would act like a magic bullet, killing the pathogen while leaving the host relatively unaffected, fit Park's scheme neatly. Gaylord used his experience with the mouse tumor literature to offer the investigators several other "chemotherapeutic" substances with which to experiment.[19]

Reflecting centuries of battling syphilis, mercury and other heavy metals were among the first substances examined for fish thyroid chemotherapeutic properties. Gaylord and his bureau colleagues quickly recognized that dosage was critical. So too was the number of times that the agent needed to be administered to provide evidence of efficacy. Much to their pleasure, both arsenic and mercury in appropriate measures seemed to reduce, even eliminate, the tumors. That discovery placed them squarely in Park's camp. They proclaimed "that the action of iodine upon" the fish thyroid tumors was "not due to its physiological relation to the thyroid gland." Since other heavy metals possessed "curative qualities," there must be "some quality which [iodine] shares in common with the metals." Indeed, that discovery rendered "the theory of Marine and Lenhart" that tumors in fish were simply thyroid goiters "untenable."[20]

Their primary conclusion was that fish thyroid disease was "a malignant neoplasm." Although they reported that "no evidence has yet been produced to indicate the direct transmission . . . from individual to individual," that did not dissuade them from offering their diagnosis. They argued via analogy and offered Rous as confirmation. "Peyton Rous" had demonstrated, they declared, "that a virus of cancer is no longer hypothetical." He had proven the existence "in three varieties in chickens of a filterable virus capable of producing type-true neoplasms," maintained Gaylord and the bureau. This unidentified chicken cancer agent possessed various properties that made it difficult to detect or to rule out, and the authors delineated its unusual behaviors. Rous's initial agent passed through a medium grade filter. It succumbed at a higher temperature than did chicken cells themselves and was not quickly injured by freezing. It could be preserved by drying and could withstand grinding. It could live for several months and, when injected, produce the characteristic disease. Each of these attributes could pertain to the fish disease. "It is needless to point out that the agent of [trout thyroid disease] is also filterable, which should strengthen the theory that the [causative] agent is a living organism and not a soluble toxin."[21]

To ensure that no scientist lacked access to their conclusions, Gaylord and the bureau published them in German and French, as well as in English. The *New York Times* gave a detailed summary of the publication, but few other newspapers followed suit. Marine offered two further studies in 1914, both of which demonstrated means to prevent epidemic goiter and to remediate it once it had occurred. George M. Gould, editor of *American Medicine* in 1914, also found himself especially frustrated by Gaylord's massive study. "It is rather disappointing that six years have not produced something conclusive," he said of Gaylord's efforts. The federal government and New York state have "given many thousands of dollars to preserve trout fishing," he insisted, but now he hoped they "will square [themselves] with Heaven by giving ten times more to find out the cause of cancer in mere men."[22]

But perhaps the strongest statement made against Gaylord's increasingly tenuous hypothesis came from the New York State Conservation Commission. It had been stung by Gaylord's assertion that it did little to assist him in his fish cancer quest. The commission vehemently disagreed, provided evidence that it had successfully taken up the matter, and took to the newspapers to make its case. Relying on the studies of Marine and Lenhart, the commission cited the report of Tarleton Bean, the state's fish culturist, showing that simply by changing conditions at its hatcheries, the disease could be arrested. Six of the eight facilities in New York were now disease-free, Bean declared. Despite its success in curtailing the hatchery malady, the commission maintained that Gaylord had continually demanded that the state erect a fish experiment station near Buffalo to carry on his fish cancer work. Gaylord proposed to identify means to rid hatcheries of the disease that Bean already had declared remitted. A second letter told a more questionable tale. Gaylord argued that "after giving the matter careful consideration the only person" suitable for heading the Buffalo-located effort "is Bradley J. Gaylord, my oldest son." Gaylord closed by stating that he expected the commission to pay his son's salary and to offer the Buffalo physician a stipend for his time.[23]

Charges of nepotism and greed clouded the matter, but the fact remained that the state commission, like virtually all researchers, no longer believed that the disease Gaylord highlighted was cancer. His failed experiments, Marine and Lenhart's work, and the success that hatcheries had simply by implementing the preventives and curatives outlined by the Ohio researchers virtually ended the controversy. Gaylord issued a final paper in 1916 with "additional evidence" in support of his position—he found fish cancer/goiter in some species raised in the wild and argued that iodine acted in water, not as a nutritional supplement for fish, but rather as a bacteriostatic agent, killing the circulating cancer pathogens. This paper was ignored. Fish cancer was a dead subject.[24]

A similar uproar attended work with crown gall disease. Crown gall was long known to botanists and horticulturists. It attacked tree roots just above the soil line and was characterized by growth of large, often proliferating nodules. Erwin F. Smith, pathologist in charge of the USDA's Laboratory of Plant Pathology, began work on the disease in 1892, searching for its cause. Fungi and plasmodia stood as his initial focus, and Smith was unable to detect such a parasite in conjunction with the disease.[25]

Smith then turned elsewhere but about 1900 became immersed in a dispute with German plant pathologists over whether bacteria—taxonomized as a plant—could produce plant diseases.[26] He took the affirmative, explored several plant diseases to prove his point, and eventually settled on olive tubercle. Growing on olive trees, the disease produced small projections or nodes similar in form to those produced in humans and animals by the disease tuberculosis. He even called olive tubercle disease a tuberculosis, to assert that it produced tubercles, but he also recognized that it was likely caused by an agent different from animal/human tuberculosis. From Koch's work, Smith knew that human/animal tuberculosis was caused by a bacterium enveloped by a wax-like coating. He set out to uncover the olive tubercle disease agent, which he hypothesized was also a bacterium. Others had pursued the culprit—fungi and slime molds were most frequent targets—but apparently had not chosen to investigate if it were a bacteria-borne disease. Smith rigorously applied Koch's postulates and found the causative microbe, a bacteria, which he described in meticulous taxonomic detail.[27]

Smith turned to the galls at about the time he prepared to publish his olive tubercle conclusions. Quickly Smith extended his predilection for analogy. No longer dealing with the olive tubercle, which he had labeled a plant tuberculosis, he now referred to the galls as "plant-tumors." The naturally occurring gall on the class of plants that included chrysanthemums became the first gall he selected. He described the disease's parameters as if it were cancerous. "The tumors grow rapidly only in young fleshy organs," Smith wrote. It "attacks both roots and shoots. It frequently induces abnormal growths on the wounded parts of young cuttings." The disease's "power to produce hyperplasia is not confined to the marguerite." Smith also maintained that, when the material from the chrysanthemum gall was introduced into other plants, it produced "well-developed small tumors on the stems of tobacco, tomato and potato plants and on the roots of sugar beets." He completed his chrysanthemum gall work by isolating the bacterial culprit, plating it in pure culture, and reintroducing it into a healthy plant. It yielded the characteristic galls in the recipient. Smith was then able to separate the pathogen and plant it in pure culture.[28]

Implicit in Smith's olive tubercle and gall work was the identification of plant disease in a way parallel to animal disease. Rather than pursue a plant specific course, Smith focused on establishing a single ideology and nomenclature for plants and animals. In this way, knowledge of plants was reinforced by what was known about animals and vice versa. Rather than examine something de novo, Smith started with the a priori assumption of correlation between the anatomical and pathological realm of plants and animals. This approach almost guaranteed a certain type of conclusion no matter the question asked.

In the course of his chrysanthemum gall work, Smith noticed that the tumors were reminiscent of those associated with crown gall, especially the variety that attacked peach trees. Since peaches were an economically important crop, Smith decided next to focus his research there. His initial effort was to determine the disease agent, which he did fairly expeditiously. But the true heart of the research was to "prove" that crown gall was actually plant cancer, that the tumors on roots were comparable to tumors on pancreases or lungs.

His magnum opus was a February 1911 USDA Bureau of Plant Industry bulletin. Appearing under the title *Crown-Gall of Plants: Its Cause and Remedy*,[29] the bulletin provided an extensive history of all Smith's previous gall work. It also took great care to explore the taxonomic relationship of crown gall to other galls and root diseases. Smith even did a similar thing to the types of bacteria that produced the various gall or root diseases. This also included the best means to propagate each for laboratory work. But the pièce de résistance of the work was a nearly twenty-page discussion of the similarity—comparability—between the plant cancer known as crown gall and animal cancer.

Smith persistently offered a "suggested relationship to animal tumors." Crown gall was, he wrote, like "a sarcoma." It was not a teratoma because it did not "have a restrictive growth comparable to a defective normal growth." It was not an "edema" nor an "inflammation" nor a "degeneration." Smith took the offensive. "Cancer occurs in a variety of animals, and no good reason has been advanced why they should not occur in plants." Galls "are tumors, morbid new tissue developments tending to weaken and destroy the plant." Like cancer in animals, "crown-galls are of indefinite structure and indeterminate growth." The intertwined nature of plant tumors "strongly suggest[s] malignant tumor tissue of animals." Crown galls possessed "well marked metastases . . . secondary tumors, arising from within, at some distance from the primary tumor." The causative factor located itself within a plant tumor cell, and then that infected cell traversed "through the stems to a distance of several feet from the primary tumor before a second external tumor develops." As in animal cancers, "a certain degree of immunity can be induced in the plants by repeated inoculations" and "spontaneous recovery is quite frequent" in crown gall cases. Plant cancer arose in areas of irritation or inflammation. It had a tendency "to appear in callous or scar tissue" and "to return after excision" by the plant surgeon's knife.

Despite these many, marked similarities, most animal pathologists refused to recognize crown gall and similar plant tumors as comparable to cancer in animals. Smith had many explanations for the refusal, but among the most prevalent was the causation question. A significant number of animal and human cancer investigators cited the repeated failure of investigators to identity a cancer germ as evidence against the microbial origin of human and animal cancer. Conversely, to these men and women, the identification of a crown gall–producing bacterial agent demonstrated conclusively that the plant disease was definitely not cancer. Smith faced this objection in his research. Three times—in 1909, 1910, and 1911—he addressed the American Association for Cancer Research with his crown gall conclusions. Each time members of the group argued that plant and animal life and organization were sufficiently different to render the analogy unwieldy and cited crown gall's bacterial cause as irrefutable evidence that the disease did not constitute cancer.

Smith thought that position incorrect and ahistorical and offered his own work to press his point. Before 1900, plant pathologists recognized that a piece of a crown gall–infested root implanted in a healthy tree would create the tumorous cancer there. During the same period, animal scientists did similar things with mouse tissue and produced cancer in otherwise healthy individuals. What bound these two approaches together was that neither group could "explain the reason why."

In the case of the plant pathologists, many expressed skepticism about "the existence of a parasite." The reason was clear: "After repeated careful searches by a good many people no such organism had been demonstrated." These experiments, many of which identified suspect microorganisms, led to the proposed culprits being plated in pure culture and introduced into health roots but yielded "nothing comparable to the growth from which they had been taken."

Researchers pursued this course without success for a decade or more. Smith offered explanations for the repeated failure. In some cases, tumor tissue was incubated so long that it degraded and became invaded by other organisms. The crown gall pathogen proved quite delicate; an external pathogen killed it quite easily. When these invading microorganisms were placed in tree roots, they did not produce the disease. An alternate explanation stemmed from difficulty in plating. Common nutrients in agar dishes would barely sustain the crown gall organism. Examinations of the dish would likely not reveal measurable growth until weeks after the bacteria were plated. Thirdly, even after six years of experimentation, Smith could not find a suitable stain for the bacteria. Whatever accepted any of the stains that Smith employed looked simply like cellular detritus. Apparently the bacteria grew well under the precise chemical conditions of tree roots but was barely sustainable otherwise; isolating it for identification proved almost Sisyphean. Also, the bacteria adopted different shapes, forms, and characters when it was subjected to hostile but survivable conditions. Put more simply, it did not look or act like itself. The way Smith and his fellow researchers initially identified the bacteria of crown gall was not by its anatomy but by physiology. Even if they could not see it or find it, they knew it was there because it produced the disease.

Smith found his crown gall difficulties prophetic. They made it "reasonable to suppose that similar difficulties would be encountered in isolating the parasites of animal organisms." The past served as prologue. He labeled his experience as consistent with "past difficulties encountered in determining the causes of tuberculosis, leprosy and syphilis."

Smith then drew up "suggestions" for animal pathologists "who believe malignant animal tumors to be of parasitic origin, but have not been able to demonstrate" it. He urged investigators to begin a "renewed search" for microorganisms "either independent of specific cells or confined to them and using them as a means of dissemination." Smith reminded his audience that the invaders could be "active" in "very small numbers only" since, like the crown gall germ, they could change shape or be diminished in a swarm of hardier organisms. If the cancer-causing microbe was destroyed by extraneous organisms, then all attempts to produce the disease using only the remaining microscopic bodies would certainly fail. A similar fate would befall those who introduced ground plant cells. Initially infested with crown gall bacteria, they now stood free of those pathogens. Other agents had killed those fragile creatures.

Crown gall had taught Smith something he hoped his animal pathologist compatriots would learn. Investigators were "under no obligation to consider all malignant tumors as etiologically identical." What Smith meant here was that animal researchers had "normalized" their research on mouse tumors. Most of what they knew they had deduced from these laboratory animals. Any other species might provide a differing portrait, different etiological particulars. Certainly the plant cancer otherwise known as crown gall presented a radically contrary route. It was likely that cancer in other animal species could be equally idiosyncratic.

Smith's pronouncement of crown gall's peculiarity, at least when compared to mouse tumor, did not stop him from using animal diseases as analogous to what could happen in various animal cancers. For example, difficulties among lab workers finding suitable media on which to grow syphilis and yaws, or even the streptococcus associated with endocarditis, long delayed their identification as specific disease-causing pathogens. Something as simple as a small difference in pH or hypersensitivity to salt or some other common nutrient could prove inhospitable to the cancer germ. Similar problems of the conditions and chemicals of staining or washing, again common in some animal disease, might mask the microbe of cancer.

Crown gall could be spread from plant species to plant species, a fact that Smith recognized. He acknowledged that fact and suggested that the less complicated nature of plant structures accounted for this "cross-inoculability." But he also maintained that the "doctrine of non-cross-inoculability of animal tumors may be based on insufficient evidence." Smith noted successes in inoculating rabbit sarcoma in a hare and dog tumors in a fox as proof that such interspecies transfer did occur in the animal kingdom. Smith merely hypothesized that this fact might be more extensive that supposed.[30]

Smith's report was aimed at laboratory investigators. But what had been drafted so clearly as a scientific document became a public sensation a month before its official release. The *New York Times* was especially enthralled with the work's implications. "The Department of Agriculture has advanced a theory that cancer in human beings is caused by a disease in plants," a piece in the *Times* began. Since "these plant growths are truly cancers, then it is extremely probable that micro-organisms of some sort are also the inciting cause of sarcoma and carcinoma." Thinking that plants also got cancer was not such a foreign notion, the *Times* maintained, because "tubercular diseases occur in plants as well as animals." The Logansport [Ind.] *Pharos* agreed. Tumors produced by crown gall are "anatomically and otherwise strikingly like those found in certain malignant animal tumors." Given the cancer research's "uncertain state, . . . any clew whatsoever becomes of importance." A parasite similar to that causing crown gall probably "lies at the bottom of the malignant phenomenon" among animals. The San Antonio *Light and Gazette* asserted that "experts of the United States Department of Agriculture" revealed a cancer in plants "very similar, perhaps identical, with that which afflicts human beings." This discovery "is of vast importance to humanity." Cancer remained "still an insoluble problem to science." The disease "is now recognized as the greatest menace to mankind. It is even feared that it may be the means of' destroying all human life on earth." The *Light and Gazette* juxtaposed tuberculosis with cancer. Tuberculosis caused more deaths, but cancer "is a greater menace." Science knew "how to cure tuberculosis. We do not know how to cure cancer."

The *Light and Gazette* also acknowledged Gaylord's studies as part of the cancer continuum. Fish developed cancer "to a remarkable extent." In fact, the paper continued, some researchers had suggested fish as "the source of all cancer in man." Now, plants, "still further down in the scale of life," had been proven to harbor cancer, a disease caused by a distinct pathogen. That knowledge meant, metaphorically speaking, that the "spectre of cancer seems to leer at us from the smiling cluster of grapes" and other fruits and vegetables. Though a sobering thought that the foods eaten by humans caused their disease, the discovery was of great moment: "It is expected to lead to the isolation of the germ in human cancer." The *Light and Gazette* acknowledged that many animal and human cancer researchers did not believe the disease to be borne by a pathogen. The paper dismissed that contention as folly with one sentence. "Up to the present time," the paper declared, that denial "might have applied equally well to plant cancer."[31]

Smith pressed the case in 1912 with two more influential publications. Both consciously made the case that crown gall was analogous to human cancer. His *Science* publication was an address he delivered as the outgoing president of the Botanical Society of America to a joint session of that organization and the AAAS Section on Bacteriology. This address rested on a single premise. His crown gall studies transformed cancer research. His findings demanded that "closed doors in cancer research must now be opened and studies on the etiology of the disease must be [reconsidered] with a view to finding a parasite within the cancer cell, and separating it therefrom by an improved technic of isolation." The old theory that "the cancer cell is the only parasite" and that cancer could not be transmitted "unless the living cancer cell [was] present" must "now be abandoned." If his audience was not convinced by his work, Smith pointed to "the discovery by Peyton Rous that sarcoma of chickens may be produced in the absence of cancer cells." There the "cancerous fluid [was] filtered free from all traces of living cancer cells." "Nothing else than a living microorganism, minute enough to pass through the walls of the rather coarse filter," must cause the disease.

He shifted focus to support his contention. What happened in the development of crown gall provided "a striking analogy to what occurs in malignant animal tumors." Crown gall's characteristics included "an enormous multitude" of specific cells "in opposition to the best interests of the organism," a tumor with no "plainly visible parasites," growth at the periphery of the tumor, a structure for the transfer of food and gas between the tumor and the organism, and "strands" from the primary tumor "from which secondary tumors develop." Both primary animal and plant cancers tend to develop "in bruises, wounds or irritated places."

Both show "complete recovery if all the tumor tissue is extirpated" and both exhibit cases "of spontaneous recovery." The sole significant difference, Smith argued, was that we know the cancer-causing parasite in plants, but we have not as yet identified, isolated, infected, and reisolated it for animals.

Smith did not claim that the crown gall pathogen caused human cancer. Warm-blooded animals were too hot for that fragile bacteria to flourish. Smith turned his attention to cold-blooded animals and, recognizing the work of the Germans and then Gaylord, decided on brook trout as a suitable cold-blooded animal on which to test whether his bacteria might cause cancer in these lower animals. His initial experimental results were intriguing. He found a number of ulcers and nodules near where he had inoculated his bacteria. Smith took some of these injuries, converted them into slides, and took the specimens "to one of the most distinguished research workers on cancer in this country." The expert proclaimed that "if we had this in man we should call it sarcoma."

Buoyed by this result, Smith pledged to extend his brook trout efforts.[32] His second major publication appeared before he could make much headway. It mostly contained micrographs and histological drawings demonstrating the parallels between animal and plant cancer. It repeated many of the contentions he had used in his presidential address, such as an extensive discussion of Rous's chicken sarcoma efforts, and also marshaled a few other facts. For example, he cited a speech by Jensen, the mouse tumor authority, arguing that sugar beets suffered from a malady virtually indistinguishable from cancer in animals. Smith also mentioned an experiment that grafted a dog tumor to a fox. "Only fox cells grew," which implied that a parasitic agent accompanied the transfer.[33]

Smith's new work received less sensational, more reverential press reports. The *New York Times* linked Smith's crown gall and Rous's chicken sarcoma to declare that "apparently, [cancer] is transferred by an ultra-microscopic germ." The San Antonio *Light* maintained that "human pathologists are watching the progress of his scientific work among the plants with great interest, believing that it may hold the solution of a problem with which they have battled so long in vain." The *Washington Post* took a longer view. Until recently, investigators failed to consider "that there might be an analogous disease of plants" to human cancer. But now plant pathologists had discovered "plant cancers" and found that they "are due to a micro organism[*sic*]." Since the disease "appears to be the same in plants and humans," the *Post* concluded that human cancer "may also be due to some parasitic organism."[34]

Leonard Keene Hirshberg, a Johns Hopkins medical school graduate who wrote for the daily press, offered a bold prediction. Citing Smith's and Rous's work, he found them of a single piece. If plant cancer and animal cancer were both caused by microbes, Hirshberg analogized, then human cancer too was certainly the product of a microorganism. He did not stop there, however. He assured his readers that by 1915 "all insurance companies . . . will be expected to pay indemnity to all policy holders who succumb to cancer." Hirshberg's reasoning was clear. "Malignant growths are the result of infections in wounds."[35]

Medical organizations heralded Smith's work. The AMA provided Smith a certificate of honor for his plant cancer work in 1913. The *BMJ* offered a more grudging but nonetheless upbeat assessment. Smith maintained that crown gall was "a key to unlock the cancer situation." The journal demurred, arguing that the work was preliminary; "we do not think the key has yet moved to the lock." Despite its hesitations, *BMJ* conceded that Smith's experiments were a "thoroughly good and painstaking bit of research." It was his conclusions that gave *BMJ* pause. While the editors could not endorse them at this point, they remained certain that his statements would "stimulate other workers to enter upon this field of investigation."[36]

JAMA was more enthusiastic, at least in part because Simmons linked Smith's work to other efforts. He praised Rous as having "shown conclusively" that chicken sarcoma was caused "by a living virus" and referenced Gaylord's trout studies as another study demonstrating that "a malignant tumor can be propagated by cell-free material." Smith's work fit within that context. If further investigations bore out Smith's proclamation, "then to him will belong the credit of having discovered first the precise cause of a cancerous growth." In any case, "the view of the infectious cause of cancer in general is strengthened by [Smith's] work."

Simmons argued that Smith's conclusions, in light of Rous's and Gaylord's experiments, "warrant the adoption" as "a tentative or working hypothesis" that "cancer is infectious." This position will "stimulate and guide" future cancer research. E. W. Taylor, editor of the *Boston Journal of Medicine and Surgery*, summed up what he recognized as the significance of Smith's work. "All neoplasms, of men, animals and plants, may be due to parasitic organisms which induce abnormal, riotous and anarchic proliferation of the particular type of cell in which they find lodgment." While Smith work "is of course hypothetical, . . . the analogy of the argument is . . . stimulating and suggestive." The fact that it pointed to a parasitic cause for cancer meant that "the recent researches of Ehrlich and Von Wassermann" were vital. Taylor foretold of a time that investigators "may in time be able to deal with malignant diseases as successfully as we do . . . other undoubted infectious processes," some of "whose causative agent is as yet unknown."[37]

Smith's and Gaylord's research brought forth numerous references to Rous's chicken sarcoma work. Investigators employed it as a model from which to consider their results. Smith also referred extensively to Gaylord's trout studies as he tried to place his crown gall plant work firmly in the context of cancer generally. This association enabled him to argue that animal and plant cancer proved primarily similar, a contention accepted by his nation's leading cancer research group. Both Smith's and Gaylord's studies broke new ground. They depended on a sense of imagination for which it might have been very difficult to get a hearing a decade earlier. Their emergence in the public/professional discourse about 1910 was due to the fruitlessness and confusion of the years before 1910. Frustration and failure seemed to have opened rather than closed minds. Investigators proved willing to brook and produce new theories, many much more tenuous than what had been offered only a decade earlier. With the new speculations came an increased dependence on analogy. The more distant researchers went from the status quo, the more necessary they found analogies to be. Flights of scientific fancy required a mooring. Analogies to ground the work and to make it appear as something familiar helped ensure a hearing among their peers. Analogy was both corroborative and interpretive. It provided evidence of why something was so, while channeling thought down a well-known path.

7

The Euphoria and Despair of Chemotherapy, 1910–1915

E. W. Taylor's reference to the recent work of Ehrlich and Wassermann, who was Ehrlich's laboratory associate, did not refer to Ehrlich's immunology or mouse cancer work or Wassermann's test for syphilis. Instead, it was to chemotherapy, a new, exciting discovery of the first decade of the twentieth century. Atoxyl, salvarsan and later neo-salvarsan were all laboratory-produced chemicals that rid the human body of syphilis. A disease almost as feared as cancer, syphilis ravaged the body and the mind, often culminating in death. There had been no cure.

Anti-syphilitic chemotherapy changed all that. Manufactured in a laboratory, chemically modified substances designed to cure disease opened new vistas, new possibilities. Newspapers and medical journals heaped praise on Ehrlich's atoxyl and then salvarsan chemotherapy. Physicians quickly hailed the drugs as effective and relatively non-toxic. Ehrlich acquired celebrity that few researchers ever attain. Over a thousand medical men traveled to Koenigsberg in 1910 just to hear Ehrlich discuss his newest chemotherapeutic creation. Three police officers "made a path for him" to enter the hall. Several members of the royal family attended, as did "representatives of all countries."[1] For investigators, the reception accorded Ehrlich was virtually unprecedented.

With fame came opportunities and obligations. It was not long before commentators began to suggest that human cancer might be susceptible to a chemotherapeutic remedy. Both Park and Gaylord had argued that mercury, iodine, and arsenic proved effective against thyroid trout cancer. But chemotherapy's urgent embrace indicated something more. It suggested broad agreement about how chemotherapy might work and what it might do.

Ehrlich's chemotherapeutic theory depended on existence of a physical pathogen and three-dimensional chemistry. It echoed his immunity musings. In Ehrlich's parlance, a chemotherapeutic agent—a chemical—bonded with the offending microbe and left surrounding cells unscathed. Chemically modified shapes, created by varying the structures of aromatic hydrocarbons, would bind themselves to specific loci in the pathogen's conformation. A bound pathogen would be tied up at the exact site where it otherwise would have affixed itself to healthy cells and caused disease.

The relevant body cell would therefore be left free of pathogenic invasion, enabling this cell to perform its life-sustaining tasks. Ehrlich called his synthesized agents chemical side chains and argued that they acted like meticulously targeted "magic bullets," received only by the desired place in the microorganism's anatomy.

Ehrlich designed possible chemotherapeutic agents by creating numerous, closely related compounds, each of which was sufficiently varied as to possess a slightly different three-dimensional shape. Beyond that, the process depended upon deduction. In the case of his syphilis work, he began with the aniline dyes. Two assessments guided his work. Ehrlich believed that the three-dimensional configurations of the aniline dyes accounted for their different colors. He knew also these dyes to be receptive to living cells; they were the basis of histological staining. Ehrlich's selection of the heavy metal arsenic proved more tenuous. He knew that the metal had exhibited some effect against trypanosomes, which he believed closely related to spirochetes. His 606th manipulation produced salvarsan, and his 914th conformation begot neo-salvarsan.[2]

The medical and public celebration of chemotherapy often did not extend to Ehrlich's explanation for the phenomenon. Newspapers took care to call the drug "a specific;" it was designed for a particular type of microbe. The Rockefeller Institute's Samuel Meltzer hailed salvarsan as the world's second specific—the naturally occurring quinine for malaria was the first—and the first chemically formulated one. It was "epoch making," opening "up a wide range of possibilities in medicine." Sir Almroth Wright, Britain's leading bacteriologist and immunologist, termed chemotherapy "the internal administration of antiseptics," a model considerably broader than Ehrlich's magic bullet. Charles H Chetwood, a New York physician specializing in venereal disease, labeled salvarsan a "sensational contribution to medical progress." Hugo Schweitzer, a New York chemist who would later head Bayer Company in the United States, proclaimed in *Science* in 1910 that Ehrlich's discovery had produced "intense excitement" and "interest" among medical men. Schweitzer thought that chemotherapeutic agents would render many diseases passé. He even predicted that "cancer, the cause of which has been ascribed by some investigators to organisms resembling the spirochete of syphilis," soon would be "amenable to chemotherapy."[3]

Schweitzer's reference to the close association among cancer and spirochetes proved no idle chatter. Czerny put the theory into practice almost immediately by testing salvarsan's cancer-fighting prowess. A longtime devotee of the microorganism explanation for cancer and among the first to apply chemotherapy to the disease, Czerny gave twelve patients several doses of the drug. He reported them much improved. Czerny was particularly encouraged by salvarsan's effects on sarcomas. It lessened markedly those tumors, and he promised to continue his trials until his patients became cured or "much debilitated."[4]

In late 1910, Emil Fischer, Nobel prize-winning chemist and then professor of chemistry at Berlin, adopted a theory similar to Ehrlich's for his cancer chemotherapy experiments. Fischer had received his prize for stereochemistry. He had demonstrated that a group of physiologically active substances, which he called the purines, all shared similar base conformations. They different only in their add-on groups or the order in which their essential elements were configured. With form at the forefront of his thinking, Fischer attempted to devise a chemical to fight cancer. Following in Ehrlich's footsteps, he started with a photoactive substance that readily was accepted into biological tissue. This aniline dye-arsenic derivative was manipulated many times and tested by Georg Klemperer, who had succeeded Leyden at the Berlin charity cancer hospital established by that fervent advocate of the parasitic cause for cancer. These experiments yielded a substance that they called elarson, and the two researchers quickly patented it. They also patented its phosphorus complement and a series of arsenic- or phosphorous-based compounds that were structurally similar, in case any of these closely related drugs proved significantly more effective than elarson.[5]

While Fischer and Klemperer were quietly synthesizing and testing arsenic and phosphorous compounds and as Czerny performed additional experiments, Wassermann made a fantastic announcement. In an event reported throughout the western world, Wassermann, now at the University of Berlin, declared that he had developed a chemotherapeutic agent that preliminary results showed effective against cancer. His long association with Ehrlich gave him considerable credibility, as did the test for syphilis that even then bore his name. The method by which he discovered his curative mimicked that of Ehrlich. He developed a notion of what happened on the cellular level and then set about synthesizing numerous closely related compounds to determine which affected the tumor but left surrounding cells virtually unaffected.

Despite all the hoopla, Wassermann's cancer chemotherapy bore less in common with Ehrlich's theories than might be imagined. Unlike Ehrlich, who targeted pathogens and sought to bind them so they would not attack healthy tissue, Wassermann aimed at cancer cells. Wassermann remained unconvinced by the work of Rous, Gaylord, and Smith. He adamantly maintained that cancer was "organic." By that he meant that it was the consequence of a biological process confined to the individual; it was not the result of an external living agent.[6]

He set his mind to finding a chemical that would be deadly to cancer cells and relatively innocuous to regular body cells. He first experimented with biological agents, such as snake venom, but to no avail. He then drew on previous experience. Wassermann had undertaken a series of experiments a year or so earlier in which he explored whether cancer cells lived longer in blood serum derived from healthy persons or from cancer victims. In the course of these investigations, Wassermann subjected the freshly excised tumors to salts of tellurium and selenium. He found that living cells incorporated the oxygen from these compounds and deposited reduced elements near the nucleus, where maximum cellular activity occurred. Toxic to those cells, tellurium and selenium soon combined with the cells to form black and red precipitates. Wassermann applied those results quickly. He injected the salts into tumors of cancerous mice and found that tumor size greatly diminished. They became soft and eventually liquefied. He then gave another set of cancerous mice intravenous injections, requiring the material to travel through the blood stream. No change in the cancerous tumors was noted.

Wassermann understood that the fastest growing cells, cells such as cancer cells, possessed the greatest affinity for the tellurates and selenates. Armed with this knowledge, Wassermann's problem was this: he had a substance that, when injected directly into a tumor, caused the tumor to lessen and dissolve. But that method was not feasible to treat cancer on a broad scale. That method could not account for cells outside the tumor, cells that could produce metastases. Intravenous inoculation was the only recourse, and that reality focused his consideration on how to take advantage of the relatively minor differences between healthy and cancerous cells. Wassermann again centered his thinking on the key distinction of cancer's rapid growth. This required oxygen beyond that necessary for regular cell maintenance and repair, and Wassermann targeted the cancer cell's voracious oxygen consumption as the characteristic to exploit, to have the salts selectively settle in tumor tissue. The common aniline dye eosin, long used in histological staining, was avidly accepted by red blood cells. These oxygen bearers became Wassermann's delivery system or, as he noted, his "railroad tracks" to the tumor. His tests quickly convinced him of eosin's virtue. When eosin was injected into normal tissue, the tissue turned red. But when given intravenously, healthy tissue appeared slightly pink while tumors became a bold red. Clearly cancer cells accepted the eosin voraciously.

Wassermann then began the extensive systematic slight manipulations that had marked Ehrlich's salvarsan work. Finding a balance of selenium/eosin compounds—he eliminated tellurium—that would not markedly interfere with normal functioning but would ultimately bind and kill cancer cells remained the goal. Wassermann used five different breeds of mice to test the preparations—four liable to different tumors and the other to sarcoma—finally choosing a combination that could be injected into each of the breeds for three straight days and that would dissolve tumors within ten days.

In cases where the tumor had reached cherry or larger size, the mice died at about the same time the tumors disappeared. Wassermann did not attribute their demise to his chemotherapeutic substance but rather to the then liquefied tumor entering the blood and poisoning the otherwise cured animals. Hansemann, professor of pathological anatomy at Berlin and a long-standing proponent of cancer as an indigenous creation, supported Wassermann's contention. He argued that the liquid tumor material went to the spleen and was destroyed there, unless it overwhelmed the animal body and caused its death. With the exception of some of the dissolved substance being absorbed by the liver, Hansemann could find no other evidence of an organ being affected by the tumor by-products or the chemotherapeutic agent.

Both Hansemann and Wassermann cautioned that mouse anatomy and mouse cancer differed from human anatomy and human cancer. Both also concluded that the time was not yet ripe for human testing. Dosage issues and means to prevent tumor products from overwhelming patients need to be resolved before humans could be involved.[7]

Researchers immediately hailed Wassermann for his innovation, while warning against unbridled euphoria. The matter was more complicated than a simple celebration of discovery, however. Investigators honored themselves and their method as much as they championed what the German had done. *JAMA* saluted Wassermann as "one of the best investigators known in modern medicine" and argued that his method showed "the promise of great things." It mattered not if "this particular compound will favorably influence human cancer," *JAMA* incredulously maintained. "No one can doubt that this is a definite step." A "long series of most arduous investigations" must be "patiently continued with the least possible distraction" before cancer could be conquered. Bashford placed Wassermann's efforts in a long "line of thought" that characterized the modern research laboratory. Based upon systematic investigation rationally pursued in a closed environment, Wassermann's efforts "open up one of the most hopeful prospects [for] our ultimately being able to treat the disease in man." He urged "continuation of rational experiment into the mysteries of the nature of cancer," arguing that the past "ten years of investigation by my colleagues and myself" were but prologue to an even more glorious "next ten years of experiment." Czerny offered a longer view. The vast new suggestions for cancer's cure required investigators "to sift and study each medicament and method" rationally. If

England and Germany built "one Dreadnought less each and invest[ed]" the money into research facilities, Czerny predicted that "the cancer problem would . . . be solved in fifty years." Taylor was less circumspect. "Whether or no Wassermann's observations really indicate an important clue to the successful treatment" of cancer was almost irrelevant. "The really important aspect of his work is as a demonstration of method in research." It venerates laboratory research, which he claimed constituted a "new and rational mode of empiricism." Its "further application" to "medical problems presents very great and brilliant possibilities of accomplishment."[8]

Accentuating method and effectively elevating it above substance was no accident. With a decade of repeated failure and prostration behind them, men and women engaged in laboratory research found that establishing the preeminence of their method and by extension themselves was paramount. It defined them, provided them legitimacy, and offered them access to funds. The laboratory and its people needed continued sustenance. Their meager successes did not meet their initial promise. Researchers at these facilities proved unable to establish a joint vision of what cancer was, even as they took opportunity after opportunity to proclaim a shared method for its pursuit.

Establishing cancer hospitals and staffing them with laboratory personnel provided a temporary reprieve from public scrutiny. These units could test whether a proposed cure for cancer was in fact a cure. But the desultory years immediately prior to 1910, characterized by a tremendous profusion of utterly chaotic and often contradictory cancer studies from across the globe, more than negated whatever benefits the hospitals produced. Laboratories had every right to feel threatened.

Lack of easily articulated successes required explanation to their constituencies. That responsibility fell directly on the shoulders of laboratory directors. They reported to the public, trumpeting the slightest encouraging sign while beating down expectations. They continually reminded the populace of the enormity and desperation of the cancer problem, finding no doubt that a healthy dose of fear loosened purses. Gaylord, Ehrlich, Leyden, Czerny, Ewing, Bashford, and the other directors became cancer's face. They had the critical but thankless task of traveling into public venues and proclaiming victory as they suffered almost constant defeat.

In this endeavor, laboratory directors continued the program of the last years before 1910. They brazenly substituted more nebulous progress for definitive success and explained that their method accounted for their virtue. They doggedly maintained that their laboratories were systematic and precise and, therefore, ultimate triumph was inescapable. Investigators reasoned from what they knew and applied it to what they did not know. This was the enterprise of making something so. If and when an investigation yielded unanticipated results, researchers modified techniques in a predictable manner without changing the investigation's essential character and tested again. That approach to reality was viable in theory; it was suitable for a fixed, steady-state environment. But since the amount and types of variations were practically infinite in these open biological complexes, the method proved anything but systematic. Possibilities were endless and their "systematic" exploration merely a charade. That did not mean that employable results could not be uncovered. They could be, and they were. Rather it is to argue that the hubristic methodological assumptions that produced cancer laboratories—that you can rationally test things that you don't know by relying on things you do know—were anything but axiomatic or even markedly superior to other methodological applications.[9]

The method of the cancer laboratory exactly replicated Ehrlich's salvarsan and Wassermann's selenium-eosine chemotherapeutic notions. Indeed, they were all cut from the same cloth. Ehrlich's histological staining assumptions were analogous to his immunity theory, and his chemotherapy theory incorporated both. Wassermann merely adapted staining theory and chemotherapeutic specificity to his efforts. The two scientists then engaged in long testing processes. They began by finding a substance that apparently performed the desired action in vitro. They then took that substance and worked ad nauseam to manipulate it to function that way in vivo without harming other living tissue. Each of these manipulations required extensive animal testing and then a recalibration in light of the result. In each case, researchers repeatedly went back to the metaphorical well. They persisted in applying the basic assumption that they would inevitably create the desired substance with little more than their fundamental conviction (or, in the case of later investigators, because of Ehrlich's or Wassermann's results) that this was the correct way to proceed. And they venerated it, raising it to a state where the pursuit justified whatever ends they achieved.

Shortly after Wassermann announced his chemotherapeutic cancer agent, Ehrlich unveiled another cancer-fighting substance. Called nigrosin, the drug was an aniline dye derivative that Ehrlich systematically manipulated until he was satisfied that it fought the scourge. Its differential absorption pattern characteristically turned tumors black and left healthy mouse tissue its natural color. Reports claimed that early tests of nigrosin proved 100 percent effective in destroying tumors.

Ehrlich refused to predict when nigrosin might be given to humans, arguing that that day was far in the future. The chemotherapeutic search that produced nigrosin depended on differential absorption of the agent by cancerous and non-cancerous tissue, not the killing of a microbe. Its fundamental thrust was similar to that of Wassermann. In the wake of the nigrosin announcement, the two investigators pledged to join together in a grand German cancer chemotherapy effort. These two giants of laboratory medicine pooled resources, began a combined chemotherapeutic quest, and generated considerable worldwide notoriety.[10]

Despite their now prominent advocacy of cancer as a disease indigenous to the living being—not the consequence of an external parasite—their union had little effect on propagating that viewpoint among cancer researchers. Reports surfaced that there were filterable ultramicroscopic trypanosomes and spirochetes, as well as the barely visible varieties that caused sleeping sickness and syphilis. Apparently there existed a continuum of parasitic agents from the visible to the beyond visible. Could the same hold true for cancer?[11] Investigators, especially in the United States, had an even more poignant referent. They cited Rous's chicken sarcoma work as confirming the disease's external origin. Rous's findings "place the parasitic causation of cancer upon a new basis," argued William James Morton, a New York City cancer specialist and son of the anesthesia pioneer. He urged researchers to focus chemotherapeutic studies on killing the cancer-producing parasite, not dissolving tumor cells. Rous himself participated in the discussion. He argued that his chicken sarcoma researches had explicitly refuted the theory behind Wassermann's cancer chemotherapy and Ehrlich's recent adoption. Cancer was not "organic." Nor did transmission of the disease between two individuals require transplantation of cellular material. "Such evidence is void," Rous proclaimed. His work proved conclusively that cancer could be contracted like an infection and was "transmissible independent of cells." Flexner referred to his protégé's dramatic statements as "conservative and guarded" and offered a more impassioned opinion. A slew of diseases are now known to be "caused by germs of ultra-microscopic dimensions," Flexner argued. We "possess no criterion for their presence other" than the most important one, "the power to produce infection." A list of diseases caused by these tiny invaders would be multiplied if we knew where and how to look for them, if we had methods to test "their symbiotic relations or co-operative effects with the usual bacteria and protozoa." In light of Rous's work, he saw an "analogy" between those many diseases and cancer. He was virtually certain that cancer was simply the product of "ultra-microscopic microorganisms."

Flexner knew of what he spoke, sort of. His research on poliomyelitis colored his view of cancer and chemotherapy. In polio as in cancer, "it can hardly be doubted that they are living organisms." They can be transmitted "from animal to animal, in which they produce infection, through an infinite series." These two analogous diseases, he maintained, would both prove susceptible to specific chemotherapeutic agents, but he warned that even then the matter would not be resolved. The problem was that the causative entities were living organisms, subject to, in Darwin's words, "infinite variation." Mutation rates differed from parasitic organism to organism, but Flexner recognized that the mutation process was inevitable and natural. It accounted for relapses in certain diseases. And he predicted that it would be shown that a particular chemotherapeutic agent would prove deadly to the initial pathogen but likely harmless to its subsequent mutations.[12]

Flexner and Rous provided potent voices in opposition to the internalist theory of cancer causation, a theory of which Bashford was the most noted celebrant. Introduction of the idea of regular, continual, prolific mutation further complicated the issue. How did one pinpoint a pathogen when its normal course was to change, to configure itself in a different way? What tests would be definitive if, through mutation, pathogens varied their basic characters—form, function, growing conditions, nutrients, and a whole host more? Whatever test was run might immediately be rendered obsolete upon its conclusion through the natural evolutionary process of infinite variation. How could things be made so in a world where change was continual, ongoing, and most explicitly not directed? Random variation was the enemy of systematic exploration; it refused to hew to that template. To researchers, that template was essential. It was the means to make something so.

Shortly after Flexner and Rous issued their rousing defense of the parasitic theory of cancer, three German investigators published an extensive new approach to cancer chemotherapy. They too focused on cancer's ability to grow quickly, but rather than concern themselves with increased need for respiration, they restricted themselves to cell division. The rapid growth and autolysis of cancer tumors produced a chemistry different from normal cells. The trio targeted the different enzymes involved in tumor chemistry, especially that which was responsible for autolysis. They sought to redress the balance between growth and destruction, to change the equilibrium in favor of destruction. They searched for "some substance which will act [primarily] in the presence of the enzymes in question and increase the degeneration to such an extent that all the tumour [*sic*] cells will be destroyed."

Metals—silver, gold, copper, platinum, mercury, and others—seemed excellent candidates. These metals and their salts were considered proficient catalytic agents for various enzyme reactions, and the German researchers initially tested their utility by injecting their salts directly into tumors. They understood, of course, that the chemotherapeutic substances they chose would have to be given intravenously, but quickly found that they would need to vary their agents' nature. Solutions were unusable. When metal salts dissolved in solution, the fine chemical particles dissociated into ions. The entire animal body indiscriminately absorbed these ionic metals; healthy cells took them as readily as the usually glutinous tumor cells.

Colloidal suspensions came next. Made by striking an arc in a cold water bath between two electrodes of the metal you hoped to suspend, the metal would initially vaporize and then quickly condense into minute suspended droplets in the cold water. When exposed to a chemotherapeutic agent in this form, the tumors accepted the substance and combined with it to leave a precipitated mass. The metallic colloids went from "insoluble to more or less full-continuous precipitation." The Germans tested their suspensions on several animal species, always with good results. Nonetheless, they warned against any "utopian notions" that their approach would soon be applicable for human cancer.[13]

Use of metals to combat cancer gained currency. Gaylord published an article in *Berliner Klinische Wochenschrift*, a leading German medical journal, claiming that his mercury and iodine research with trout helped spawn the approach. Charles E. Walker, director of research at Glasgow Cancer Hospital, did some work with selenium colloids. He was especially interested in understanding the mechanisms by which his agent worked.[14]

A more interesting case was that of a French physician, J. Gaube du Gers. He reported to the Parisian Society of Medical Practitioners that he had perfected a method of "decancerization," a "radical disappearance . . . of all cancerous manifestation." Gers had long noticed that a particular mineral water "gave good results in cancerous afflictions of the tongue." He analyzed the water's trace minerals and found it high in copper. Deciding that that must be the active ingredient, he took some of the metal and through "a series of laboratory experiments" rendered it a colloidal suspension that could be injected into patients. Terming his colloid "copper protoxide," he claimed he made the drug by reducing copper salts with albumosic acid. The resulting substance was so delicate that it had to be kept in yellow vials in the dark to prevent decomposition. Each dosage contained "171 hundredths of a milligram of pure copper." Gers injected his curative in "the loins" every two to fifteen days. The tumor shrank almost immediately. A few months later, no evidence of the disease could be found in his fourteen patients. He proclaimed his preparation successful "so long as the patient is not actually dying."

Gers manufactured his chemotherapeutic agent for sale and published two broadsides puffing his cure. Neither *Decancerisation* nor *La Cuprase et Le Cancer* received significant medical attention; only one French medical journal even mentioned the theory. But Gers's paper to the medical practitioners' society was cabled to the United States and excerpts appeared in several daily papers, including the *Washington Post*. In several of these abstractions, editors confused Gers's name. He was referred to as Haube Dugers and Haube Rugers among other bastardizations.[15]

Gers clearly rested outside the conventional cancer research nexus. Yet it was testimony to the desperation that cancer laboratory investigators faced that at least one stoic researcher felt it appropriate to acknowledge the work of this obvious quack. Leo Loeb, director of the new Barnard Cancer Laboratory and Hospital, which was associated with Washington University in St. Louis, leaned on Gers's communication as he began his colloidal copper studies. Loeb was no cancer research neophyte. The brother of Jacques Loeb, the younger Loeb had spent time in the laboratories of Bashford, Gaylord, and Ewing. He had even headed the University of Pennsylvania's cancer laboratory before moving to the grand new St. Louis facility. At every stop Loeb proved his research mettle. He had already made noteworthy contributions in tissue growth and transplantation, the serial transplantation of tumors, and resistance and immunity to cancer. He was a charter member of the AACR.[16]

Loeb began his colloidal copper exegesis by firmly establishing his research in a long tradition of laboratory investigation. He pointed to the "experimental study of tumor growth" as a consequence of "a systematic analysis" of the environment in which tumor cells developed and grew and maintained that those pioneering efforts "laid the foundation for rational investigation aiming at the cure of cancer." He then selected what he considered relevant antecedents: Wassermann for his cancer chemotherapy work, the three German investigators because of their experiments with colloids of various metals, and finally Gers, copper's prominent proponent. Ironically, Loeb acknowledged in his paper no direct knowledge of Gers's labors nor even access to the Frenchman's two broadsides. Loeb relied on American newspaper accounts and brief references in popular and peripheral medical publications to locate Gers's claims in the history that Loeb was creating for himself.

Loeb's initial paper recounted how he had tried colloidal copper directly in mouse tumors and then switched to injecting the material into the animals' circulatory system. Having determined what he thought was the lethal dosage for that animal, he extrapolated what would be comparable for a human and began testing on hospital patients a few months after the studies by Wassermann, the three Germans, and Gers were announced. Loeb's results showed significant tumor reduction and relatively few disruptions to normal tissue. He recommended continuance of a course of daily copper colloid injections until tumors disappeared.

While announcing these impressive results, Loeb reminded his readers that his treatment was "still in the experimental stage." If any researcher wanted to try the experiment on patients, Loeb warned them to do so only in "institutions in which all means for scientific observation is available." Put simply, Loeb recommended the drug be given only in combination cancer labs/hospitals where the various workers followed the methods of scientific research. Results from those institutions would presumably be comparable and the efficacy of the remedy resolved. Things would become so.

Loeb made two additional claims in this initial paper. First, he maintained that he rushed into publication not for glory or to establish priority but only because news of his work had leaked to the press. By rushing to present his research in the manner of laboratory investigator—a rigorous, scientific manner—Loeb could demonstrate that he had fulfilled the methodological conventions that characterized his cohort. Second, Loeb offered a controversial conclusion. He contended that his mouse-human dosage and efficacy comparisons—the basis of his work— constituted "very strong additional evidence . . . that there exists no essential difference between cancer of rodents and human cancer."[17]

If carried to its extreme, Loeb's outlandish and wildly speculative mouse-human cancer continuum promised to change the character of cancer research. It made the mouse so. What happened in the mouse was by definition consistent with what happened in human cancer. Loeb's statement was distinct from arguing that mice were synonymous with humans, of course. Yet, if put into practice, it simplified the situation by removing humans from the equation.

Within weeks of Loeb's announcement, American newspapers were ablaze with stories about the great event. In some cases, the periodicals quoted verbatim from Loeb's medical paper. Few newspapers sensationalized the story beyond identifying Loeb as a prominent researcher whose work demanded attention.[18] Loeb continued his experiments and presented two additional papers on cancer and colloidal copper in the first months of 1913. The first reported on a "gradual decrease in the effect of injections" over time. Signs of tumor diminution were soon followed by cancerous regrowth. While Loeb argued that "the degree of response to the treatment varies somewhat in different cases," he also concluded that "the action of the intravenous injections of colloidal copper is too slow to render it probable that in the large majority of cases a cure will be accomplished by this mode of treatment." Mouse experiments confirmed that conclusion. Not only did mouse tumors rebound even as treatment persisted, but they often proliferated once the substance was discontinued.

Loeb tried adding casein and then lecithin to his colloidal suspension before finally pausing his copper experiments. Despite lack of success, Loeb refused to consider the research a failure. "Secondary difficulties" could "be overcome," he stated emphatically. Besides, others needed to take into consideration that he had tested only three substances. It was folly to think that the first three materials tried would "represent the most potent ones which can be found." Confident of ultimate triumph, he deemed it "in the interests of science and of practical medicine, to follow to the upmost these lines of investigation."[19]

Loeb then undertook a series of investigations to determine why his injections lost their effectiveness over time. An analogy guided Loeb's experiments. He reasoned that the colloidal substance was akin to the introduction of a foreign pathogen; the animal body responded by attacking the invader. White blood cells and antibodies were mobilized to stop the intruder. Put simply, immunity to the colloid negated its cancer fighting properties. Loeb also speculated that the tumor itself might have its own immunity mechanism; it might also unleash some biological substance to bind the colloid before it reached the tumor.

As Loeb carried out these mouse experiments, he thought of what made salvarsan successful and neo-salvarsan even more so. Salvarsan required only a few doses to rid the body of syphilis, while neo-salvarsan needed but one. The body did not have opportunity to develop immunity. As a consequence of this determination, Loeb hypothesized that "it will be necessary to counteract . . . immunization" by using chemotherapeutic agents "so strong that a few injections destroy the whole tumor." That would be the future of cancer chemotherapy, a situation that lay far in the distance. Even then Loeb thought the situation dicey. If such a potent drug existed, it would "in all probability . . . be too dangerous for the organism as a whole." The tumor and the patient would die.[20]

Loeb envisioned a situation that bordered on hopelessness. Cancer chemotherapy seemed considerably more challenging than initially supposed. It did not appear likely to resolve the cancer problem. For the foreseeable future, chemotherapy likely was a dead end.

8

Better Living through Biochemistry

Experimental vs. Spontaneous Cancer, 1910–1915

In 1911, Henry Butlin, Hunterian Professor and past president of the Royal College of Surgeons, revived his notion that the cancer cell itself constituted a parasite. First proposed by Butlin in 1905 but mentioned as a possibility by a few others a year or two earlier, his proposition maintained that cancer expressed protozoon-like characteristics. He even named the alleged beast "Unicellula cancri." Butlin maintained that each cancer acted like "a new creation of animal being," and was "governed by natural laws just as clear and just as defined as those which govern single-cell organisms . . . recognized by naturalists."

Butlin's renewed and far more extensive identification of cancer as a unicellular microbe was similar to Smith's crown gall argument in a most important way. It took something known—the entire natural history and biology of protozoa—threw it "into a common receptacle," and argued that cancer at every point in its existence functioned precisely in the same manner as at least one protozoon. For all intents and purposes, Butlin maintained that a cancer cell was a distinct and new organism.

Butlin explained the evolution of this new organism. Some agent or force transformed a normal body cell. In most cases, the deformed cell died or was killed by healthy cells. But in some instances, the "power of selection" enabled the new "organism" to survive and proliferate. That was why cancers differed in form, cell type, avidity for particular tissue, tenacity, and the like.[1]

Butlin's hypothesis spawned considerable discussion in the United Kingdom and notice outside. Both the editors of the *BMJ* and *The Lancet* offered comments. Letters to the editor were voluminous.[2] Butlin even maintained that his ideational creation conformed to Koch's postulates. The cancer cell was associated with the disease. It could be isolated from the disease and grown on media. It could produce the disease in a healthy animal and again be isolated.

Butlin's insistence that cancerous cells adhered to Koch's postulates relied on the very recent work of Carrel, who had shown that living tissue could be grown on artificial media. But it was Carrel's Rockefeller Institute colleague, Rous, whose chicken sarcoma work loomed over the era. Accepting Rous's proposition that a physical entity free from cancerous cells caused cancer seemed to many researchers to fly in the face of years of careful investigating. Study after study, test after test, had disproved or at least heaped vast suspicion on every proposed external living being. Yet Rous's chicken sarcomas always bred true; each of the three filterable agents produced a distinctive cancer.

Howard W. Nowell, a Boston University pathologist and laboratory investigator, offered reconciliation. He claimed that cancer cells produced a poisonous substance that irritated other cells and caused them to mutate into renegade cells, or new cancer cells. When isolated, this poison passed through biological filters and caused the disease when injected in healthy individuals through a self-sustaining irritating/poisoning process.

In this formulation, no living microorganism was necessary. All that mattered was the poisonous fluid. If a toxin-like substance produced the disease, then anti-toxins could cure it or immunity could prevent it. Perhaps it was because of this promise that such a ludicrous theory gained such significant attention. Although it flew in the face of almost all that was known about the biology and chemistry of cancer, Nowell's research papers appeared prominently in *Zentralblatt für Allgemeine Pathologie und Pathologische Anatomie*, a leading German pathology journal, and the *Boston Journal of Medicine and Surgery*, home to the work of America's foremost cancer researchers. *JAMA* and *New York Medical Journal* reported on the work. These major professional publications were joined by the *New York Times*, which ran three major articles featuring Nowell's claptrap.[3]

Such a prominent display of such silly material simply reaffirmed how incredibly muddled the cancer situation had become. Failure to find a microorganism that clearly hewed to the model established by Koch proved unsettling. Inability to find a means beyond surgery to cure the disease was immensely disappointing. Rous's ultramicroscopic microbes demanded a reexamination of all that was known. Almost everything that had been trending toward becoming so reverted once again to suspect, in need of a second, third, and fourth look. It was as if a great part of forty years of cancer research was for naught. Little was conclusively determined, and less seemed secure.

European investigators took a far more draconian approach. Rather than attempt to explain away Rous's findings, Bashford and several other ICRF investigators, as well as a number of German pathologists, summarily dismissed them. These Europeans declared that the sarcomas that Rous's ultramicroscopic germ induced were not in fact cancer but common benign cellular changes or granulomas. They patently rejected the idea of a parasitic cause of cancer and so defined his "discovery" as not cancer. Rather than confront the material that Rous had presented, they simply dismissed it, preferring to remain secure in what they had always known and done. Stubbornly refusing to brook any possibility outside their long-established frame of reference, these investigators devoted only the slightest mention to Rous's work. Rather than examine possibilities seeking to prove it in error, they simply disregarded it as false and untenable. The editor of the *BMJ* outlined the case succinctly. Claiming it "a very debatable point" to consider the Rous sarcoma "a malignant tumour at all," he maintained that this growth did not act like a true malignancy. It was transmissible "by tissue grafts but also by injections of expressed virus." If that were not enough to damn it, the editor then argued the case in the negative. "Too little is known of the granulomata of birds," he concluded, even to rule out "that the Rous tumour is not an infective granuloma." Rather than pursue the matter in the laboratory, the editor recommended dropping the Rous sarcoma entirely from cancer research consideration. To "experiment with it may only lead further into the wilderness" of ignorance.[4]

That posture surely ran contrary to the spirit of inquiry that researchers claimed had always categorized their work. But that spirit of inquiry had hardly ever been open or free. Restrictiveness and exclusivity had functioned as the dual pillars of that spirit. Laboratories stood as artificial, manufactured environments. Scientific research was predicated on restriction of variables, not replication of intrinsically manifest complex systems. Investigators demanded that only persons expert in laboratory methods pursue research in laboratories or cancer hospitals, so as to frame everything from a single perspective.

That rigorous but rigid reasoning circumscribed possibilities even as it promised the opportunity of confirmation. Holding such an inflexible position surely encouraged investigations along the lines of those previously undertaken. Studies of mouse and other immunities, ways of transplanting tumors, and other unsettled but intensely examined questions focused attention. At the heart of this persistence was their core, their raison d'être, the undocumented assumption—article of faith, really—that this research would bring investigators closer to the truth, to finding cancer's cause and/or cure.[5]

To these laboratory men and women, it remained the only way to proceed.

Rous's study constituted a fork in the road. It could be dismissed and the status quo ante pursued. Or it could be acknowledged, which demanded a reexamination of virtually everything laboratory researchers thought they knew. Neither position was particularly palatable.[6]

Hansemann offered another challenge. He longed for a return to "the scientific period of cancer research"—the era of the pathologists—and he blamed Koch for its decline. Although Koch made "distinguished discoveries," he was not a pathologist but an "outsider." That made "cloudy waters" and "all different people thought they had the right to fish in it." Now "everyone," not just pathologists, "thinks he is qualified to make great discoveries in the field of the etiology of the cancer, because he is an outsider." "Discovery" after "discovery" was announced and soon refuted, only to be followed by yet another declaration of certainty. Without a common referent, there was "no etiology of cancer."

The mechanism that enabled interlopers to invade cancer research was experimental cancer, especially the Jensen mouse. These mice have gobbled up "immense funds." "In our science," Hansemann wrote, few if any matters have "received such funding as these mice tumors." Hansemann called this biological research poppycock and suggested that, for the question of human cancer, their yield was "actually nothing at all." Mouse cancer and human cancer were not analogous. Persons who tried to make that connection were delusional. He called on researchers to recognize that you "cannot make science with sentimentalities" and to rely on only "scientific deduction." Hansemann declared that investigators continuing the folly were doing nothing to advance human cancer research and must "acknowledge, from the beginning," that mouse experiments "are not transferable to the human."[7]

Within this milieu emerged another thread to debate. Was cancer that emerged spontaneously in living beings somehow fundamentally distinct from that transferred among laboratory animals? A concomitant issue also galvanized attention. Was cancer in human beings similar/identical to that in laboratory animals, and if not, what different parameters mattered? In this framework, transplanted cancers in animals were identified as "experimental cancer," as distinct from the presumably naturally occurring variety, often referred to as "spontaneous cancer."[8]

The possibility that something differentiated experimental cancer from spontaneous cancer caused some consternation, but it also yielded new directions. In the case of humans, this possibility focused attention on what was natural—spontaneous—among human groups, what practices, customs, and habits were undertaken by collectives that rendered them distinct. This was life as lived, where cultures, environments, and biology intersected.

The intersection now drawing scrutiny occurred not in the formalized, constricted, artificial laboratory but in the home, the workplace, the physical location. Measuring these new metrics was not especially complex—correlating them with what constituted normality was more challenging—but it required access. And that change of investigative venue itself changed the equation.

Reconceptualizing human cancer as perhaps fundamentally different and dissimilar to that disease in animals reintroduced medical practitioners into the cancer causation equation. Medical men tended humans, not four-legged creatures. They ministered to cancer patients and, in this process, grew to know their subjects intimately. They went to homes, sat at bedsides, took medical histories, noted the peculiarities of person and group, and were primed to reveal what was normal and what was not. They could characterize pathology, activity, and occurrence.

Measuring distinctive social and cultural markers required access to human lives, perceptiveness, and a sense of order, but it did not necessitate laboratory training. Indeed, those very techniques essential to laboratory investigation were not applicable to assess the peculiarities of human populations. Control, the restriction of process in an artificial environment to but one free variable—one degree of freedom—was absent. And with this absence came the lack of centrality, essentialness, and exclusivity that cancer laboratories had carved out for themselves and their researchers. The intense labors of the past decade to demarcate cancer research in that way had come apart.

The failure of laboratory workers to achieve the end for which their facilities were created certainly contributed to their loss of authority. Their inability to gain control over the cancer question—to make things so by realizing a common, single perspective—had even brought their method into doubt. Physicians also influenced the situation. Medical men had chafed at having been disregarded in the search for cancer's cause. Before the advent of cancer labs, practitioners had been avid participants in the quest, their skills and access critical factors. Rise of the laboratories and the supplanting of humans by experimental animals had rendered them significantly less vital, a situation that now seemed ameliorable, maybe even reversible.[9]

In one sense, the tumult caused by Rous's discovery and the collapse of the confidence that experimental animal cancer was fundamentally similar to spontaneous human cancers restored old categories and areas of inquiry to the cancer investigative nexus. Questions, apparently settled, reemerged as crucial possibilities. Social statistics, long dismissed by laboratory researchers as unreliable—the German cancer effort, controlled by the insurance industry and its actuary tables, had remained the exception—regained center stage. Demographic, cultural, and other discriminations revealed the particulars of human life as lived and as practiced. In rapid succession, physicians using sophisticated and (more commonly) rudimentary statistics reported on cancer rates among the "primitive" tribes of Africa, persons of Iberian descent, and African Americans. They compared cancer rates in Paris with the rest of France, correlated age of domicile with incidence of cancer in Amsterdam, contrasted cancer rates among Norwegian inmates in prisons, workhouses, and leper asylums, and noted elevated occurrences of cancer of the cheek among the betel nut chewing population of the Philippines. Statistical medical men also detected higher incidence of cancer in places suffering elevated rates of tuberculosis, influenza, and diabetes and attempted to identify the loci of cancer tumors with other external factors.

Nor was that all. Medical men provided numerical "proof" that there were cancer families, houses, and neighborhoods. They compared cancer rates near riverbeds with those in hills. They noted low cancer numbers in areas near limestone formations and the opposite in tree-lined properties. William B. Coley capsulated this new approach. "Laboratory studies alone," he maintained, "can never solve this great problem of the cause of cancer." Its attack must come "from all sides—the clinical as well as the laboratory."[10]

In the course of these numeric and statistical discriminations, physicians sometimes noticed correlations between occupations and cancer rates. The possibilities of such a relationship was not new. More than a century earlier, Percivall Potts noticed that chimney sweeps suffered from scrotal cancer in unexpectedly high numbers. But while he argued that soot and cancer of the scrotum were related in chimney sweeps, he did not explore that relationship, especially why it struck only some sweeps.[11]

The discovery of an epidemic of ulcerations of the skin and other significant growths among coal-derived pitch industries was different. As part of the British social welfare state of the early twentieth century, around 1910, the Home Office set out to regulate those industries to reduce cancer risks. In a very Potts-like way, the initial proposal set about to reduce not exposure but irritation. The Home Office planned to mandate showers near these works so that laborers could wash off the noxious material before it caused irritation, which was closely associated with ulcerations and, ultimately, cancer production. Two distinct pitch-related processes garnered attention.

The first, gasworks pitch, was the residue left when coal was heated in a deficit atmosphere to generate coal gas for lighting. The second, blast furnace pitch, resulted when coal was heated to drive out impurities—a temperature significantly lower than with coal gas production—and create coke briquettes. These briquettes proved much less friable than coal and provided temperatures necessary to fuel the blast furnace–based steel industry.

Physicians used their observational skills to detail a relationship between gasworks pitch and what was even then sometimes called precancerous skin disruptions. They also noticed that contact with blast furnace pitch seemed to yield far fewer skin anomalies. Before the Home Office issued any permanent regulation, a laboratory researcher intervened. Hugh Campbell Ross was the brother of Sir Ronald Ross, the 1902 Nobel Laureate in medicine for his malaria work and vice-president of the Royal Society of Medicine. In 1908, Hugh Ross served as director of special cancer research at the University of Liverpool-Royal Southern Hospital, a new facility joining laboratory with hospital investigation. Looking at cell division for clues to cancer's mechanism, he detected a chemical substance that functioned as "an excitor of reproduction for human lymphocytes" and hypothesized that a "similar substance [might be] associated with cancer."[12]

A relationship between chemical substances and that disease's rapid, unchecked cellular division became the subject of his book *Induced Cell-Reproduction and Cancer* in 1910. He identified a class of chemical accelerators, including some found in cancerous tumors, that drastically altered the speed of mitosis and argued that they accounted for cancer's unrestrained growth. Ross's conclusions alarmed the professors of botany, zoology, biochemistry, and physiology at the University of Liverpool, who deemed them speculative, wrote broadsides separating themselves from the work, and claimed that Ross had used their good name to push his unorthodox view. Their objection was clear. Ross posited an external regulator to mitosis, which in good Virchowian terms was known to be guided within the cell by the nucleus. Included among these skeptics was C. S. Sherrington, who would serve as president of the Royal Society. Ross's brother, Ronald, countered the assessment of these naysayers by publishing under his name a synopses of his brother's work in the *Proceedings of the Royal Medical Society* and in *Nature*.[13]

Hugh Ross followed up these investigations with a more nuanced, more strident book, *Further Researches into Induced Cell-Reproduction and Cancer*. Ronald wrote the introduction, a diatribe against Hugh's detractors. In effect, Ronald used his scientific reputation to certify his brother's work. The reviewer in the *Bulletin of the Johns Hopkins Hospital* was offended by

Ronald's adoption of this antiquated reputational approach and demanded that Ross's work be subjected to close scientific scrutiny and laboratory examination to pass muster. H. T. K. in the *American Journal of Medical Sciences* was more adamant. He claimed that Ross's revised work exhibited "the same deficiency in detailed report of individual experiments, the same general type of illy founded conclusions, the same disregard of other work in physical biology, and the same diffuse pedantic style of presentation" as his earlier work. Ronald's rebuttal came soon after. He dismissed Hugh's critics as unscientific, as locked in "a priori objections." They refused to give his experiments the attention they demanded. This was similar, Ronald remarked, to the treatment received by Galileo. The famous astronomer's critics "denied the possibility of Jupiter having satellites, but . . . refused to look at them through Galileo's telescope."[14]

While controversy swirled around Hugh Ross's research, its particulars were straightforward. He argued that two classes of compounds controlled cell reproduction. Auxetics caused accelerated mitosis, and augmentors enhanced the action of the auxetics. Auxetics generally were "extracts of organs," but augmentors—the "propellants" and "proliferants"—were more complicated. They could be "produced in the body by injury" but more generally were unleashed by a force external to the being. Put baldly, Ross argued that mitosis was not something entirely indigenous to and regulated by the cell but, rather, something very much external to that unit.

Ross thus outlined a theory of cell division that immediately had implications for the mechanisms of cancer causation. Injury or external factors caused organs and other body cells to produce auxetics and augmentors, which resulted in cancer, or auxetics and augmentors were introduced from the outside and set off the whole process. He had this mechanistic theory in mind when he turned his attention to the pitch question. He first took gasworks pitch, mixed it in an agar medium, and placed drops of blood in the plate. After ten minutes he noticed rapid lymphocyte cell division. Subsequent experiments showed him that gasworks pitch contained a potent auxetic and an equally active augmentor.

He then replicated his experiments with blast furnace pitch. He found that cell division in his cultures occurred at a normal rate. His microanalysis of the pitch constituents revealed a weak auxetic but no augmentor; blast furnace pitch did not cause rapid, uncontrolled cell division, a chemical explanation for what physicians had noted empirically. He then broadened his experiments to test soot and other industrial chemicals and found them to contain both auxetics and augmentors, though not nearly in the quantities of gasworks pitch. To Ross, his experiments showing that gas pitch was especially virulent, while blast furnace pitch seemed almost completely benign, provided "strong evidence that the chemical agents which cause augmented cell division of lymphocytes" were critical to "the causation of cancer."

Ross undertook a final experiment. He wanted to see if he could extract the auxetics and augmentors from his gasworks pitch and render it safe. This he felt would be of "great value to cancer research." New regulations undercut this proposed research protocol, however. The Home Office had issued a regulation that would require all persons coming in contact with gasworks pitch to shower at the end of each shift to wash away any of the material that touched their skin.[15]

Ross's cancer theory did not go unchallenged. Two major objections were raised. First, researchers questioned Ross's live cultures and what could be discerned from them. Ross acknowledged difficulties in keeping his cultures viable for a period greater than ten minutes, the minimum time he deemed necessary to run his human lymphocyte experiment. When he placed his specimens under the microscope to deduce rates of cellular growth, the cells appeared so mangled that his critics thought them unidentifiable, certainly unverifiable. Second, his mechanistic chemical mitosis seemed to violate much of what was known about the process of cell division. It reduced the process to a chemistry-based stimulus response phenomenon, akin to amoebal action.

These sorts of objections caused Ross to take his leave of the Liverpool consortium and to find a new home as the director of research at the John Howard McFadden Researches, an England-based endeavor of a Philadelphia philanthropist. There, he expanded his inquiries, finding that "arsenic, manure, betel nut, tobacco and its smoke, 'khangri' charcoal, some aniline dyes, and petroleum . . . contain auxetic or augmentor" agents. These external agents held chemical substances that, when in contact with some susceptible site, resulted in rapid cellular division. These "commodities themselves do not actually cause cancer; they merely render the tissues prone to it, which seems to occur in a specific manner," Ross argued. He then outlined the process. "The commodities always in the first instance produce cell-proliferation usually in the nature of warty growth; and it is not until an open ulcer has appeared, generally at the base of the wart, that malignancy supervenes." Cancer, he concluded, was "a combination of two causes," a "predisposing cause" and "an exciting cause." Ross concluded that even x-rays and radium operated to predispose individuals to cancer. They caused "cell-death, even amounting to ulceration, which in turn sets free auxetics resulting in cell-proliferation, which is prone to become malignant."[16]

Ross's auxetics and augmentors continued to be quite controversial. But while investigators debated his chemical cell division mechanism, many did begin to examine the possible role in cancer of various substances outside the cell. Recognition that chemicals played a fundamental part in many biological processes led to examinations of these chemicals as part of the cancer process. To be sure, laboratory chemists had devoted some time to analyzing the chemistry of malignant growths. They had compared cancerous tumors to normal tissue, identified their constituents, measured by-products, including those that lysed healthy cells, applied toxins in an attempt to debilitate them, and suggested the composition of serums to neutralize their chemical manifestations.[17]

This research changed dramatically in the era of nutrition. The investigations of Thomas Osborne and Lafayette Mendel at Yale and of Casimir Funk, then at the Lister Institute for Preventive Medicine (the facility that superintended Ross and the McFadden Researches), opened a new chemically based cancer research vista. Rather than focus of the simple results of combustion, decomposition, and excretion to mark the gross chemical composition of a successful diet, these researchers and others identified significant differences in the types of chemical compounds and trace materials needed to produce growth and maintenance.[18]

To persons interested in the cancer question, possibilities quickly emerged. In the largest sense, growth was reduced to chemical combinations and diet was the gateway. Variations in diet caused variations in growth of normal cells. How susceptible might be cells that proliferated dramatically and without apparent direction? Might regulating the growth of an individual also regulate the growth of runaway cells? Were there particular food constituents—chemicals—that produced or supported rapid, persistent growth? These questions were quite different from the speculations surrounding trout and human cancer of a few years earlier. In those investigations, trout was considered either the source of a poison or an infection that caused cancer; the fish's chemical constituents and how they affected growth was never the issue.

The noted British physician Alexander Haig was among the first to propose that certain chemicals be eliminated from the human diet to battle cancer. Haig produced a uric acid–free diet, heavy in fruits and vegetables, to stop the scourge. Research of this sort proved tricky for medical practitioners. Some attempted to compare two groups of people with different diets; vegetarians versus meat eaters gained favor. But beyond that simple dichotomy, things became very murky. Convincing healthy persons to remove chemical substances from their diet was difficult. Research protocols necessarily dealt only with cancer patients. But it would have been unethical, perhaps even unconscionable, to experiment on patients immediately after the onset of disease. Surgery was the best—only—option for cure. Immediate action mattered. It could not be withheld.[19]

The only human research subjects remaining were patients after failed operations and inoperable cases. That cohort of terminal cases posed its own limitations. Experimenting with persons near death skewed what could be learned through varying diets, adding some nutrients and reducing others. Working with experimental cancer offered more possibilities. Mice and other laboratory animals could be sacrificed without recrimination, except among the antivivisectionists. Yet even experimental cancer possessed restrictions. Cancer induced in laboratory animals might be subject to different laws from spontaneous human cancer. Experimental cancer had its own peculiar constituency. It was the province of trained laboratory investigators, not medical practitioners.

Researchers examining diet in cancer often referred to metabolic change. They wondered if a change in metabolism—by metabolism they usually meant rate of growth—would cause cancer to slow down, speed up, or even perish. Metabolic cancer researchers stood as distinct from those investigators willing to remove single nutrients required for growth from experimental rations. This latter group explored whether the absence of a single nutrient could spell cancer's death. Diet might kill cancer.

Peyton Rous was among those interested in exploring metabolism to conquer cancer. He justified this avenue of exploration by referring to the essentials of basic human physiology. Wounds healed more slowly in under- and malnourished people. Bedside observation had shown that cancer's course seemed to slow in old, sickly people. But Rous was also aware of the uniquenesses of experimental cancer. To that end, he aimed to establish a research protocol that crossed several types of tumor nexuses. Rather than work with just one cancer, such as that standardized in the Jensen mouse, Rous ran his experiments with both mice and rats, used several different tumor strains, and employed several breeds of each animal. As important, he made sure that his tumors were well established. He wanted his tests to determine not if severely restricted diets would prevent or terminate transplantation among laboratory animals, but rather what the course of the disease would be when commencing a diet well after external tumors were integrated in the hosts. Rous chose to measure several states: metastases, occurrence of subsequent spontaneous tumors, metastases of these spontaneous tumors, gradual reduction of diets, and radical immediate restriction of diets.

Rous established this broad, diverse research agenda because of earlier reported research results. Investigators had noted considerable success limiting tumor growth through guiding metabolic change. Rous found that point of view not sustainable when his wider lens was employed. He claimed that, in his experiments, results "varied from series to series of animals;" when carried to their natural termination, his experiments precluded any universal definitive statement. Yet his study did offer one solid conclusion. He pronounced "strongly . . . that generalizations from work with transplanted tumors as regards the effect of diet on spontaneous growths are unwarranted." Previous researchers' claims of success proved false once Rous expanded the frame of reference. A slowing of growth was initially seen when diet was restricted among some animals with transplanted tumors. However, those growths often resumed or exceeded their previous healthy growth rates once the animals became acclimated to the new diets. Spontaneous tumors operated otherwise. They showed little if any change when diet was reduced, drastically or otherwise. Metastatic rates also were undiminished.[20]

Rous published a more limited study a short while later, this time working with spontaneous cancer in mice. But this cancer too was not truly spontaneous. Rous used a strain of mice known to develop adenocarcinomas of the breast at about thirty-five days. He divided his tumorous mice into two groups, fed one a normal ration and the other a ration barely adequate to sustain life. For both groups, he took each mouse's primary cancer, cut two incisions, and transplanted parts of the tumor. He waited another thirty-five days to see the results of the transfers. Of the fully fed mice, 68 percent took the graft and sprouted tumors. Only 41 percent of the surviving underfed mice developed similar growths.

Rous quickly noted what he measured. He measured only what percentage of mice took transplants within the "normal" thirty-five days. Persistence of the experiment beyond that date showed that the diminished diet mice caught up to the others. There was virtually no long-term difference among the two groups.

Rous's experiments did little to suggest how reduction of diet might work to battle cancer, but they did deepen suspicion of the applicability of experimental cancer treatments when dealing with human tumors. In fact, Ewing maintained as part of the discussion of Rous's paper that human cancers behaved differently. "There is a sanitarium in this state where cancer is treated with remarkable results, chiefly by starvation," he contended. This approach to human cancer constituted nothing less than "a new field into modern cancer research."[21] In a very real sense, Rous's experimental results begged the question of just how useful animal testing was when it came to the human disease. They also pointed to the long-standing difficulty in designing an experiment that would prove definitive. A conclusive protocol might require investigators to create situations to account for things that they did not yet know, as a means to rule some of those things out.

Such was perilous work. Rous's apparent success depended on contrasts among several different states. Work with specific dietary factors functioned just the opposite. Investigators eliminated or added one variable—or thought they were changing a single variable—in hopes of learning if cancer growth would be encumbered or enhanced. The University of California's T. Brailsford Robertson was among those embracing the research. Operating out of a physiological laboratory endowed by the family of a sugar magnate, Robertson wanted to test the impact of cholesterol on tumor growth. Robertson knew this would be a problem. He recognized that the body transformed other substances into cholesterol, that even if he fed his rats a totally cholesterol-free diet, the animal would manufacture the substance. To overcome this obstacle and to see expressly cholesterol's affect on cancer, he chose to inject tumors from two unrelated rat populations with significant quantities of the substance. In every instance, he found that the tumor grew rapaciously. Cholesterol speeded cancer's growth. Robertson also found yet another result: cholesterol apparently increased the likelihood and number of metastatic sites developing from the primary tumor.[22]

Injecting material directly into tumors hardly resembled a feeding experiment or anything that humans normally did. Silas Palmer Beebe and Elizabeth Van Alstyne, two chemistry specialists at Cornell's Loomis/Huntington laboratory, sought to explore the popular notion that the "dietetic habits of a group of people" bore "some relation" to the number of cancer cases that will develop and would have "some influence upon the character and progress of the disease." The nutrient they chose to restrict was carbohydrate, and the investigators focused on the transplantation of tumors. Starting with tumor-laden rats from Gaylord's laboratory, they found that these cancers, when transplanted, both established themselves in their new animals and grew at a similar rate under both carbohydrate-loaded and carbohydrate-free diets. But they also found that initial transplants were far less successful in animals long fed carbohydrate-free diets. This was an exciting discovery. Yet the investigators were quite circumspect about what these experimental cancer-based researches meant for human cancer. "It cannot be said," they reported, that these experiments indicated "that tumor incidence is higher in . . . people eating rich, carbohydrate diet than on a flesh diet." It could "be maintained, however, that susceptibility and immunity to tumor implantation are not entirely independent of the diet."[23]

The two Cornell investigators followed that study up with another, this time focusing on butter fat. Noting that Osborne and Mendel had shown that butter fat speeded normal growth, the two cancer researchers found that tumors grew at a remarkably accelerated rate when butter was a large component of the rat's diet. Growth was so pronounced that some tumors weighed twice the normal weight of the animal. From that experiment, they argued that a "diet favorable to the growth of animal tissue is also favorable to the growth of tumor tissue." They also weighed in on another issue. Since they determined that growth and diet were intimately related, they found it "difficult to reconcile such observations with the theory that these tumors have an infectious origin." Ability to manipulation growth in living things through diet had, to Beebe and Van Alstyne, suggested that unchecked growth also originated within beings. Yet in the end, caution overtook exuberance. Their paper ended with a reminder to their professional colleagues that all their efforts were "based on experiments with the Buffalo sarcoma." They remained "unprepared to say what results may be obtained with other types of tumors."[24]

Funk undertook a far more extensive agenda and was less circumspect. A pioneer in this new nutritional model, Funk tried diet to answer many questions. He even attempted to determine if diet could account for Ehrlich's "x" factor, his explanation of why trans-species tumor transplantation always failed. Funk's solution was simple but grisly. He ground up the parts of mice that were the loci of the original mouse tumor, fed that material to rats, and then grafted on the mouse tumor. He claimed modest success for this technique; he was able to pass the tumor through five generations and to keep it alive for over five weeks.[25]

These numbers were unprecedented in interspecies tumor transfer. Yet it remained unclear exactly what they implied. Did it mean that eating beef containing cancerous cow tumors, for instance, would help establish an environment for an indigenous cow tumor to be grown on another species? If that were so, what did that indicate about the human food supply and what might transpire from a beef eater's casual contact with animals suffering cancer? Were ranchers and farmers inherently in danger? What about Gaylord's tumorous trout? Did fishermen and fisherwomen have reason to be concerned? And what of Smith's plant cancer? Were gardeners in mortal danger?

Funk was especially taken with Rous's discovery that chicken sarcoma could be "propagated by cell-free filtrates," because it more nearly approximated the behavior of cancer in humans. In experimentally produced rat and mouse cancer, tumors rarely metastasized and were generally encapsulated. To our mind, both were a consequence of the nature of transplantation, the establishing of a foreign body in another member of the species. Chicken sarcoma was different. The action of "tumors of fowls seem to resemble human rather than any other experimental tumors."

The metastasis and encapsulation issues ruled out rats and mice as appropriate experimental animals. But that was not Funk's sole consideration. He set his cancer research agenda as determining "the composition of the diet and particularly the influence of vitamins" on tumors. More to the point, he demanded that his results must "be transferred to other animals and to humans." What had to happen "inescapably" was to identify for experiment an animal "in which the lack of vitamins yields a pathology similar to that in humans."

Funk chose young chickens for his work. He received from Rous a healthy amount of a strain of chicken sarcoma filtrate from which to experiment. Funk inoculated his chickens and placed them on several different vitamin-deficient diets. He had difficulty keeping his birds alive long enough to measure the impact of his nutritional changes but found that tumors and chickens with certain deficiency diets grew much more slowly than his controls. To his surprise, he found that using polished or unpolished rice—the key determinant in beriberi and its remediation—did not alter tumor growth.

Stepping back from his research, Funk hypothesized that a cancer cell, like a healthy cell, depended on chemical substances—vitamins—in the diet to achieve proper growth. He recognized, however, that cancer cells were not normal; they did not grow naturally in every being. He felt cancer needed an external chemical factor to fuel its breakaway development. There must be another as yet unidentified growth factor—an auxiliary factor—that contributed to tumor growth. Funk suggested that that factor was ingested and then modified in chickens to spark tumor development. He reached this conclusion after undertaking another series of experiments. He removed the pituitary gland from some of his cancer-suffering animals. Chickens with this gland and their tumors grew swiftly. Without this gland, chickens were not able to use the unidentified nutrient and showed only stilted growth.[26]

Funk deduced the pituitary gland or another of the ductless glands produced the modifying substance that spurred cancer to develop. He was not alone. Hormones, the ductless glands, and other similar excretions and secretions increasingly became implicated in cancer. Robertson, for example, seconded Funk's assessment that the pituitary gland held a central cancer-producing role. He noted the gland's role in acromegaly and gigantism and examined whether chemical substances produced there acted as a growth propellant. The way he investigated this phenomenon proved quite unusual. He took ox pituitary glands, ground them up, and injected the material directly into the tumors of rats. What he found was perplexing. The injected tumors grew at twice the rate, but those tumors did not metastasize at the rate of normal tumors. Indeed, at the end of his thirty-seven-day experiment, the injected tumors showed no metastases.

Robertson then theorized that the ox tissue, rather than its pituitary chemicals, might have caused the accelerated growth. To rule that out, he concocted an ox-derived liver emulsion to measure against the pituitary complement. No acceleration occurred.[27]

The work of Robertson and Funk stood as examples of a new cancer philosophy. Cancer had gotten much more complicated. No longer simply the product of a microbe or a latent condition, cancer now seemed the consequence of at least a two-pronged situation. There was regularly an auxiliary cause and an necessary cause. Put slightly differently, a cancer agent was necessary but usually not sufficient to produce the disease. Something else had to pave the way for that agent to act. To many investigators, that something was thought to be chemical. And those chemicals were the product of the endocrine or other glands.

This new research beachhead attracted many adherents, especially those conversant with chemistry and biochemistry. With emphasis on body chemistry and diet, chemists and biochemists assumed new organizational vitality within cancer laboratories. Working at the physiological laboratory of Philadelphia's American Oncologic Hospital, J. E. Sweet headed a team that sought to determine if castration would increase cancer transplants into mice. As his marker of what constituted the epitome of success and specificity, Sweet used Rous's inoculation work with the Plymouth Rock hen, which gave virtually 100 percent positives. Sweet acknowledged that he chose the testes because of work showing an intimate relationship between them and the other ductless glands. He understood the thyroid in terms of growth, as he did the pituitary.

It was this last criterion, that of growth promotant, that appeared most compelling. Tuberculosis provided the model. There, Sweet contended the "best treatment" was "not directed primarily against the disease process," even though investigators had known the tuberculosis-causing microbe for over thirty years. Most effective therapy was "directed towards the stimulation of the normal protective functions of the body," and he expected that cancer would necessarily follow that pattern.

Sweet found that castration significantly increased transplantation among mice, and that the testes produced a substance that inhibited cancer transfers.[28] His conclusion stood in direct contrast to those issued by the Columbia University Cancer Laboratory and funded by Crocker money even before the facility opened. This research constituted the first broad-based investigation of the impact of the ductless glands on cancer. G. L. Rohdenburg, F. D. Bullock, and P. J. Johnston surveyed the various isolated studies to see how previous investigators identified the effect of a secretion from a single gland on tumor growth. The Columbia researchers quickly dismissed that piecemeal approach and adopted a comprehensive perspective. They started with 190 rats, put aside a small group as controls, cut out one or more glands in some, and injected extracts into others, in the hope of developing a complete portrait. They even injected several hormones into human patients to compare to the animal tests.

Their conclusions were provocative. While they acknowledged that 190 rats hardly constituted a definitive study, they nonetheless argued that removal of the thyroid, thymus, and testes, either collectively or individually, decreased susceptibility to cancer in those breeds usually vulnerable to the disease. Conversely, they concluded that removal of the same glands in immune animals significantly enhanced their ability to develop the disease. Injecting these animals with extracts of "thymus, spleen, pancreas, pituitary, and testes" created a chemically restored immunity. Results showed, the Columbia researchers maintained, that many of these tissues "contain some common element, possibly . . . a hormone, which is capable of producing immunity."[29]

Rohdenburg and the others, fortified by Calkins, who had long worked in Gaylord's lab, took a new approach the following year. They took their chemical cancer explanation far beyond the ductless glands to construct a model for cancer consonant with the new dualistic consideration and their biochemical musing. First, they demonstrated that any number of naturally occurring biological chemicals could radically affect the rate of mitosis in a series of organisms from protozoa to rats. They rushed to publish their work even as their research had "not produced a tumor—we should like to say that we have not yet produced a tumor"—because it was so suggestive. "By known means," the researchers created "characteristic changes in normal tissues which might well represent, and which may yet turn out to be, precancerous conditions."

Such a profound claim encouraged them to consider the philosophical implications of their experiments. They wanted to "emphasize the difference between the genesis of cancer and its continued growth." To that end, the group ran through all the conventional explanations for cancer genesis, finding each flawed in some way. "What induces the unusual division of apparently normal cells," the Columbia contingent asked, and they stood ready with an answer. It was "a result of abnormal, local, metabolic conditions, brought about by injury, by chronic irritation, by parasites, or by other causes." Quite simply, they did not know what caused cancer, but they did know that cancerous tumor formation was a two-step process. The critical formative moment was creation by one or more of the methods listed above of the "products of autolysis . . . which stimulate the division energy of latent cells." The organism's regulatory processes—substances secreted by the ductless and other glands, tissues, and organs—usually maintained the status quo, "but with continued irritation the division energy outruns the regulation of the organism and a tumor results." Tumor growth was accomplished "through the activity of the cumulative products of cell autolysis." In that way, "the degeneration of cancer cells . . . produce the stimulating agents for further and more widespread development."[30]

In this scheme, autolysis, the product of some abnormal stimulus, unleashed chemicals—promotants—that caused what had been healthy cells to run amuck. These chemicals overwhelmed the body's natural regulatory mechanisms, which caused more cells to lyse. The lysing released more propellant substances and cancer ensued. Several German investigators offered a different role for autolysates. They found that these chemicals, when collected and injected directly into the tumor, lysed the tumor itself. Rather than promote tumor growth, autolysate chemical substances performed as they always had, as the chemical mechanism governing cell destruction. These substances were thought of as either idiopathic or useful for a specific cancerous tumor type. Ferdinand Blumenthal, who followed Klemperer as the director of what was initially Leyden's cancer laboratory, was a passionate advocate of autolysates. A longtime member of Comite Für Krebsforschung, and editor of *Zeitschrift für Krebsforschung*, Blumenthal claimed that "nothing in his experience to date proved so effectual" against the disease. Autolysates derived from an individual mouse's cancer "melted away" a duck-egged sized tumor "after a single subcutaneous injection." Blumenthal's manner of autolysate preparation began with the tumor itself. He cut up the mass, ground it in a mortar, and combined the ground substance with water and chloroform. More chloroform was added to the emulsion, which was then put in a stoppered bottle. The bottle was placed in an incubator at 39 degrees for three full days. The supernatant fluid was then decanted and injected near tumors.

Blumenthal found a 35 percent cure rate, with over 80 percent of his cases significantly improved.[31] Hans Lunckenbein, a prominent German gynecologist and cancer researcher, carried the chemical case a step further. He argued that cancer functioned as if it had an independent existence from the being it inhabited. It produced its own ferments—chemicals—which lysed the proteins of the host cells to fuel its growth. The host, in turn, defended itself through production of special chemicals that attacked the tumor cell proteins. Since the malignant cells were essentially foreign, the defensive ferments did not decompose host tissue. This destructive war continued until a spontaneous recovery or death of the host occurred.

Lunckenbein proposed to move the equilibrium point of this epic battle. He sought to manipulate cancer cells in such a way as to stimulate the host's manufacture of the precise tumor-proteid lysing chemical fermenting agents. Like Blumenthal, Lunckenbein started with the tumor. He pulverized it, put it in a sterile salt solution, and let it stand for three days. It was then filtered and heated for one hour at 36 degrees centigrade to ensure that all cancer cells that might have passed through the filter were killed and only the proteinaceous chemicals remained. This material was then given intravenously to the host, whereby new specific defensive ferments would be unleashed and the tumor devoured.[32]

An Italian investigator, Gaetano Fichera, proposed an observation-based, chemical-dependent theory. Holder of the surgical pathology chair at the University of Cagliari, Fichera noted that cancer was almost unknown in fetuses and the very young. Operating from a chemical framework and in a way reminiscent of Beard, he supposed that the paucity of cancer cases among these groups stemmed from a chemical suppressant that naturally existed in fetal and infant tissue. These "substances, which are generated by the special tissues during the process of autolysis," then "when injected into the organism act on tumors" to dissolve them.

Fetuses were rich in this tumor suppressant, which apparently diminished as the being developed. Fichera chose not to confront the experimental vs. natural cancer issue and went directly to human patients. Each of his thirty-six cancerous subjects was deemed inoperable. All received Fichera's special concoction. The Italian pathologist took parts of fetuses, mixed them with a sterile salt solution, and added thymol or phenol. He covered the preparation with a sterilized layer of toluene and placed the preparation in an incubator set at 37 degrees centigrade for two months. That final step was necessary to ensure that the autolysates fully developed and were freed from the cells that had produced/contained them.

Only then was the material ready for testing. Fichera reported that fourteen of his patients quickly discontinued treatment "for various personal reasons" and four more had just begun the fetal autolytic process at the time of publication. That left him with a group of eighteen with "malignant tumours, varying in substance and position." Several even had "multiple and voluminous metastases." Of this cohort, eight found "no marked benefit" from his fetal autolytic substance. In half of the remaining ten cases, "the neoplastic tissues have completely disappeared." The other five showed significant and continual improvement. Fichera noted that, after the products of fetal autolysis decomposed the tumors, phagocytes swarmed to clean up the detritus.

Fichera argued that his experimental results confirmed his fetal autolysate hypothesis and constituted nothing more than good laboratory science. He had merely brought into focus a "physio-pathological phenomena, explicable by general laws." He was especially proud that his work held an "analogy of the structural characters . . . with those noted by various authors." Orth's work on spontaneous involution of tumors in humans received direct mention. Perhaps the leading pathologist of his day, Orth held Virchow's chair in Berlin. Claiming one's research paralleled Orth's investigations enhanced credibility, the initial measure on the road to certainty for his theory of "the direct and elective action of the autolysates" against cancer. Fichera added another stipulation to his theory. Physicians employing his cure should not worry about introducing an autolytic dosage so strong that it would dissolve the tumor too quickly and unleash poisons so fast that they would kill the human host. His reasoning was clear. The fetal autolysates, which were harmless to normal healthy cells, would neutralize the cancerous cells and their chemical substances before they could prove toxic beyond the point of confrontation. "This single set of active principles" acted, according to Fichera, "successfully in different ways" depending on "whether they had to deal with normal cellular elements or neoplastic elements."

Fichera concluded his paper by acknowledging that he rushed into print because he found his results so compelling. Even as he did so, he took care to acknowledge that his work could not pass muster as "a statistical comparison." Such a study required "numerous cases" and a far more rigorous consideration if indeed "the last neoplastic cells had been destroyed" by fetal autolysates.[33]

Fichera's introspective, scientifically valid statement did not immunize him or any of the other autolysate research from professional criticism. Rohdenburg and his associates jumped on failure of the sort pinpointed in Fichera's apologia to decry the entire notion of autolytic products influencing tumor growth. They recognized that each of these diverse theories was bound together in one particular regard; all relied on intracellular enzymes or chemical products for explanation. The Columbia contingent designed experiments to test these specific suppositions. They identified thirty-three different, researcher-proposed chemical products of autolysis that reputedly lysed cancer. Lots of ten mice, as well as controls, were established and each lot member was implanted within a specific fast growing, invasive tumor that Columbia had developed. They gave each lot a different hypothetical autolytic chemical. The investigators dispensed these chemical interventions in a standardized dosage size, at a standard frequency, and for a standard period of time.

At intervals of ten, seventeen, and twenty-four days, a specific number of the animals from each lot were slaughtered and compared to the controls. In thirty-one lots, "none of the various groups showed any variation from the normal course of growth." Microscopic examinations confirmed initial assessments. The two remaining groups showed a slight ability to retard cancer growth. Rohdenburg quadrupled the lot size in these two instances and ran the experiments again. This time "the supposed retarding influence disappeared." "Use of larger numbers" of animals had demonstrated "again the fallacy of regarding slight variations in small numbers of animals as of any importance."

The Columbia investigators pleaded with their research colleagues to know what results they were reporting and to know if they were meaningful. "Minor variations, or even differences of 10 or 20 per cent, in small groups of treated animals" are likely inconsequential. They are almost certainly "due to accidental and uncontrollable variation in the growth of neoplasm." This kind of error "can be eliminated only by the employment of a much larger number of animals than are recorded in any of the published papers."

The group also claimed that several proponents of autolysates were ignorant about the basic knowledge of the tumor they used in their research. Its members cited one study that included the Buffalo rat sarcoma in its experimental design. That investigator reported substantial success in his experiments, unaware that that tumor "spontaneously recedes in from 5 to 40 per cent of all inoculated animals." In general, the Columbia experimenters warned that significant variations in tumor growth rates occurred even "in parallel series of animals from the same source and under exactly similar conditions of inoculation site, dose of tumor, food, and age of animals."

Their final statements were devastating. They posited that their fellow researchers either lacked "common knowledge" of animal biology or "blithely disregarded" such knowledge. They closed by noting that, while they based their study disproving the utility of autolysates only on animal experiments, they were confident that its conclusions held for human trials. In fact, dosing human cancer sufferers with autolysates "can be expected to produce nothing but the psychic exaltation common" to every new proposed cure.[34]

The Columbia group's criticism was unusual in its specificity and tone. It sought to eliminate what it deemed inadequate research. It was this research that set investigators and others carelessly down various primrose paths. Research built upon faulty premises was not just wrong but pernicious. It wasted effort and money, not only in its conduct but also in its falsification. It inhibited the quest for knowledge and cost lives.

The Columbia critique begged the entire question of research reportage. What constituted significance enough to merit professional announcement? In the case of publication, that decision tended to rest entirely on the investigator and the journal editor. They decided when a result needed to be offered for scrutiny to that periodical's readers. And scrutiny there was because professional journals and societies were venues in which researchers and others voiced their suggestions, criticisms and disagreements. Announcing one's experimental result was less an end than an invitation for comment from parties interested in the work and its possible implications.

Creation of specialized organizations of cancer researchers in country after country in the first decade of the century had done little to restrict the debate. Each of these specialty societies had hoped to be the primary body for vetting cancer research that had occurred in its country. They never gained that sway. Just as medical practitioners, repositories of observational experience, persisted in claiming a vital cancer research role, their periodicals and societies remained keenly interested in new research announcements and insights.

Public vehicles also avidly participated in this knowledge exchange. Patients—cancer sufferers—were the ultimate consumers of this information. They chose to seek remediation from a variety of sources—surgeons, doctors of various stripes and abilities, research institutions, and patent medicine vendors. In the United States, for instance, a tradition of yellow journalism—sensationalism—combined with the muckraking journalists of the early twentieth century elevated newspapers and the new ten-cent magazines to prominence; they served as locations from which various cancer claims and contentions were shared. In these publications, scrutiny of the scientific validity of any argument was further attenuated.

The entire question of research announcement ultimately resided in the making something so argument. Mechanisms to establish something as so proved ineffectual in doing just that. As a consequence, debate and dispute continued as they had been, as incredibly difficult to resolve.

The withering attack of Rohdenburg and his colleagues itself failed to meet the template it was passionately recommending. Put bluntly, this attack did not disprove what it maintained it was disproving. First, it used one species—mice—and then only one type of tumor that struck mice in a precise location. That tumor was especially invasive; it was not normal. Second, the researchers mounting the attack used the autolysates as if they were chemical products; they did not meander through the various different and often unique steps that each of their targets had undertaken to achieve their presumably biologically active substances. Third, they maintained in their mice precisely the same conditions of dosage, frequency, and duration for each of the supposed autolytic substance tests. That stood in marked contrast to the protocols of the protagonists.

None of the above was to suggest that Rodhenburg's critique was invalid. What it did demonstrate, however, was just how difficult it remained to make something so. Concentrating on chemical substances revealed by the emerging concepts of vitamins and the mechanisms of the endocrine glands, dealing with the repercussions and uncertainty of the Rous discovery, and complicating the matrix through which cancer emerged did not yield light, only more puzzlement and confusion. Older techniques were reintroduced into the cancer quest, and groups formerly marginalized reemerged as vital forces. Progress did not simply seem elusive. It increasingly started to look like a delusion.

9

Losing Control

An Inflamed Cancer Research Dilemma, 1911–1915

The cancer investigations into the chemistry of biological processes sought to identify the substances and equations at work in malignancies. Success would have enabled researchers to interrupt or intercept the disease or disease processes, thereby eliminating it as a menace. Embedded in some of these determinations was the notion that cancer development was a two-fold phenomenon. Cancer needed an auxiliary cause, something that prepared the site to accept cancer, and a necessary cause, a microbe or indigenous internal event. Both seemed essential for cancer to result. The duality of cancer causation embraced two separate types of approach. Investigators could seek the predisposing agents and incidents or the necessary casual mechanism.

Frustration and failure in the search for the cancer-producing culprit for thirty-five years had given pause. Almost nothing seemed final; few contentions went unchallenged. Positions among laboratory scientists had hardened, some set in stone. If "progress" was to be made, searching for the predisposing (auxiliary) causes appeared more immediately profitable. Just as necessary as the essential cause, predisposing conditions, situations, and substances lacked the vested interests that poisoned the microbe-organic debate. Investigations could be freer, more wide ranging, less restricted. The world, not the laboratory, was their oyster. Their investigations would have to rule out or implicate the panoply of activities that characterized life and living.

More diffuse explorations yielded more diffuse results. More diverse groups undertook these studies. Many of the researchers into cancer's predisposing events had a reverence for and dependence on numbers—statistics—that their laboratory counterparts lacked. Simple statistics could demonstrate differential rates of cancer production according to behavior. They could uncover variables from real life otherwise hidden from sight.

What they could not do was adjudicate the already contentious discussion about the merits of using experimental animals in cancer research. Was animal cancer the same as the disease in humanity? Put more precisely, did the rules and parameters of cancer in a specific animal or animals generally translate directly to humans? Nor did they come to bear on the equally heated debate on the validity of experimental cancer. Did cancer that was artificially produced hew to the same criteria or even the same sort of criteria as a case that was spontaneously produced?

Heightened emphasis on predisposition lessened the laboratory researchers' grip. Studying everyday human existence was outside their ken. Some modified portfolios to seek auxiliary causes, but in that endeavor they contended with others lacking their veneration of artificially constrained environments. Certainly laboratory men and women continued to weigh in on all matters related to cancer propagation. They did so with decreasing success. The entire quest for predisposition rejected artificiality. It targeted natural activities, the activities of life and living. Experiments conducted in laboratories provided correlations and analogies, but observations and measurements done outside were much richer and often more nuanced. And without the artificial exclusivity of the laboratory, researchers held few natural advantages in other investigative milieus.

○●

In 1913, Johannes Andreas Grib Fibiger published a study that would lead to the Nobel Prize some thirteen years later. Professor of pathological anatomy at the University of Copenhagen and president of the IACI in the year of his momentous publication, Fibiger's study complicated an already confused situation surrounding cancer's cause. It started simply enough. As part of an investigation into tuberculosis, Fibiger preformed autopsies on three rats that shared the same cage. Much to his surprise, he found that the stomachs of each of these animals were riddled with a thick tumorous mass so large that the stomachs were "almost obliterated." The rest of the alimentary tract showed no signs of malignancy, although a few suspicious patches appeared on the lungs.

Intrigued by these three virtually identical occurrences, Fibiger tried to inoculate other rats with the tumorous tissue. That failed to spark the disease in the inoculants. He ground up the tumor and fed it to other rats. That too did not produce growths. Fibiger then subjected the tumors themselves to microscopic analyses. He found that the epithelium was so disrupted and the cell growth so prolific that it broke through the stomach muscle and the tissue beneath the muscle. Closer examination showed that a series of cell-nests and cysts accompanied the disrupted tissue as it pierced the rat's fundus, the part of the stomach characterized by squamous cells. Fibiger then returned to an even finer analysis of the epithelium. There he found numerous oval holes and complex bodies, the latter characteristically associated with egg laying parasites.

What Fibiger did next was instructive. He mined these holes and sites for the debris within and then used these small pieces of residual tissue to reconstruct the kind of animal that made them. He identified his invader as a nematode, a roundworm. Three-quarters of an inch in length, the extremely thin parasite produced odd-shaped eggs containing coiled embryos. These eggs lay free between epithelial layers.

Fibiger set out to determine how frequently rats had similar tumors in their stomachs and how often their stomachs were invaded by nematodes. Each of these activities required minute microscopic analyses of rat stomachs. His initial autopsy results were negative, so he continued the process, sacrificing 1,144 rats in all. He found no instance of the peculiar tumors he saw in his first three rats, although he did detect among eleven animals some small ulcerative conditions. In twelve of the rats, a nematode had invaded the stomach muscle, and in ten more, a nematode was found free in the cavity. Further description demonstrated that the nematodes in the musculature were similar to the nematodes of trichinosis, and those in the stomach chamber were the type that produced roundworm infestation in humans and pigs. Neither resembled the nematodes of the three caged rats.

At that point Fibiger shifted his inquiry and decided to trace where the three caged rats were bred. Dorpat, in what is now Estonia, proved to be their place of origin, and Fibiger focused on "the life-cycle and habitats of the peculiar nematode" that had infested the cancerous rats. He examined Osman Galeb's 1879 doctoral dissertation at the University of Paris and learned that rats in Europe regularly consumed a particular species of cockroach. These cockroaches bore a filarial, a kind of nematode. Fibiger than contracted for a shipment of wild rats from Estonia and proceeded to dissect them and examine their stomachs. He found cockroaches but no cancer. Feeding live cockroaches to the Estonia rats also failed to produce the disease.

A subsequent shipment of Estonian rats, this time from a sugar refinery, presented a different portrait. Of the sixty-one rats examined, twenty were entirely normal with no parasites. But the other forty showed nematodes identical to the ones in the three caged animals. Eighteen of the forty showed cancerous and precancerous changes in the stomach. Nine exhibited very advanced tumors consistent with the initial group.

Examination of the nematodes in these diseased animals proved identical to those in the original rats. But the cockroaches were a different species from the species mentioned by Galeb. They were a cockroach not usually found in Europe but indigenous to North America. Fibiger hypothesized that the refinery cockroaches had come initially from the West Indies as an unanticipated traveler in the sugar trade. Fibiger incorporated this information into his next experiment. He took fifty-seven indigenous Danish rats and fed them cockroaches caught at the Estonian sugar refinery for from five to twenty days. All were allowed to succumb naturally. On necropsy, Fibiger found three with neither nematodes nor tumors. The other fifty-four had nematodes, and thirty-six of these had cancerous or profound cancerous changes in their stomachs. The nematodes were identical to the nematodes reconstructed from the original caged rats, complete with eggs and coiled embryos.

Fibiger concluded that "no doubt" existed "that the tumor formations were dependent on a particular nematode carried by" a particular species of cockroach. But he did not end the investigation there. He took the eggs excreted by the infected rats, fed them to or inoculated healthy rats. In neither case was the disease produced. He then undertook a detailed microscopic examination of the cockroaches themselves. He found no parasites in any part of the alimentary canal, but in many of the striated muscles of the animals, Fibiger detected encapsulated nematode embryos. To ensure that some other parasite ought not to be implicated in the cancer-nematode-cockroach-rat continuum, Fibiger took those cockroaches in which the nematode linked to rat cancer did not naturally occur and fed them eggs found in the susceptible cockroach species. Microscopic examination showed that these nematodes developed in the appropriate muscles just as they did in the sugar refinery variety. Fibiger then fed the newly infected roaches to Danish rats. Nearly half developed the characteristic lesions and produced eggs in their feces. He then performed a final experiment. He took the variety of cockroach found in the refinery, made sure it was nematode free and then fed it to Danish lab rats. None of those animals developed cancer.[1]

Fibiger worked out the life history of his nematode and the cancer-producing pathological changes that he claimed they caused. He had accomplished two noteworthy things. He had joined a specific agent—a parasite—in a specific locality to a specific tumor, the very definition of causality among his scientific peers. Even more impressive was that he experimentally created the disease in the laboratory. These signal events met the challenge of Koch's postulates. He found a causal agent, isolated it, grew it, inserted it to again cause the disease, and ultimately isolated it again.

Fibiger's impressive exposition of the worm-insect, vector-cancer nexus made the study almost impossible to ignore.[2] Yet it provided more smoke than light. To many investigators, application of Fibiger's work to the human condition was obvious. An historical context emerged for Fibiger's study. Amédée Borrel's early century research at the Pasteur Institute was resurrected. He had found nematodes associated with cancer in mice and used the proximity of the worms to the tumors in these animals to account for "the frequency of tumours of the digestive tract" in humans. Nematode infestation had been hypothesized by Borrel to explain "why cancer is common in damp countries, in places where manure heaps are badly kept close to human habitations, and in places where irrigation of sewerage is carried on."[3]

Knud Magnus Haaland, who worked with Borrel, Ehrlich, and finally Bashford, had offered a more measured perspective. His 1911 Imperial Cancer Research Fund study was published in the *Proceedings of the Royal Society*. The Norwegian confronted what he called spontaneous cancer—as distinct from experimental cancer—in laboratory mice. In each instance of these 288 cases, he tried to determine what preceded the disease. He noted, for instance, that old age was closely linked to spontaneous cases, but he concentrated on incidences of chronic inflammation. Nematode invasion accompanied many of these inflammations, which seemed directly to portend pathological changes that resulted in cancer. Put simply, Haaland argued that inflammation changed the character of extant cells; it created "new cell strains with powers of continuous growth."[4]

Both researchers had connected their animal experiments with cancer in humankind. Borrel tackled the human cancer question directly a few years later, reporting that his microscopic investigations had often uncovered nematodes in association with human cancers, especially epithelial tumors. "What is the role of the nematode," Borrel had written in closing. Is it "able to bring itself malignant transformations of cells or is it only an inoculum?" Does it alter "the structure of normal tissues" or is it the "vehicle for introducing the real cancer pathogen?" Borrel chose not to parse that difficult question, but he did note that the nematodes located in tumor cells "seemed unlikely to be a coincidence." Haaland offered a more menacing proposition. "Cancer in the mouse is essentially the same process as in man," he argued.[5] Fibiger quibbled with the specific implications of Haaland's conclusion. He termed it "doubtful that the precise nematode [implicated in rat stomach] cancer holds a pathogenic role in human cancers." That, however, did not mean that he thought his study had few human cancer implications. He cited research by other investigators on a different nematode, Trichinella, that placed that parasite in or near human tumors. The nematode responsible for trichinosis, Fibiger maintained that the medical literature was full of cancer cases in which the attending physician noted that the patients suffered chronic infestations of that worm. Cancer of the breast seemed especially suspect. Speculating further, he maintained it likely that nematodes caused some human cancer cases. Harkening back to his initial caged rat discovery, he predicted that when investigators examine the cause of "cancer epidemics among humans," the "connecting link between the sufferers will often be nematodes."[6]

Fibiger's extremely convincing research and profoundly troubling statements of Borrel, Haaland, and himself could not go without comment. The research and conclusions so well fit the questions that had guided cancer research for several decades—what particular microorganism caused cancer? That microbiological/germ theory view was the referent, the model for so much action as investigators had labored to prove or disprove it. Here was an instance of it coming to fruition. Fibiger's investigations demanded direct engagement.

Gaylord was among the first to consider Fibiger's pioneering effort. Unlike many of his colleagues, he saw in Fibiger's work the mature expression of a consistent research line that included Borrel and incorporated Rous. Each investigator had identified an infectious cancerous agent that reached its target by "some round-about route, . . . possibly an intermediate host." Fibiger's study stood as "a hopeful and colossal field for research." Its human implications were unassailable. "The significance of so-called 'cancer houses' . . . takes on a new light," he argued. The "possibilities of limiting the spread of certain kinds of cancer and of beginning a rational attack upon the distribution of the disease" has increased immeasurably.

Gaylord's comments on Fibiger's work no doubt reflected his unswerving commitment to a pathological agent as the cause of cancer. He had championed a cancerous parasite to account for the epidemic of trout cancer in hatcheries and for the epidemic of cancer among caged mice. But Gaylord's bias should not undercut what made Fibiger's work so attractive. Gaylord had called the study "easily appreciated."[7] That was the investigation's most alluring element. It was relatively pure, reproducible, unanticipated, and seemingly straightforward. In all those senses, it seemed a natural complement to Rous's chicken sarcoma efforts. Both seemed virtually unassailable, scrupulously consistent with the highest principles of the methods of science. Both seemed to expose or contradict what researchers already understood.

Bashford was having none of that. He praised Fibiger on his meticulous research, even as he noted "that the association of round and other worms with cancerous growths has long been known." But he insisted that "the presence of worms must not be interpreted . . . that they are the cause of cancer." Rather than produce the disease, he asserted that "they probably act as chronic irritants," a legion of which has been "associated with the development of cancer."

Among the most fervent opponents of a pathogenic explanation for cancer, Bashford maintained that a litany of irritants had been identified. Irritants could be "animate or inanimate," a "mere direct physical injury as in fracture of bone," or they could be "chemical as in paraffin, petroleum, tar, arsenic, and aniline." Irritants implicated in cancer included things "actinic as in the case of the short hot claypipe, the Kangri, the X-ray or brands" to mark animals. Sites of repeated use and old injury, as in places long exposed to heat, "an old lupus scar," or a place of previous infection or infestation all were associated with cancer and, to Bashford, no less involved or important in the cancerous process. Even spots on the backs of experimental animals "subjected to the repeated irritation produced by transplantation" experiments "have been demonstrated in propagated tumours." Only one thing was certain. These diverse irritants possessed in common only that that they came in contact with living cells. It was the cells "capacity . . . to undergo variations in structure and in powers of growth" that marked something cancerous.

Bashford thought the "growths produced experimentally by Fibiger" offered no clarity. They "present just as much difficulty in the elucidation" of the cancer process "as do all other natural growths." Despite the fact that he accorded Fibiger no place in the cancer causing debate, Bashford nonetheless congratulated the Dane for his "pertinacity as an investigator." He had isolated "an apparent irritant" and therefore produced "cancer experimentally" by "carefully imitating the natural process" of "mediate intervention of a parasite."[8]

Bashford's reduction of Fibiger's work to just an aspect of the cancer process reflected an increasingly common assessment. Cancer's cause was much more complicated than any of these researchers had believed a decade earlier. Investigators and others writing in the medico-scientific literature entered into a new series of debates. In addition to the consideration of the relationship between experimental and spontaneous cancers and between animal and human cancers, they also began to question whether cancer was routinely a multivariate disease. Did various conditions and substances make "the soil" suitable for cancer to grow?

Dawson Williams, the editor of the *British Medical Journal*, concurred with Bashford but added the Indian habit of betel nut chewing to the list of "predisposing or mediate factors that preside at [cancer's] onset." He then set about to justify why investigators had not contemplated "mediate" causes in any great detail before this time. "It is but natural," he maintained, "that the mind of man in constructing hypotheses on which to base a prospective investigation should choose the most easy generalization from sets of known phenomena." Cancer," Williams continued, "is anarchistic to the economy. It is multiplication of cells derived from parent tissue normal to the body; springing from it, it grows without heed to the order of things, lawless in its origin, lawless in its progress." Cancer's irrationality, as set out by Williams, had made it impossible for purveyors of laboratory methods to resolve the disease's cause. They thought rationally. They observed. They tested hypotheses. Their grounding was in laws, natural rules for biological action. "Cellular disloyalty" was illogical.

The cancer situation was incredibly complicated. One might argue, Williams continued, that if we remove the mediate cause of cancer, then the "cancerous process would not ensue." That appeared logical, but Williams recognized "that in the great majority of cancers no history of definite preceding, nor histological evidence of accompanying irritation can be obtained." Those cancer cases might arise without warning, a situation beyond modern science. But Williams had a different prescription for instances of severe irritation. He demanded preventive surgery, removal of the irritated tissue. Only through this "treatment of a predisposing condition" that "so clearly may succeed to cancer" can medicine prevent "such a grave sequela."[9]

Rohdenburg and Bullock thought the problem even more complex still. They examined numerous infestations in rats and tried to determine if they could establish a rule to predict cell proliferations. Much to their chagrin, some of the instances of the grossest, most severe irritations did not result in cancerous growths. There seemed no logically consistent guide to correlate depth or quantity of irritation and injury with cancer occurrence.

In the course of these investigations, the two Columbia University professors noted something unanticipated. They saw cancers more regularly arise from areas of long-standing injury, chronic inflammation or irritation. Therefore, they proposed that it was not the injury itself that usually predisposed cells to become cancerous but rather the duration of that insult. Sites of "chronic irritation" had "the power of inducing inflammatory changes tending to cancer formation."[10]

Czerny offered his own variant. Now the doyen of German cancer research, he surveyed his forty years in the field and attempted to provide a taxonomy of what he had learned. He, too, thought predisposition essential to the disease but believed it could be "either congenital or acquired." Rather than simply prepare the body for cancer, Czerny also maintained that the predisposition could be in the other direction. A substance that would "defend the body against cancer might be absent" or caused to be gone; freedom from cancer was the natural state of affairs. Only when an inhibitor went missing was an invader able to propagate the disease. If that were not confusion enough, Czerny thought it possible that "a debilitating disease may form a suitable field" for a carcinoma to flourish.

That constituted only one class of preparations. Also necessary was to prepare a disease seat. A site of "trauma, injury, inflammation, a scar or other congenital malformation" could provide cancer's home. Beyond that, "a real cancer organism must exist." It might be from a "group of the so far unknown ultramicroscopic organisms." It undoubtedly would be "brought to the human subject by an intermediate carrier." These carriers could be the "bedbug . . . other bloodsucking parasites or one of the family of the small round worms carried by cockroaches." Like "all other infectious diseases, the virulence of the exciter is of great import." A "healthy body can overcome a small number of exciters."[11]

Czerny's outline and his express dependence on predisposition was both old-fashioned and cutting edged. Cancer to this leader of the German cancer research community was likely a multivariate process. Predisposition dictated why and how some individuals got the disease, while others remained disease free. Czerny used that understanding to bolster support for the idea that cancer was caused by a parasitic agent. Predisposition explained why people did *not* get cancer. It suggested why there were "cancer houses and neighborhoods," places of dense cancer occurrence, as well as isolated incidents of cancer. In sum, it buttressed the possibility that infection/infestation was a matter of circumstance, behavior, or some other action. It "explained" why universal patterns were so difficult to find and reinforced the work of Rous and Fibiger, both of whom proved that cancer was a disease caused by a microorganism.

Czerny was not alone in his attempt to formulate a taxonomy of inflammation/irritation as it related to predisposition. William B. Coley, surgeon at the New York Cancer Hospital, long an asylum for the disease-afflicted indigent, compiled data over several decades in an effort to demonstrate that previous injury was closely correlated to cancer occurrence. His more than 1,200 cases showed previous insult in more than a quarter of instances. An AACR member, Coley initially divided the disease by cancer locus and between carcinoma and sarcoma but found that each subunit had injury-related cancer in a range from 25 percent to 36 percent. He concluded that that his statistics also showed no marked difference between a one-time and repeated injury. To that end, he adopted "trauma" to subsume all sort of physical damage. Coley made it clear that while he favored the pathogenic explanation for cancer, his results did not "depend upon the acceptance of any one of the various hypotheses as to the etiology of cancer." Traumatic onset of cancer was "equally well explained whether we accept the extrinsic or intrinsic origin of malignant tumors."[12]

Tying injury to cancer onset forced Coley to broach a medico-legal question, that of liability. If an occasional or continual injury resulted in preparing the soil for cancer, was not the party causing the injury legally responsible for unleashing the disease? That had been a matter of great moment nearly a decade earlier in France and especially Germany, where insurance companies helped bankroll the Comité für Krebsforschung, the first specialty group dedicated to determining cancer's origin. By 1911, there had been more than a handful of cases linking industrial injury to cancer genesis that had worked their way through the German courts. Indeed, medical researchers had begun arguing that a single trauma was just as surely linked to cancer as was chronic and persistent irritation. Insurance companies vigorously defended their industrial clients but not always successfully. The case of the man who had a block of ice dropped on his lumbar region at work was ruled in favor of plaintiff. He had developed cancer there four months later and soon succumbed to the metastatic disease. His family recovered the indemnity.[13]

Even in the United States, juries identified injury with cancer. In Kentucky, a woman was thrown from a streetcar, and her umbrella handle bruised her breast. After listening to much medical testimony, the jury concluded that the "injury did not cause the cancer," but it brought "about a condition in the breast which would result in it when a cancer would not have otherwise existed." This was true because "any chronic inflammatory condition in the breast was liable to bring about cancer." That the victim "was a strong, healthy woman, without an ache or a pain until her injury . . .tended strongly to confirm the conclusion of the physicians that the malignant cancer was the result of the bruised condition of the breast which she received in the fall." Again, the family received damages, a verdict that was upheld by the court of appeals.[14]

Adolph Theilhaber, professor of obstetrics at a private hospital in Munich and Councilor to the Bavarian Court, added statistical substance to that impressionistic sentiment. He used his extensive experience treating cancer hospital patients to identify a pattern between the development of a bruise and the onset of cancer. Of the five hundred such cases he had studied, Theilhaber found that the vast majority of tumors—nearly four hundred—originated within the first year of the contusion. Of these cases, 220 began within three months of the initial bruising. Bruises that led to cancer were most common in patients aged from forty to seventy, but the sarcoma rate exceeded the carcinoma rate in persons under forty. Bruise-related cancers developed about equally in the breast and the leg.

It was breast cancer that galvanized Theilhaber. He noted that bruises often resulted in hard lumps in the breast and that those sites would eventually turn malignant. To prevent the disease, he prescribed hyperemia, the dissipation of the hematoma through increased blood flow generated by passing streams of warm air over the bruised area. Theilhaber applied the same treatment after breast cancer surgery to prevent recurrence, since "all large scars afford a predisposition to malignant disease." He also extended his conclusion to recommend "energetic measures against inflammation" at "all points of the body" to prevent cancer later at those spots. Within a few short months of further consideration, he was willing to suggest that atrophy "almost always" must precede cancer and that atrophy in obstetrics or gynecology cases was the consequence of "old scars, chronic inflammation or destruction of soft tissue from trauma, such as childbirth."

But Theilhaber did not end his discussion there. He maintained that cancer occurred "almost always in places where anatomical damage or a severe disruption of the metabolic processes had already existed for some time." More to the point, Theilhaber determined that specific diseases commonly preceded cancer and apparently prepared sites for the scourge's invasion. His recipe for cancer researchers was bold. Examine the changes that take place when these cancer-associated diseases strike and the cause of the disease would likely soon be revealed. On top of that, Theilhaber also posed another possible cancer link—repeated abuse and exposure of a body part to a noxious influence. "The cases of lesions among workers in lignite" mines, the classic "tarred factory seborrhea," lupus eruptions, "chronic eczema, Paget's disease, [and] psoriasis" were all skin cancer precursors. Cancers of the mouth, lip, tongue, cheeks, pharynx, and esophagus were associated with earlier incidents of "heavy smoking, alcoholic beverages, syphilis." Stomach cancer was preceded "by chronic gastritis, intestinal cancer observed after chronic colic, [and] rectal cancer after hemorrhoids." Liver cancer usually followed cirrhosis, and lung cancers observed among metal workers in mills and laborers in tobacco factories were probably due to chronic inflammation, ulcers and scarring as a result of inhalation of foreign bodies."[15]

Life—habits, customs, and circumstances—played a key role in the propagation of cancer. Theilhaber's analysis was fundamentally similar to Bashford's, even though Bashford restricted his examples to quaint customs among indigenous peoples. Modern and "primitive" life both emerged as fundamentally dangerous, because activities undertaken in both milieus exposed humans to cancer liability; they did not cause cancer, but they prepared the way for cancer. That realization further complicated the cancer quest. Researchers had adamantly denied and meticulously had proven that these behaviors did not cause cancer. Now they seemed to be a fundamental facet of the cancer equation, albeit in a way far different from the way their proponents had suggested.

Researchers were no closer to identifying the cancer agent. Predisposition simply made the situation more murky. Indeed, predisposing elements seemed ubiquitous, hardly the sort of clear cut, deterministic process that scientists embraced. Their approach treasured simple, straightforward analyses, direct measurements of unambiguous situations. Complexity proved difficult to test and to control.

The question of heredity accompanied the more general reexamination of the influence of human life and culture on the development of cancer. Cancer houses, cancer neighborhoods, cancer families, and other anecdotal evidence linking the disease to heredity had long appeared in the professional literature. *JAMA*'s Simmons considered these practitioner-derived, bedside-recorded clinical histories "unreliable information" and maintained that, so long as researchers depended on them, "there was little prospect" of "learning much about the influence of heredity." Investigators had one touchstone upon which to rely. The pioneer statistician Karl Pearson, head of the England's Galton Laboratory, had pursued a "reliable and well-controlled" investigation and concluded that "no evidence whatever" existed "that persons with a history of cancer in relatives were predisposed to cancer."[16]

Animal experiments had complicated the situation. Mice had long been selected and bred because they seemed more susceptible to certain strains and types of implanted or transplanted cancer. Rather than serve as a potent demonstration of heredity's power, however, these procedures seemed irrelevant to resolving the question of importance of heredity in a natural state. Implantation was artificial, experimental. The data researchers possessed was on animals, not humans. The mice strains were rigorously inbred, an extreme laboratory-controlled situation not encountered in nature.

A specific situation provided the impetus for early heredity-cancer researchers. The claim of Gaylord and others that cancer epidemics swept through certain cages of experimental mice and that those epidemics proved the existence of a cancer pathogen provided the justification. E. E. Tyzzer, a Harvard Cancer Commission scientist, was among the first to examine the proposition. He saw far larger implications. While he recognized that no proof existed that tumor development among humans was "due to a specific inherited character," he was struck that the medical literature contained numerous reports of cancer ravaging human families. His experimental work had been with mice and transplanted tumors. He understood that certain families of mice more readily accepted transplants and wondered if they also developed spontaneous cancer at an accelerated rate.

Tyzzer asserted that a hereditary propensity to develop tumors would be a simple inherited character and, that as such, it should conform to Mendelian principles. He further speculated that the trait would not be dominant, because "then the breeding of an insusceptible individual with one having a tumor would result in hybrids in all of which the tumor character would be dominant." Cancer susceptibility in Tyzzer's formulation was not favored by nature.

Tyzzer's initial experiments dealt with three distinct mouse families that long had proven fertile soil for Jensen and Stamm II tumor transplants. In fact, he started his breeding experiments with animals in which he had already transplanted cancer. Only in that way could he be sure that his subjects would not be immune to the disease. He bred his animals within families but across generations—mother-son and grandfather-granddaughter crosses. Two families lived in pristine environments. The third rested in "two large cages, which are seldom cleaned and then not very thoroughly," ideal "conditions . . . for cage infection"

The Harvard scientist soon found his study would not give him the answer he sought. Only twenty of the mice developed cancer spontaneously. Coupled with the multiple living arrangements and the myriad of crossing possibilities, Tyzzer recognized he had incorporated far too many variables in his research design. He was unable "to prove or to disprove that the development of a tumor is dependent upon the presence of an inherited character."

Tyzzer streamlined, updated, and continued his study for another two years. His new experimental protocol identified the locus of spontaneous tumors, increased the number of cases analyzed to eighty-three, and autopsied each cancer-diagnosed mouse. Much to his surprise, only a handful of the cancers were mammary tumors. Fully as many mice suffered lymphoma as breast cancer. About two-thirds of the affected animals developed lung cancer.

Again Tyzzer confronted his experimental design and again he found it less than ideal. He certainly did not anticipate the great preponderance of lung cancer among his mice. Nor did he expect to find such a small number of breast cancers. Nothing seemed to approach Mendelian ratios. He remained convinced that heredity likely played a factor in cancer but was willing to stipulate only that hereditary characters probably "become apparent only late in life during the period of the decadence of the individual." He offered a final caveat. These "characters may possibly become apparent only under certain conditions."[17]

Tyzzer's research offered no certainty. It directly contradicted what was known about human cancer rates. In humans, lung cancer was considered quite rare. Mammary, uterine, and vaginal cancer made up a significant portion of human cancers, surpassed only by digestive tract cancers, which were almost unknown in mice. Bashford, who had also recognized the caged mice cancer epidemics as a potential demonstration of heredity, not a microorganism, also investigated. Although he had not noted any epidemic of cancer among his mice, he took what he knew about relative incidences of cancer and reconfigured his laboratory's huge store of mice by age. Results showed "crops of tumours coincid[ing] with the ageing of groups of mice" that gave every indication "that epidemics raged in those cages." That conclusion was false, simply a manifestation of the tendency of mice to develop cancers as they reached old age. It was these types of "apparent aggregations" of aged mice that were "wrongly called epidemics by too enthusiastic advocates of a parasitic origin of cancer." In reality, cancer in mice "continues to obey the laws of age- and sex-distribution." Bashford maintained that neither infection nor heredity were in evidence.

Bashford then turned his attention to heredity in human cancer. Acknowledging that his statements were "imperfect and largely hypothetical," he maintained that human cancers were not manifestations of "innate racial peculiarities" but "extrinsic irritants," the customs and habits of living. Family histories showed nothing that would "imply hereditary transmission." The "isolated incidences recorded in the literature" demonstrated only "how rare this phenomenon really is." These conglomerations were merely statistical certainties, "what would be expected to happen in the case of so frequent a cause of death as cancer." That distribution was anticipated; it could be "theoretically calculated according to the law of probabilities." He ended by remarking that "nothing [existed] but negative evidence of the part played by inherited constitutional conditions" in human cancer aggregations. Conversely, there was considerable "positive evidence of the important part acquired constitutional conditions"—habits and activities—played in cancer's development.[18]

Two years later, Bashford and others at the ICRF reported further mouse cancer-heredity experiments. They concentrated on 1,600 female mice of a similar age, arguing that male cancers among all laboratory bred mice were "so small" that they were statistically insignificant. All mice were housed in the same facility, albeit in separate, thoroughly well kept cages. Autopsies were performed on all mice. They concluded that females whose mothers or grandmothers had had cancer developed the disease at slightly more than twice the rate of those whose immediate progenitors had remained disease free.

In this context, the Bashford group viewed ancestry as just another cancer-related factor. The "actual initiation of cancer" was the "terminal phase of a long-continued process of localized chronic irritation." That explained why the disease struck mice generally and why it struck the breast. Ancestry accounted for a "predisposing condition" of "some peculiarity of the cells of the tissues where cancer develops." That peculiarity meant that "under the wear and tear of life" the "regenerative and proliferate changes" accompanying "the inception of the disease" were either "more prone to take place" or occurred "with greater intensity."[19]

In this framework, every individual in any population could develop cancer. It simply required more irritation to erupt in those individuals lacking a hereditary proclivity. Even before Bashford published his initial comments in 1909, however, a much more extensive laboratory study of spontaneous mouse cancer was well under way. A mouse breeder, Abbie Lathrop, had noticed that three of her mice had developed similar skin tumors in similar sites without implantation. She had the cancers verified as virtually identical and found among investigators an interest in these animals. Leo Loeb was particularly interested. Earlier in the century, he detected a specific eye cancer among cows on a particular ranch. Although he published his discovery and speculated about its significance, he did not follow up that work. Cows proved too expensive to serve as cancer laboratory animals and the occurrence seemed anomalous.

Lathrop's discovery resonated with Loeb. The issue of spontaneous outbreaks of cancer among mice housed in the same or nearby cages again served as impetus, as investigators sought to account for these not infrequent outbreaks. Loeb hoped to rule out infection as cause and recognized in Lathrop's mice another possible factor: heredity.

That led to an extensive collaboration between the two. By 1913, after more than three years of investigation, they had garnered data enough to publish their first two papers. The two researchers had divided Lathrop's mice into "strains or families" and kept those families isolated from each other. All animals encountered similar climates and received the same nutritional complement.

Despite those constants, the families showed remarkable diversity in incidences of breast cancer. In some families, breast cancer effected 82 percent of the population. In others, it was merely 3.5 percent. Even more impressive was that tumor rates persisted from generation to generation; breast cancer rates seemed locked within families. Average age at onset was also fixed by family, as descendants manifested cancer at a similar age as their familial forerunners.

Lathrop and Loeb's investigation also incorporated cross-breeding. When they crossed high tumor producing families with families with very low cancer rates, the duo found that the offspring would always manifest high cancer occurrences. Sex of the parent did not matter. Males apparently carried propensity for breast cancer at the same rate as females. They also proved that hybridized mice suckled by low incidence mothers still developed the disease at the rate of their fathers' families. This last stipulation suggested that cancer germs were not passed from mother to daughter through milk or uterine infection.

Lathrop and Loeb ran one final series of experiments before they published their work. They placed low tumor rate mice in uncleaned, unaltered "boxes in which mice with spontaneous tumors had lived a long time," to see if some residual infectious agent resided there. No noticeable uptick in cancer rates occurred. They then placed other mice from tumor resistant families to live "in the same box with mice spontaneously affected with cancer." Again, the low tumor mice showed no cancer increase. The investigators concluded that "hereditary factors" played "a great part in the incidence of cancer among mice and that hereditary transmission is to a great extent responsible for the so-called endemic occurrence of cancer among animals." While admitting that Fibiger's work showed that "parasitic worms" could be a factor "of an infectious character" in cancer, they nonetheless maintained that heredity was central. In fact, Loeb and Lathrop alluded to the work of Maud Slye at the University of Chicago, who had conducted experiments at the same time as the two authors and who had also concluded that the "incidence of cancer varies in different strains of mice."[20]

Lathrop and Loeb's experiments did not settle the heredity issue. They explicitly restricted their research to mouse cancer and made no comparisons to other animals or humankind. Slye differed in that she saw her work as directly translatable to the human experience. In fact, she argued that determining if a tendency to cancer was inherited could lead to "the cure of the race." She noted reports of human "cancer communities" and predicted that heredity accounted for these outbreaks. Individuals in these communities carried "in the germ plasm" the power derived from their "progenitors and transmitted in turn to [their] posterity, to produce an individual whose tissues under a given provocation shall proliferate in the structureless and wild manner of malignant growth." As significant, Slye suggested that this hereditary tendency was passed from generation to generation by unit characters, simple Mendelian traits.

Such a proposition could easily be measured, but not for the human race. Millennia of "mixed hybridization" made delineating human family lineage difficult. Coupled with the long human life span, the unsuitability of pursuing controlled breeding experiments and the uncertainty of fatherhood led Slye to focus instead on mice. Among her first tasks was to demonstrate comparability. She asserted that spontaneous cancer attacked the same structures in mice as in humans but also noted that it did so at different rates. For example, she argued that lung cancer was the second most common form of mouse cancer—Tyzzer had it first—but rare in humans. Conversely, cancer of the alimentary cancer and head and neck cancer were among the leading human cancers—Slye excluded "female" cancers here—but almost unknown among mice.

Mice offered no other limitations, ethical or otherwise. Yet they too posed difficulties for determining Mendelian ratios. Cancer was a disease of old age. Mice that failed to achieve that state never had the chance to express the disease. Epizootics ran rampant among laboratory mice. So too did parasites. Each cataclysmic event promised to skew her cancer statistics and upset the search for the Mendelian ideal. To help mitigate this impediment (and in contrast to Tyzzer), Slye autopsied each of her animals upon its natural death. In that way she could record incipient cancers, not visible during life.

In the years before 1915, Slye autopsied over 10,000 mice and encountered slightly more than 1,000 cases of spontaneous cancer. Her conclusions were striking: "Cancers almost without exception have occurred in strains of known cancerous ancestry . . . in exact accordance with the laws of heredity governing the transmission of any other [unit] character." She also found that crossing an animal from a cancer-producing family with one from a cancer-immune group produced only cancer-prone individuals. She likened this occurrence to what had happened in the distant human past. "One long forgotten cancerous individual of the human species" formed "the basis of a whole cancerous community where through generations of intermarriages" vast segments of humanity acquired "the potentiality of cancer."

Slye argued that for that potential to materialize, "overirritation" where the cancer would blossom must occur. In cancerous strains, for instance, suckling of the young "results in the location of cancer in the mammary gland tissue." Similar suckling in a "non-cancerous strain produces no cancer." Males who fight repeatedly and are subject to injury develop tumors in those sites if from cancer strains, but these injuries "never had this result in a mouse of non-tumorous strain."

Preventing overirritation held critical implications for humanity. "Elimination as far as possible of all form of overirritation . . . should go far to eliminate the provocation of cancer" in humans of "high cancer ancestry," she maintained. But she also posed a more dramatic proposition, banishing the disease entirely. Coupling minimizing overirritation with "eugenic control of mating" would "eventuate in a considerable decrease in the frequency of human cancer." With such a eugenics policy in place, humanity could ultimately rid itself of the scourge.

Despite Slye's protestation of human parallelism, she did not ignore the question that had initially stimulated mouse studies, that of caged mice epidemics. In some experiments, she kept mice from tumor-free strains in a single cage with cancerous mice. In others, Slye placed mice from cancer-free strains in the cages where cancerous mice had died "with all the debris and old food soiled by the dead mouse." She suckled cancer-free strains on cancerous mothers and vice versa. She even systematically fed "portions of the cancer and of the viscera of dead cancerous mice" to cancer-immune mice. She "never" had a case result from that practice.

Slye's work attracted notice but it did not provide much lucidity. Despite her protestations otherwise, Slye provided no evidence for considering cancer susceptibility as unit characters following Mendelian ratios. In fact, both Richard Weil at Columbia's Crocker and C. C. Little of the Harvard's Cancer Commission maintained that Slye's entire project was suspect because of her ignorance of what constituted Mendelianism. It also failed to demonstrate that cancer in mice was comparable to human cancers. Cornell's Ewing argued that the "extensive in-breeding" that characterized Slye's inheritance studies was "unknown among human beings" and that made her results dubious.[21] Sites of the disease differed between the two life forms, as did cancer rates. At best, her work added support for the idea that heredity might well be involved in cancer in some complicated way and that cage epidemics apparently were not caused by an easily identifiable parasite.

X-rays offered further complexity. In their initial incarnation, researchers deemed these mysterious waves a godsend. Subsequent assessments of their therapeutic effects were decidedly more negative. The rays seem only to influence surface tumors and then not necessarily in positive ways. For every cancer case that reported improvement, there existed several instances where open sores formed or the scourge persisted unabated. Edward Reginald Morton, fellow of the Royal College of Surgeons, Edinburgh, maintained that the professional reaction to x-rays followed a predictable, well-established pattern. Unbridled enthusiasm and "extravagant claims" for a new curative were always followed by a corresponding sense of futility. Only later, when passions subsided, could the truth be known. Such was the time for x-rays. Only now, Morton continued, could researchers "arrive at some semblance of the truth." Worthington Seaton Russell, research fellow at the New York Skin and Cancer Hospital, agreed. He claimed that "a few ultra-enthusiasts" and the "lay press" heralded the introduction of x-rays "as the long-sought-for cure for cancer." Patients immediately demanded "that it be used on them. Incalculable harm was the result." Others tried to "counteract the wave of enthusiasm that swept over the country" by noting that x-rays were not "specifics in cancer." Now the situation would be different. Russell declared, "We await the final and conclusive verdict from those workers who proceed with scientific caution" and care.[22]

Researchers held these rationalist sentiments because the method of employing radiation had markedly changed. First generation x-ray tubes were relatively inexpensive; any well-heeled medical man could own and operate one. Practitioners and other clinicians reported case after case but without the sense of control that would permit meaningful comparison. Consequentially, chaos and disagreement over x-rays' virtues and vices remained. While practitioners persisted in using this easily available methodology,[23] introduction of radium revolutionized radiological experimentation. It did so not simply by offering the possibility of repeatable precision, but also by restricting use.

Radium was dear and very expensive. Its scarcity and cost prevented most practitioners and clinicians from gaining access to the substance. In the United States, for example, Congress held hearings to determine how to increase the nation's radium supply and to see if a radium trust hampered its mining and subsequent medical distribution. The metallic salts so appealed to investigators because their effects could be quantified. Radium salts in small test tube–like devices produced emanations, and the radioactive-yielding tubes could be inserted directly into or near the cancerous spot. Surrounding tissue could be draped in protective lead. As critical, these radium tubes allowed investigators to standardize dosages of radium and, therefore, of radioactive power generally. That was no small matter. Standardizing exposure meant that experiments could be replicated, mastery assumed, and conclusions plotted out.[24]

Everyone wanted radium, but only those with connections or plentiful funding could acquire the salts. In several places, special consortiums of medical researchers were created to test radium's therapeutic value. The London Radium Institute, for instance, was the brainchild of King Edward.

It compiled a staff of investigators to determine in which cancer cases the new substance was efficacious. Manchester also established its own facility.[25]

The various already extant cancer research institutes and cancer research hospitals clamored to undertake these radium tests. They had been formed expressly to present the consequences of scientific inquiry and to employ them to battle cancer. In the United Kingdom, the Middlesex, Edinburgh, and Liverpool cancer laboratories all ran their own experiments. Wassermann and Ehrlich in Germany initiated studies. The Harvard Cancer Commission also spearheaded a radium assessment project. Columbia's Crocker Institute would quickly embrace the radium mantle. It even entered into a partnership with James Douglas, a major producer of radium, to guarantee the Columbia investigators a plentiful supply of the radioactive material.[26]

Almost all cancer research laboratories, along with the new specialized institutes, sought the parameters of radium's cancer-fighting properties. At least one major laboratory took a markedly different tack. The Middlesex Cancer Research Laboratory, under the direction of Walter Sydney Lazarus-Barlow, perhaps the most well-appointed cancer researcher in the British Isles after Bashford, quickly incorporated radioactivity as a phenomena into its cancer genesis research. Its first major x-ray project was to decide if radioactivity was in any way involved in the biological event known as cancer. Lazarus-Barlow configured a gold leaf electroscope to determine if cancerous cells naturally spawned radiation in a quantity different from healthy tissue. In experiments that extended over two years, Lazarus-Barlow used ten electroscopes to measure the radioactive content of tumors from four different human organs, which he measured against healthy tissue from the same individuals. He failed to achieve unambiguous results. His instrumentation posed a large problem. It proved so sensitive that it needed continual manipulation and correction. Perhaps because of this mechanical dilemma, he reported no significant difference between malignant and normal tissue.

Lazarus-Barlow's lab did not exit the work, however. It also entered into the vigorous debate over whether radiation speeded or slowed cell division in animals. The subsequent Middlesex experimental results helped explain why the issue had been such a flashpoint. Middlesex investigators found both sides correct. Small doses of radiation enhanced cell division, but larger quantities slowed it, even causing it to cease. A modest dosage apparently fostered "the formation of monstrosities and of irregular divisions," which led these London-based workers to conclude that radioactive substances possessed several "distinct properties."[27]

Measuring the difference in intensity between x-rays generated by machine and naturally occurring radium emanations constituted the last step in this initial set of investigations. The researchers assumed that radiation was convertible; differences lay in strength, little else. That assumption enabled them to draw up conversion charts that gave them the dominion necessary to more nearly control future experiments. They first demonstrated that x-rays possessed “a marked bactericidal action” to a wide range of microorganisms, as the living forms absorbed the radioactive “fluid.” Middlesex researchers broadened experiments to include other known pathogens—nematodes, larvae, and other insidious agents. In each case, the pathogens incorporated the radioactivity, which hindered their multiplication. Finally, the group tested the two radiation types on the vitality of mouse cancer cells undergoing transplantation. Both absorbed the rays and prohibited the transplanted tissue from proliferating.

Lazarus-Barlow modified and extended his electroscopic experiments further in 1911. He measured the radioactivity emanating from healthy organ tissue and tumors, both from the same mice, and compared these findings to similar organ measurements in healthy mice. His results suggested that both the healthy and cancerous tissue of a stricken mouse produced significantly greater radiation than the tissue of a cancer-free mouse. Lazarus-Barlow took that result to mean that his earlier research design had been imperfect. It used both cancerous and healthy tissue from the *same* mouse. He now concluded that cancer-ravaged animals showed excessive radiation throughout their being, not just in diseased organs. Lazarus-Barlow then moved the experiment in another direction. He tried to determine if he could see a special radiation bump in conditions that were commonly thought as precursors to cancer. He deemed gallstones as the gallbladder cancer’s antecedent, and his radioactivity measurements proved conclusive. Gallbladders with gallstones exhibited similar radiation levels to cancerous gallbladders.[28]

Rather than extend those experiments to other conditions and other organs, Lazarus-Barlow in 1914 combined these insights to offer a grand new theory of “the cause and cure of cancer.” Decrying the then-common tendency to consider cancer as needing a necessary and an auxiliary cause, he eschewed any attempt to divide up what he considered a single malady. Among researchers today, he argued, the alleged “causes of cancer have multiplied to such an extent that . . . the sole ‘cause’ to which universal assent is given is ‘chronic irritation.’” Such a view was totally wrongheaded. “In radiations, and particularly radium radiations, we have an agency which might well serve as a cause of cancer to the exclusion of all others.” That cause was radioactivity itself.

His reasoning was simple. Radium was widely distributed in nature, and therefore it was omnipresent. It invaded all environments and afflicted every species. Small amounts were a demonstrable cellular accelerant; the substance caused cells to divide more quickly, the essential manifestation of cancer. Parasitic agents, such as bacteria, roundworms, and other parasites, absorbed the radioactive material within their cell structure, enabling virtually any one of them to be the conduit through which a considerable excess concentration of radiation entered the human body. Radium/radiations were closely associated with the disease. Radium was found in much higher concentrations in cancerous and precancerous tissue than in other tissues. Lazarus-Barlow also cited studies that indicated that prolonged exposure to radium frequently resulted in cancer.

The Middlesex researcher took these experimental conclusions together and used them to configure nothing less than a reconceptualization of the idea of cancer. The accumulated facts—those enumerated in the previous paragraph—Lazarus-Barlow contended, support "my proposition that radiations . . . initiate the changes which culminate in the production of that which we, as medical men, term 'cancer.'" The power of radiation, especially radium emanations, proved awesome. Minute quantities of radium produced, in less than twenty-four hours, "one hundred thousand alpha particles, beta particles, and gamma particles travelling with initial velocities" of up to "180,000 miles a second." To Lazarus-Barlow, it was "inconceivable that such a force should fail to produce changes in any cells upon which it acts." Radiation invaded cells, its accelerating properties producing dramatic, permanent change. The blatant radioactive assault had profound evolutionary consequences. "The laws of evolution indicate that from formerly normal cells a race of cells must gradually arise in which rapidity of division dominates all other functions." That is the reality of cancer. Put baldly, radioactive emanations "constitute the etiological factor of all new growths."

Lazarus-Barlow then reinterpreted and re-explained how several of the habits and activities thought to create chronic irritation and therefore induce cancer were in truth the consequence of radioactivity. Clay pipes, paraffin, soot, and betel nuts led to cancer not because of heat, chemical inflammation, or soreness but because of radioactivity. Cells were accelerated by radioactivity contained within these substances. He brought a similar argument to bear on the concept of cancer houses and neighborhoods. The pestilential domiciles and environments spawned cancer because their raw materials—the wood and the soil—contained quantities of radioactive substances in excess of other areas. It was that quality of radioactivity, nothing else, that marked the spot as potentially cancerous.

Radium caused cancer, but Lazarus-Barlow understood it also cured the disease. Investigators recognized both that radiation in sufficient dosages could kill all cells and that different cells and tissue types accepted the x-rays differentially. Cure, then, was simply a matter of targeting radiation to destroy cancer cells and leave normal tissue unimpeded. In that sense, Lazarus-Barlow's thinking and the thinking of like-minded men was analogous to Ehrlich's chemotherapeutic agents—magic bullets. Cure required a good pathologist to determine the type of cells afflicted and to monitor the dosage necessary to render them dead. Healthy cells would be relatively unaffected by the selective radiation.

Lazarus-Barlow did not rest there. He also claimed that radiating a tumor out of existence immunized the being against a subsequent case of the disease. This extrapolation from any number of mouse experiments demonstrated that an active case of a disease must exist to create lifelong active immunity. He hypothesized that curing cancer would grant the patient that benison but imagined that that immunity would only extend to the type and site of cancer that had been cured.[29]

Producing active immunity, coupled with the selective action of the targeted radiation, indicated that radiotherapy should be preferred over surgery. Lazarus-Barlow counseled against that, at least until further experiments confirmed his theory. Even with his caveat, Lazarus-Barlow's theory created a public sensation. His use of statistics from the Middlesex Hospital caused consternation. In the year prior to the full articulation of his cancer theory, the hospital reported no cured cases. But in early 1914, Lazarus-Barlow noted that about half the patients being treated for cancer that year had been cured. Most had been discharged, and many had resumed work. Others at the hospital disagreed. In particular, the hospital's surgeons claimed that they saw no discernible difference in cancer curative rates in the wake of radium treatment. Opposition by the very group likely to be most affected by radium's success dampened enthusiasm but did not kill it. Alfred Pearce Gould, a senior surgeon at the Middlesex Hospital, moderated his group's hostility. Calling radium "potent" and "wonderful," he praised the substance for differential action on living cells. Radium's "wonderful selective" affinity" was "akin to salvarsan" in cases of syphilis; radium could even "be thought of in terms with which Professor Erhlich has made us familiar." But Gould cautioned that "it would be a gross exaggeration to speak glibly of radium as the 'cure of cancer' in the sense that it will deal with any and every case of the disease." Decidedly more research was necessary to determine the parameters of radium's cancer-fighting efficacy before it had significant practical application. Until that time, surgery remained the sole effective option.[30]

Taken at face value, Lazarus-Barlow's radiation as the cause of cancer theory would have had tremendous repercussions. At the very least, it would necessitate a reexamination of virtually all previous experiments. Since radiation-containing material, whether breathed, ingested, absorbed, or situated in close proximity, seemed the sole cause of the disease, every experiment would have had to be redrafted, rerun, and reinterpreted within that context. As important, Lazarus-Barlow's theory disaggregated phenomenon. Each clay pipe, each house, each mine's coal, each microorganism could differ considerably in the quantity of radium or radioactivity contained therein. The number of experiments necessary to reconcile what was suspected with Lazarus-Barlow's new theory would be tremendous. Did Rous's filtrate contain radium? Were Gaylord's cages made with wood contaminated with radioactive materials? Did Fibiger's Estonian factory cockroaches feast on radiation-contaminated food?

Ultimately, two major protocols were necessary to conform to Lazarus-Barlow's universal cancer-causing theory. Each separate case of cancer was the starting point in the first protocol. Investigators needed to begin with the onset of disease and then work backwards to determine where the culprit radiation originated and how it found its way into the diseased individual. The second was even more problematic. To prevent the radiation-caused disease, every situation, every substance, needed perpetual radiation monitoring. Anything less was irresponsible. Situations and places would become known as contaminated by radiation, not fit for living beings. In short, Lazarus-Barlow's theory not only required prodigious effort, but it also cast aspersions on what was known.[31]

Despite his stellar reputation, Lazarus-Barlow's sensational theory of cancer production failed to capture the day. Like much other cancer work done after 1910, he presumed cancer was a most complicated phenomenon. Investigators needed to account for two things. First, they needed to explain why some people got cancer. Then they needed to explain why others with apparently similar circumstances did not develop the disease. What caused the discrepancy? What marked those who acquired the disease from those who were disease-free? Many researchers found resolution to that question in the concept of predisposition—auxiliary cause. Cancer was found in those individuals predisposed to the disease. Heredity, irritation, and radiation each seemed a possible offender. A second layer had been added to the already intensely complicated cancer causation question. Rather than narrowing possibilities, rather than zeroing in on potential culprits, the field of cancer research was expanding. Like cancer itself, cancer research was growing uncontrollably.

10

All Cancer Is Local

The End of the War and the Beginning of a New Era, 1910–1915

With the backdrop of cancer as a complex, two-phased or two-stepped disease and a belief that cancer laboratories had failed in their essential mission to resolve the cancer problem, Bashford took out against the quacks. Claiming that they fed on human misery, he railed against their patent medicine and other nostrums purported to cure cancer. To a man of science, what the quacks proposed was poppycock. If that were not enough, Bashford slammed them for refusing to submit their various preparations to laboratory analysis and scientific scrutiny. The quacks duped their unsuspecting marks, taking their money and, ultimately, their lives. By delaying responsible treatment until cancer riddled their victims' bodies, the quacks were no better than murderers. Their broadsides and other advertisements "are avowedly intended to divert the cancer sufferer from the assistance of surgery" because that practice interfered "fatally with the therapeutic" pushed by the nostrum vendors, a therapeutic that its proponents argued "otherwise might have proved efficacious."

One man in particular fueled Bashford's ire. Dr. Robert Bell drew Bashford's scorn because he was a long-established member of the English medical profession. To Bashford, Bell and his ilk mimicked the protocols and verbiage used by researchers but to fanciful and selfish ends. Bell's "kind of physiology and pathology" were "make believe." His explanations were "a jumble of words—irrelevant chatter." "Milk, nuclein, the thyroid gland, pork, butcher's meat, constipation, menstruation, cell metabolism, platform experience, and contaminated blood" appeared in juxtaposition to "one another without order or reason." Bell threw in "biblical" quotations for good measure, while always harping upon the "natural dread" of surgery.

All that disgusted Bashford, but it was the Bell's central contention that represented the most egregious affront. He "kept alive among many members of the public" the "old fallacies about cancer being a 'blood disease.'"[1] Bashford's entire career and much of the work of cancer laboratories worldwide had been dedicated to demonstrating that cancer was of local origin, site specific. It was not a constitutional disease, a disease that could be mitigated through enhanced sanitary or nutritional practice. To Bashford, cancer began at a specific site. And so long as it was restricted to that site, it could be removed. Only when it metastasized to other tissue was the prognosis unfailingly dire. To utter any other theory was preposterous, a deliberate attempt to deceive for personal gain.

Bashford was secure in his position. That confidence did not deter Bell, who remained as resolute as Bashford. He filed a libel suit before the Lord Chief Justice Alvarstone, demanding $10,000 for being branded a quack for his medical theories, theories he claimed that had been deduced from decades at the bedside of innumerable cancer sufferers. For the first several decades of his practice, Bell had recommended surgery for cancer, just like his professional brethren. But as early as 1894, he became convinced that that approach held little hope. His empirical clinical experience showed him that cancer was a constitutional disease—a blood disease—and its effects could be mitigated or prevented through dietary reform and abundant fresh air. He rarely missed an opportunity to report his findings to medical societies, reporting a cure rate for his therapeutic of about 30 percent and dismissing surgical cures as unsubstantiated; if cancer abated upon surgery, Bell maintained that the tumor removed had been misdiagnosed. The mass had not been cancerous.

Bell claimed that he could determine cancer victims and potential cancer victims simply by looking at their blood under a microscope. He was called upon to demonstrate his blood reading technique in court, ironically determining that his barrister was a prime candidate to develop the malady. A vegetable and dairy diet, coupled with copious amounts of fresh air, could cure or prevent the disease. To Bell's reckoning, the modern day predilection for diets heavy in meat set off a dangerous imbalance within the body that often ended in cancer. Only by restoring the natural order could the patient ward off or vanquish the disease.

Bell's vigorous defense included evidence that his long-standing refusal to operate for cancer actually cost him revenue. His medical theories and advice had generally been offered free of charge. London physicians who had used Bell's techniques to cure their own patients served as his most effective advocates. Several testified to the efficacy of his treatment, and all pledged allegiance to the Bell's blood theory. All pointed to cancer patients they had treated who had made full recoveries and resumed their normal routines.

Bashford's defense countered by calling several prominent medical men, including King Edward's personal physician, to testify that cancer was not a constitutional disease and that surgery had remedied many cases. Lazarus-Barlow also spoke extensively. He recounted how the Middlesex Cancer Laboratory had been charged for several years with examining the various cancer theories and remedies making their rounds in London medicine. The director maintained that, while he investigated numerous techniques and nostrums, only surgery could mitigate the disease.

Bashford testified last. He admitted that he had never treated a case of human cancer but argued they he held extensive clinical experience because he had tended to thousands of cancerous experimental animals—mice, rats, and rabbits. He claimed that his surveys of human populations had found that even meat-free areas suffered extensively from cancer, and he provided Japan as example. Bashford affirmed that Bell probably did not benefit financially from his theories but nonetheless maintained that they were "written out of vanity or through sheer ignorance." He persisted in arguing that Bell traded "on the credulity of the public" and did irreparable damage by "frightening people against operations."

Under further cross-examination, Bashford acknowledged that he did not know what caused cancer. He also confessed that he had written earlier in the year that cancer laboratory researchers had made little progress over the decade in determining cancer's cause or means to combat it. While he had initially thought that cancer would give up its mysteries quickly, he now was resigned to the fact that overcoming cancer rested well into the future. Despite that sentiment, Bashford argued that the research of cancer laboratories worldwide had ruled out the possibility of it being a constitutional disease.

Bell's lawyers closed by reminding the jury that the question was not whether Bell's theories were correct but whether he had been libeled by Bashford. Despite that tack, they asked the jury to remember what it was that made something so. They maintained that, in medicine and science, the "heterodoxy of one day" was "very often the orthodoxy of the next generation." While "intolerance and bigotry" were often raised during religious arguments, they questioned whether "was there not intolerance and bigotry among scientific people?" Whenever these twin pillars were found, they were "a thing to be repudiated." Differing professional opinions were no justification for libel.

The Lord Chief Justice's charge followed that course. He acknowledged that the court was not a "scientific theater," but believed it a "most lamentable thing" if "research, experiment, and an attempt to find some cure for this dread disease, this scourge of mankind," was disregarded "by unjust criticisms and comment upon the action of such as man as Dr. Bell." No matter what the jury concluded, he urged a medical panel to review Bell's work, "fairly examine the matter and publish the results." The jury deliberated for less than a half-hour and rendered a verdict for Bell, which was met with applause.[2]

The Bell-Bashford libel case exposed some fundamental truths about cancer and cancer research. It was incredibly difficult in the case of cancer to make things so. Thirty-five years of investigation had yielded a pittance of usable information about cancer's cause. The various laboratories found uniform agreement about even less. The case also proved a most potent demonstration of just how disconnected researchers were from medical practitioners and the public. Neither of the latter two groups cleaved to the same sense of exactitude and reproducibility as cancer laboratory investigators. All the groups claimed to adhere to the ideas of testing and examination, but a vast chasm separated the laboratory men and women from the others.

Bashford's testimony also was revealing. His profound acknowledgment of and deep disappointment about the inability of cancer laboratories to solve the puzzle of cancer suggested just how frustrated and disillusioned cancer researchers had become. Bashford reinforced that notion a few months later. Speaking at the New York Pathological Society, he noted that, in the preceding ten years "enormous amounts of money have been spent in cancer research, in the establishment of hospitals for the sufferers of cancer, in laboratories and in statistical research." All that remarkable effort had resulted in "a little progress and a little advancement in the exactitude of our knowledge of cancer." Surveying the past decade, there was "little that is apt to prove of immediate benefit to the human race," Bashford lamented. "The announced wonderful cures" trumpeted by the "medical and lay press . . . are rubbish."

Lack of success "by competent investigators has given faddists and enthusiasts of all sorts too much opportunity to air their irresponsible views," he declared. These sensational pronouncements contributed to the present confusion. Because of these outlandish claims, "people who give money for [legitimate] research demand quick results." Careful researchers were pressured to go public, "whether right or ready for publication or not." The consequence was a blizzard of pronouncements uttered "before they are mature."[3]

Bashford complained about expectations that he and other cancer researchers had helped create. Their repeated contention that cancer was the modern human plague, poised to overwhelm even tuberculosis, heightened public awareness and anxiety about the disease. Their claim that they alone held the power to remedy that situation, and to do so quickly, raised their visibility and granted them authority beyond all reason. This argument of essentialism proved necessary to achieve the station they demanded—the establishment and perpetuation of cancer research laboratories and, then, cancer hospitals. Victims of self-proclaimed expectations, when they failed to deliver what they promised on schedule, others filled that void.

Bashford was hardly alone in recognizing the failure of the cancer laboratory dream. Czerny also concluded that cancer laboratories failed to achieve their purpose. They did not lack for energy or an abiding sense of mission. What they were missing was simply what they promised: the swift, complete conquest of cancer. Every year, noted a weary Czerny months after he resigned his Heidelberg position, "we hear of new discoverers who promise more or less infallible results, but close examination of their specifics shows their worthlessness." As he ended his career, he reluctantly acknowledged "that a specific cure for cancer...perhaps never would be found." When directly asked about cancer during a public meeting in Berlin, Wassermann sadly noted that it had "resisted medical skill, chiefly because the cause" evaded researchers. Prospects seemed dim. The newly appointed director of the medical department of the Kaiser Wilhelm Society for Scientific Research wondered if it "would ever be eradicated."[4]

Wassermann, Czerny, and Bashford were perhaps the three most prominent cancer laboratory directors outside of Ehrlich. The three of them had come to the same conclusion. Institutions like theirs had failed to conquer cancer. Several American laboratory directors shared their pessimistic sentiment. Columbia's Wood pointed out that, "despite the most painstaking experimental study," the past three decades of cancer research had generated "a surprisingly small harvest." Just "a few words suffice to sum up all that we know" regarding cancer. "No simple chemical or complex organic body seems to have any permanent influence on tumor growth," he noted. Chemotherapeutic agents "have not the slightest curative power." Physical agents, such as x-rays and radium, treated only superficial lesions. Cornell's Ewing offered a similarly stark assessment. "I have to confess," he started, that "I do not contemplate the early subjugation of cancer. . . . I do not look for any startling advances or sensational discoveries, either in the etiology or therapeutics of cancer. I do not think the citadel will ever be stormed." Rous, the effective director of the Rockefeller's cancer efforts, found himself even "unable to say" if a cure for cancer would occur during "our lifetime." But he thought that more likely than the larger question of determining what actually caused cancer. No matter how distant, he remained sure that a cancer cure "will be discovered before the cause of the disease is known."[5]

Others inside and outside cancer laboratories shared the directors' pessimism. Joseph Louis Ransohoff, an orthopedic surgeon at the Cincinnati Hospital, argued that despite a worldwide web of "richly-endowed and manned" cancer laboratories, virtually no progress towards subduing the disease had been made. That goal remained "as distant as it was ten years ago." "It is not even known whether or not cancer is an infectious disease. . . . Little has been learned." Nothing had become so, but research nonetheless continued apace, "hoping, ever hoping that some day the goal may be reached." Charles E. Woodruff, editor of *American Medicine*, cut immediately to the chase. "The study of cancer is being prosecuted all over the world more vigorously than any other disease," he wrote, "Much money is being subscribed to the work." Despite these Herculean efforts, he concluded that "the cause seems no nearer discovery than it ever was." Samuel Squire Sprigge, *The Lancet*'s editor in 1911, said it simply: "The etiology of cancer is still mystery." David Von Hansemann, one of the giants of German immunology, took it to the next level. He came "to the conclusion that it will never be possible to find a specific remedy for cancer." Orth, then chairman of the Comité, concurred. "We know approximately nothing," Orth maintained. "We know nothing about the pathogen of cancer."[6]

Profound disillusionment about the fruits of cancer laboratory research, coupled with an equally frank assessment of its meager short term possibilities, marked a fundamental shift in thinking about that research. The initial mission—a swift resolution to the cancer question—was no longer tenable. Forty years of futility had effectively demonstrated the folly of that view. Cancer seemed to defy conquest. And with the demise of that objective as a realistic, imminent goal came an entirely different mission: managing cancer. Researchers managed cancer not by uncovering its cause but by preventing its inception. The focus changed to avoiding or removing those specific situations and conditions in which cancer was known to emerge. Cancer could be prevented, not subdued, managed, not conquered. That had been the genesis for the various campaigns outlined in the last two chapters. Analogy followed analogy. Researchers considered irritants, cell accelerants, and heredity. They examined the proximate cause—the auxiliary factors—rather than the specific, necessary causative agent. They reasoned back from the onset of cancer to determine the proximate cause, using statistics, examining heredity, or considering cultural habits and practices. Investigators disaggregated data, focusing instead on the individual occurrence to reveal critical factors. Both proximate and actual causes seemed necessary to produce cancer, but delineating one of those causes now seemed somewhat attainable. That dominated the research agenda.

An almost manic search for a means to diagnose cancer before it became symptomatic emerged as a fundamental thrust of the new managerial effort. The sooner that emergent cancer was detected, the more likely the behaviors or conditions that facilitated it could be discerned. This was critical because, as Roswell Park noted in frustration, incipient *"cancer as a disease"*—cancer readily susceptible to the knife—*"has absolutely no symptomology of its own."*[7] Investigators recognized precedent for examination of blood reactions to detect disease. That technique served as the basis for the Wassermann and Widal tests for syphilis and thyroid issues, respectively. Researchers postulated that an analogous situation might exist for cancer and so embarked on a two-pronged program. They adapted extant tests, hoping to see a possible agglutination or other reaction, and they tried to develop new cancer-specific tests.

Two Pavia researchers, M. Ascoli and G. Izar, developed an agglutination-based technique expressly for cancer that initially drew considerable comment. It proved extremely subtle. This practically invisible phenomenon required an ether or alcohol extract of proposed cancerous material and blood serum from the same individual. When mixed together, agglutination occurred but was visually imperceptible. The binding together of the complements altered the fluid's surface tension. The Italians developed an apparatus to detect the variation. Their initial tests indicated an 88 percent success rate.[8]

Subsequent experiments failed to sustain enthusiasm. Other methods drew adherents. Some researchers simply measured quantities of ferments in the blood. There, Beard's trypsin work provided inspiration, but Beard was not the only model cancer investigators co-opted. Attempts to develop skin tests for cancer, akin to the tuberculin test for tuberculosis, received attention. Others focused on the biological products of cancer. Measuring a cancer patient's urine for excessive sulfur was a staple of the professional literature. Still others sought a biologically sensitive means to detect the slightest variation in blood chemistry to diagnose incipient cancers. Two Yale University professors, Frank Underhill and Lorande Woodruff, found paramecium an apt experimental animal.[9]

None of these diagnostic measures bore up. Experimenters in different venues announced radically dissimilar outcomes, as differences over the most mundane facets of these tests proved the most notorious basis for dispute. Increasingly, investigators questioned the likelihood that cancer would yield to a diagnostic stemming from relatively familiar principles. This despair arose from the idea that, "with respect to complement deviation, allergy, specific precipitation and hemolysis," cancer sufferers did not seem "constantly peculiar in any way." With established principles proving disappointing, investigators considered fresh approaches, taking what was known about cancer to postulate a new means to identify the disruptions necessary to produce the disease.

Such was the approach of two German researchers, Ernst Freund and Gisa Kaminer. Rather than search for antibodies and antiserum produced when the body was exposed to cancer, they maintained that the natural state of an organism was cancer free; healthy individuals were free of some essential substance necessary for cancer to gain a foothold, or possessed some as yet unidentified substance that forbade cancer from erupting. Only when that prerequisite substance was either created by cellular action or the natural preventive was destroyed—action in either case spawned by chronic irritation or whatever precursor—could cancer find a tantalizing site upon which to nest. Indeed, Freund and Kaminer, in the spirit of the great Ehrlich, even suggested the chemical formula—it was an organic acid—and stereochemical shape of this anticipated cancer receptacle. Their initial experiment indicated that their diagnostic test produced a mere 12 percent error, a more than acceptable rate when no other diagnostic means existed.

The Freund/Kaminer method accounted for cancer's onset without pretending to understand what actually caused the disease. The test measured only the physical manifestation of susceptibility, an interesting work-around during a time of great frustration over the cancer quest. Investigators continued to disagree over the disease's cause, but they had achieved something of a consensus that it required an initiator. They disagreed about the identification of the initiator but generally believed it manifested or left a physical presence. The two Germans merely tried to explain and quantify that physical incidence.[10]

The Germans' technique seemed promising, but another diagnostic drew even more attention. It too received impetus from an examination of what cancer actually entailed, in this case that cancer at its essence was nothing more than rapid cellular division and growth. Emil Abderhalden, a Swiss biochemist, created this technique, though not originally for cancer. He was interested in pregnancy. He hoped to find some biochemical measure to determine pregnancy before its visual manifestations. He conceived of a more general phenomenon first. Abderhalden maintained that the healthy body was stable, its biochemical activities constant. That changed radically when something put the body out of harmony. It caused the body to produce what he called "defensive ferments," substances aimed at restoring harmony by countering the cause of the disorder. To his mind, pregnancy was just such an imbalance. Rapid growth of a foreign substance—the fetus—exposed the body to a new stimuli, and the body responded by unleashed a barrage of biochemical agents—digestive enzymes—to set matters right. Abderhalden claimed to be able to measure those ferments and thus to diagnose pregnancy. He and others soon adapted his test to measure the body's response to the other common form of rapid cellular growth, cancer. Indeed, pregnancy and cancer were deemed analogous because they presented similar profiles. Both were manifested by tumor-like growths. Both occurred in specific loci; cancers emerged at sites prepared for their emergence.

Initial tests on cancer patients showed a nearly 99 percent correlation. The diagnostic recognized pregnant women with similar surety. Subsequent experiments recorded positives for syphilis, acute infections, goiter, tuberculosis, and a host of other maladies. The myriad agents producing positives was a problem for the diagnosis of cancer, but the fact that the Abderhalden test measured the ferment's presence on a sliding continuum made things even more complex. Traces of the ferment were almost always present. A positive reaction came from "strong powers of digestion," essentially a greater quantity of the ferment.

Reading the Abderhalden test proved an art, not a science. And artistic sense was not distributed equally among the members of the medical and scientific community. Debates raged in the literature about just how effective the new diagnostic was. Freund, for example, claimed that the test failed for 18.4 percent of clinically pregnant women and reported that 53.1 percent of men and non-pregnant women presented false positives. Abderhalden himself attributed dubious results "to faulty techic [*sic*]." Another researcher found the test a faithful diagnostic for pregnancy only "if it was possible to exclude other conditions . . . such as cancer, tuberculosis, nephritis, exophthalmic goiter and fever from any cause." It certainly was not a panacea. Its inability to provide clear, definitive results brought cancer no closer to resolution.[11]

The lack of an effective diagnostic agent, coupled with a campaign to vanquish cancer that seemed no closer to its end than it had at its beginning, proved extremely troubling. Statisticians throughout the western world were virtually unanimous in arguing that cancer cases were increasing. Many European countries under the auspices of the IACI had created cancer commissions and similar organizations to undertake systematic compilation of cancer mortality rates. Often based on surveys filled out by practitioners, these state-based groups reported soaring rates of cancer for almost every tabulated subpopulation. Some pointed to exponential increases.[12]

Bashford was almost alone in disagreeing with the statistical assessment. As he had for at least a decade, Bashford maintained that cancer was not necessarily increasing. It was simply being reported somewhat more reliably.

Nowhere did Bashford find the situation more egregious than the United States. In 1911, only twenty-two states had any sort of death registration law. Even then procedures were rarely reliably followed. As significant, no two states conformed to the exact same reporting criteria. The Census Bureau worked to encourage states to adopt uniformity but with less than ideal results. As a consequence, the bureau produced its own tabulations, which were also deeply flawed. Bashford insisted that more dependable, more refined cancer mortality statistics would reveal a quite different pattern than the manifest increases so loudly proclaimed. Cancer might or might not be on the increase but he was certain that it had changed differentially. It surely increased among some groups, such as those engaging in what he had long considered predisposing behaviors, and declined among those who abandoned those risky activities. What was presented in the United States and elsewhere, he contended, were "vague rumors," not science. These reports were "figures," not statistics.

Always the laboratory researcher, Bashford demanded certitude, definitive, unambiguous results. Absence of such discriminating data rendered conclusions speculative. It was that belief that compelled Bashford to take out after quackery, theories and practices not supported by scientific rigor. That sense had also led Bashford to oppose England's entry into the IACI. Its data collecting propositions were, to Bashford, deeply flawed and unsustainable. The data IACI affiliates sought to gather and the uses to which it would be put would threaten scientific efforts to determine cancer's cause. Such was the case in most of the rest of Europe, where various national and state agencies gathered data, issued conclusions, and implemented imperfect research strategies derived from those bogus accumulations. Questionable, perhaps even spurious data led investigators down false paths and undermined their hard fought credibility.[13]

Intellectually isolated, Bashford battled the cancer increase crowd. Others mobilized around the death of the idea of swiftly conquered cancer. Extremely active in the United States, those questioning cancer's quick banishment also spoke of the "cancer problem," but defined it very differently than had cancer laboratory denizens. They began from the presumption that cure was elusive, perhaps a pipe dream. Even attempts to create a diagnostic were unfulfilled. Cancer seemed unconquerable, at least for the foreseeable future.

John B. Deaver, a noted Philadelphia surgeon, provided a quick recap of the unsuccessful history of cancer laboratory research. "With a rise of bacteriology there came the hope that . . . we might find the causative factor of malignant processes." It "has failed us." Investigators have found no evidence that cancer "is directly transmissible in the way than infectious diseases are." Then "protozoan disease came to the forefront." That disease agent too did not provide "solution to the cancer problem." The cause of "malignant disease . . . remains beyond our understanding." We "still are well nigh powerless when it comes to malignant tumors." Laboratory diagnosis remained elusive. We have not "discovered any specific serum or hemolytic reaction in patients suffering from cancer." Several have been "suggested, but are equal in their lack of true value." A "serum reaction for carcinoma has proven but a false hope, defective and not valuable."[14]

Charles Eucharist de Medicis Sajous, professor of therapeutics at Temple University Medical School and editor of the *New York Medical Journal*, offered a similarly damning assessment. He noted that the cancer quest had monopolized "the energies of hundreds of men . . . in attempt to find the cause and to effect a cure of whatever that cause may be." What had "been accomplished along these lines," Sajous asked. "Are we any nearer an understanding of the problem now than fifty years ago?" Again, failure to develop even a simple blood test for cancer provoked profound disappointment. "Immune reactions with serum have been attempted, but have proved of no use. The blood has been examined for the presence or absence of many substances, but unsuccessfully." The research seemed futile. "All sorts of schemes have been attempted," he noted pessimistically. "At present there is no way of telling what it is that one is dealing with."[15]

Sajous, Deaver, and like-minded medical men were deeply affected by the failure to find cancer's agent. There would be no quick resolution. There would be no decisive victory over the disease. Cancer was part of contemporary life, something to be accommodated, to be managed. Charles H. Castle, editor of the *Lancet-Clinic*, encapsulated the situation neatly. "Wanting exact knowledge"—something the laboratories had failed to provide—"what has empiricism taught us?" W. A. Bryan, professor of surgery at Vanderbilt University, operationalized that point of view. He called on his colleagues "to accept our ignorance of the cause of cancer" and to use their clinical and surgical experience to move beyond it.[16]

In that context, the twin presumptions that cancer always began as a local disease and that it usually originated at specific sites in or on the body made liable to it emerged with considerable force. Baltimore's deliciously named Joseph Bloodgood, longtime professor of surgery at Johns Hopkins, presented this unequivocal assessment. "Cancer never begins in healthy tissue," he claimed. "There is always a preexisting local defect which is benign and in which later there may be a cancerous development." That nugget of semi-truth offered an opportunity to manage or control the disease. Sajous articulated the requisite call to arms clearly, taking care to separate cancer control from the failed attempt at conquest. "The laboratory worker is busy with his research." It remained for physicians and surgeons—men "in the fighting line"—to constantly strive to identify cancer at the earliest moment "when complete removal is possible." Deaver was more adamant. He implored medical practitioners and surgeons of their duty to identify uncompromisingly "all malignant growths," reminding them that all were "purely local processes at the onset."[17]

William J. Mayo, a leading American surgeon and later a founder of the Mayo Clinic, expanded the argument to incorporate the entire human body. In his presidential address before the American Surgical Association, he agreed that physicians and surgeons must look upon local lesions as an invitation to cancer without regard to just what the "actual cause of cancer may be." Mayo maintained it equally true both on and inside the body. "The mass of evidence" demonstrated "chronic irritation in its various forms and types" stood as "the most important factor in the development of cancer" in areas "exposed to the eye." Was it not logical to "conclude that cancer on the inner surfaces of the body depends on the same precancerous conditions?" That assumption called on medical men and women to treat every internal disorder as if it constituted a precancerous condition. "Gall-stones, duodenal ulcer, fecal stones in the appendix, or intestinal lesions," as well as hyperacidity, were conditions likely to produce cancer. When confronted by these maladies, surgeons needed to remove them, a strategy that would often save lives. It prevented cancer's occurrence. James Alexander Lindsay, president of the medical section of the Royal Academy of Medicine in Ireland, readily agreed. "To procrastinate until the proof of disease is complete is a feeble policy," he wrote. It produced only "a disastrous loss of time" and, likely, life.[18]

Deaver took the matter a step further. He called on surgeons when confronted with a suspicious case history or otherwise worrisome symptomology to undertake an "autopsy in vivo." Literally a "living autopsy," Deaver's course of treatment encouraged surgeons to cut deep in the body at the slightest provocation, to rule out possible cancer or precancerous lesions. To do otherwise was inhumane. "We offer the patient a far better chance of recovery by early and perhaps useless operation than by delay and surely useless operation." Frequent exploratory surgery was a valid preventive, essential to cancer control. "We must then of necessity operate in some cases in which our diagnosis is not confirmed if we are to seize upon the favorable moment for any of those in which we have correctly appreciated the lesion present." Deaver urged surgeons to undertake radical operations, even surgeries that would result in gross anatomical deformities, as a patient's best hope. Such aggressive, often disfiguring surgery would provide cancer victims the greatest opportunity to prevent an otherwise inexorable demise. Once the disease ceased being site specific, it was incurable.[19]

Public and professional education campaigns were the natural consequence of the aforementioned sentiments. Teaching the public and physicians to recognize possible lesions as soon as possible and to understand that sudden surgical intervention might well be their only hope led to expeditious surgery and perhaps fewer cancer fatalities. Surgeons and others initiated the movement in their local and state professional societies and used the earlier anti-tuberculosis crusade as a model. The insurance industry also participated. Among the new movement's most memorable facets was the creation of the American Society for the Control of Cancer, later known as the American Cancer Society, to coordinate public and professional education campaigns nationwide. *JAMA* put it simply. The new organization's tasks were "to educate the public on the symptomology of cancer and the imperative need of early diagnosis and immediate steps."[20]

Early detection was joined by prevention as a second focus of the crusade to control cancer. Prevention lacked the specificity of early detection. No one knew the cause of cancer and its contributing factors were subject to dispute. Nonetheless, the matter was too important to ignore. In a number of works, Francis Albert Rollo Russell systematically laid out the parameters of what behaviors or practices might encourage cancer. The son of the British prime minister and a former president of the English Meteorological Society, Russell scrutinized travelogues and ethnologies and gathered various statistics from across Europe and America to highlight what he called "preventable cancer." "The habits of a nation, men, women, and children, have a great deal to do with the preparation of the 'soil,' the constitution, for cancer," Russell argued. These cultural practices comprised "unpremeditated experiments;" they constituted "an extension of science into common life." Individuals needed only to learn about and modify these deleterious actions and activities to drastically reduce the disease.[21]

A subtle undercutting of the laboratory's relationship to the public weal often accompanied these educational crusades. Control was immediate. Research was distant. Research had been tried and found wanting. Surgery at first sign of cancer was hopeful, the patients' sole lifesaving possibility. The public and professional emphasis on control elevated in importance the groups that provided the opportunity of control—physicians and surgeons—while it devalued those men and women involved in other pursuits. Cancer laboratories had become tangential. Their investigators' self-acknowledged frustration with their inability to conquer cancer set them outside the cancer control movement.

Cancer laboratories suffered repercussions from their public mea culpa. They depended directly on governments or beneficence for support. These institutions and their research hospitals were quite expensive ventures. Salaries needed to be paid regularly, and laboratory and hospital equipment continually purchased. Their impetus and funding stemmed from a promise of success in the endeavor for which they were created. Cancer labs and hospitals would identify quickly the cause of cancer, and that identification would free humanity of the scourge. Without that prospect to buttress them, the institutions would be forced to reduce their efforts, to curtail their initiatives. In effect, the quest to conquer cancer itself needed to be controlled. Its proponents were compelled to lower their sights and to offer a set of diminished expectations as they begged for public and private funding.

With the diminution in the cancer laboratories' and hospitals' panoramas came a decline in their investigators' authority. Cancer laboratory researchers had even less ability to make things so. They remained part of the scientific enterprise, of course, but without the moral authority provided by optimistic, critical prospects, they lacked the suasion necessary to convince others to defer to their dicta. They became even less adept at reining in the speculators, the ignorant, the less qualified, the unscrupulous, the quacks. Their method prevailed and provided them a sense of gravitas, but the accouterments of that method were missing and so was their ability to participate ex cathedra. They were reduced to being one voice among many, still a potent voice perhaps, but no longer a dominant presence. Without the promise of sudden victory, their research had lost its immediacy. And it was that immediacy that had provided the researchers their unique attributes. They had become cogs in the cancer machine. The editor of the *Lancet-Clinic* phrased the new synthesis in this way. "In thousands of laboratories biologists are at work," he wrote. "In many another institution the essentially clinical aspects of the disease are being studied. At innumerable bedsides experts are seeking statistical knowledge of the essential nature of cancer."[22] This multidimensional assault would control cancer.

Cancer laboratories did not go quietly into that good night. Their investigators championed the laboratory's unchanging mission, centrality, and continuance even as it had lost primacy. Such a staunch defense was essential. Now more than ever, laboratories needed to justify their continued existence. Funding—their lifeblood—depended on it. J. G. Adami, head of the cancer laboratory at McGill University, offered a typical justification. He acknowledged that "despite the labors of generations of investigators the cause of cancer was still undetermined." He also recognized that the situation would likely persist. But Adami refused to alter course. He insisted that the sole way to progress was through application of Francis Bacon's old aphorism, "vere scire est per causas scire,"—real knowledge is knowing causes—"the etiological method." This was the method of true science. He reported a familiar, if tired, litany. "The treatment and control of tuberculosis, diphtheria, and other infections during the past thirty years dated from the moment at which the causative agents were determined, or failing that (as was the case of yellow fever) dated from the time when employing rigid analogy, the nature of the disease became realized." To Adami and like-minded men and women, "detection of the cause" of a disease always "threw light upon the mode of prevention of an allied disease." There was no other "solution to the problem" than investigating "the nature of normal tissue growth, into the life history of malignant growths, and so into the cause or causes of neoplasms." Only then could cancer be conquered.[23]

Wood, too, considered cancer laboratories essential and demanded that medical practitioners impress that view on the public. He admitted "laboratory research is slow and enormously expensive" and that a way to treat cancer "may be fifty years from now; it may be longer." But he thought persistence of laboratory research essential and public criticism misplaced. "We amiably spend $10,000,000 for a battleship, which is out of date by the time it is complete, and yet criticize the scanty results which the expenditure of $5,000 produces towards discovering the cause of cancer." That was not the sole comparison Wood used. He excoriated governments for their lack of adequate support "for an enormous field of investigation, . . . one far more complex and difficult than that of contagious disease." Instead of investing in cancer's cause, most states remained "more interested in the diseases of cattle than in those of man, as the endowment of agricultural schools and stations shows." Part of the problem stemmed from the laboratories themselves. Starved for funding, they curried public favor by leaking any promising possibility long before it was confirmed. "Premature publication," Wood noted, only causes public "distrust of the final results." Notwithstanding the laboratories' culpability, Wood maintained it the physicians' and surgeons' obligation to "quiet the public clamor for immediate results." This was their position in the cancer research nexus. Doctors must explain "how slow and difficult this laboratory work is, how complex the problem presented," as researchers continued the search "to kill with chemicals a certain portion of the body and not kill the rest of it because cancer is a real part of the human body just run wild."[24]

Incorporating public outreach in the scientific nexus further distanced, and even diminished, cancer laboratory research. It now stood as only one facet of this new synthesis. It surely was no longer the most visible, the most essential, or even the most optimistic, the place where the seminal breakthrough would occur. Public information, swift visits to physicians whenever symptomology presented itself, routine visits otherwise, and the skill of an aggressive surgeon had emerged as the bulwark against cancer, at that time and for the immediate future. The AACR recognized the new formulation when the group, in 1913, called on all the nation's medical schools to remedy their "seriously deficient . . . instruction of medical students in the symptoms and early diagnosis of cancer." It did not stop there, however. The group needed also to decide "the proper methods for approaching the public on the subject of cancer." In fact, they pledged that the AACR "at the present" would "chiefly confine" its activities "to the education of the medical profession."[25]

Support—beneficence and governmental—needed to go to the campaign, not the distant prayer of some miraculous cure or revolutionary advance. That was a shocking admission for the AACR to make. It was not that research ceased to have meaning; it simply stopped having immediacy. With cure and cause believed well down the road, proximity to public agencies was lost.

Cancer research laboratories could not look to their IACI for salvation. Under German domination, the IACI increasingly downplayed cancer laboratory research and focused instead on accumulating statistics. As significant, the IACI relied on medical practitioners to create the statistical portraits. It was the statistical initiative, especially the presumption that the IACI could forge an international cancer demography, that offended Bashford. He complained that such an adventure would prove meaningless. Without sufficient understanding to frame statistical questions appropriately and without specially designed researchers to accomplish this framing, the result would likely be pernicious. Investigators and ever dear resources would be channeled down otherwise unsustainable avenues of inquiry. Cancer laboratories would be the primary institutional victim of that intellectual misappropriation.

The IACI's movement away from concentrating on cancer's cause was reflected in its official rendering of the 1910 meeting. Statistics and tumor nomenclature received "special attention" there, and "Aetiology, etc. were also discussed." Bashford's other objection—the domination of German interests to the exclusion of almost all others—also found its way into the official record. Like the English, the French also chafed at Germany's subversion of the IACI to its vision, control, and goals. The French sought to break that stranglehold, a stranglehold based on where the IACI's central office was located, and so offered a motion to rotate the IACI's headquarters (which had been at Berlin) among IACI nation states.[26] Location of the central office dictated where the organization held its regular business meetings. Those meetings set most IACI policy. Members from nearby areas always far outnumbered those from distant lands. The result was that IACI pronouncements and action reflected the interests of the German autocracy.

A "very lively discussion" took place. The IACI tabled the motion but promised to address it next year in Dresden at the International Hygienic Exposition. There, a cancer display would grace a pavilion for each IACI country. Another motion in Paris also galvanized attention, again relating to just how international the IACI was. The Italian Cancer Committee wanted all IACI proceedings and documents translated and published in Italian. Both the Spanish and Russian delegations asked that the same material be published in their native tongues. The German-dominated IACI refused the language request.[27]

The French understood the significance of taking up its central office motion in Dresden. Meeting in a city in the heart of Germany meant that the German delegation would numerically overwhelm all others and that its decision would carry the day. To forestall that event, the French demanded that the IACI formally declare its adoption of the French initiative prior to the Dresden meeting. Failure to do so would produce a boycott of the meeting by the French and their supporters. The Germans refused to yield. The French followed through on their boycott of the Dresden meeting, where the French proposal was unanimously defeated.

That was not the sole initiative considered at Dresden.[28] The Germans also unveiled and pushed through their latest attempt to create a universal statistics form under the IACI's banner. The form offered little information of interest to cancer laboratories. It compiled data only for patients said to have succumbed to cancer. It defined those persons as persons so diagnosed "even though death resulted from another cause (suicide, apoplexy, etc.)." Medical men were to stand as the information-gathering and tabulating army. The form required the usual demographic data but also stipulated trade, place of occupation, and place where the patient fell ill. Medical questions asked included if the deceased had suffered from any preexisting conditions, such as syphilis, tuberculosis, trauma, or alcoholism. Doctors were to record if women had inflammation "in the sphere of the genital organs," whether they had worn pessaries, and the number of live births and abortions. The "primary seat and nature" of each cancer was to be noted. So, too, was any "previous sickness or lesions," whether cancers of the mouth had been preceded by smoking, when the initial symptom had been noticed, and when the disease actually commenced. Physicians reported the site of initial swelling in the "cases of relapses." Medical attendants described how they treated the disease—x-rays, radium, or surgery—and for how long. They were called upon to detail how their actions changed "the local and general condition of the patient," whether an autopsy took place, and whether microscopic examination of diseased tissues occurred.[29]

These questionnaires were hardly the stuff of laboratory science. They provided an apt demonstration of Bashford's intellectual objections. The "scientific" program of the Dresden meeting provided further confirmation. Czerny detailed the results of a therapy experiment, and Fichera reported on chemotherapeutic efforts. Several presented statistical summaries of cancer cases within their domain. The group passed a measure asking all member states to keep a list of cancer victims by family, so that they could determine if heredity factored in cancer. Papers on cancer's cause were absent.[30]

Lack of discussion about the cause of cancer demonstrated how far the IACI had moved from the question that had animated the organization. Within a month of the Dresden meeting, the French Association for the Study of Cancer Research resigned its membership in the IACI.[31] Whether its vassalage under German domination or the organization's failure to adhere to its mission caused the split remained unclear. What was critical was that the grand assembly to make things so was becoming more and more irrelevant.

With the French gone and the English intractable, the Germans tightened their grip on the IACI. They reduced the number of regular meetings and granted power to the Berlin-dominated executive committee to act on the society's behalf. The IACI also felt compelled to defend itself against the French and English complaints. It did so through analogy. Its executive secretary pointed to the International Medical Congress, which had just established a permanent home in the Hague, to suggest the French objection misplaced. At the same time, Meyer singled out the International Congress on Hygiene and Demography, which concentrated on gathering statistics, as validating the union's statistical metric. Both situations were far from analogous. The medical congress located its headquarters in a place established to avoid any country's undue influence, and the hygienic organization was established primarily to foster statistics.[32]

The IACI continued to recruit new nation states as members. Chile, Argentina, and the Philippines all expressed interest in joining. Jensen nominated his native Copenhagen as the site for its next international meeting, which it scheduled for 1916. The IACI set up cancer displays at the International Medical Congress's surgical and radiological sections.[33]

These were trappings of influence, nothing more. The IACI was exceedingly late setting the agenda for its 1913 Brussels meeting. Its first attempt feebly reflected the organization's new concentration on early detection and surgery. The four areas for which the group entertained paper submissions were chemotherapy and physical treatment of cancer, statistics, care of cancerous patients, and training of cancer-care nurses. The group placed a German in charge of recruiting papers for each section. Initial submissions came only from Germany and Belgium. The organization added two topics months later: vaccination against malignant growths and public education efforts against cancer in different countries. Like the four initial questions, the two new ones did not tackle the issue that had galvanized researchers to form the IACI. The group had moved heavily into treatment.[34]

At the last minute, a seventh topic was added. At Fibiger's insistence, he wanted to present to the group his nematode work. The IACI capitulated and made the etiology of cancer its seventh question.[35] The IACI's original desire to limit the meeting to questions of control rather than cause, and its placement of these questions in the hands of local leaders, meant that few outside the immediate environs learned about the meeting. That these endeavors occurred at the last minute—and were subsequently modified two times—prohibited most involved in these issues from attending or offering to present papers. Initial notices of the meeting agenda did not appear in medical journals until a few scant months before the conclave. When the IACI did meet in early August, the group was anything but international. Almost all the presentations came from German-speaking countries. England, the United States, and France had a total of three presenters. Apparently several people who promised to attend failed to do so. In a huge break with protocol, many of presenters did double duty, talking and commenting on two disparate topics.[36]

The Brussels meeting reported little progress on the IACI's key initiatives. The IACI's statistical form was not being followed, and few if any results were being sent to the IACI. The nomenclature committee was no more successful. It agreed only to use Latin- or Greek-derived roots to name all things cancer-related and to end all types of cancerous tumors with the suffix -oma. No systematic nomenclature or definition for cellular cancer emerged.[37]

So little happened at the international meeting that almost no medical or science journal outside of Germany reported on its proceedings or even listed highlights. None of the regular foreign correspondents even commented on the sessions. The meeting had been stillborn. While not admitting disappointment, Meyer acknowledged that the Brussels conclave accomplished far less than he had hoped. He refused to concede that the cancer quest had failed. The manner by which he chose to avoid the obvious involved a significant reorientation in the organization's aim. "The fight against the formidable foe of man must not cease unless we have attained a success," Meyer maintained. No one should assume that progress wasn't being made. Much had been accomplished in all areas except the IACI's primary purpose. Achieving that objective now seemed impertinent. To fixate on it was foolhardy and inhumane. "If we would merely wait inactively until some genius has some success in the domain of cancer research regarding the cause or even the cure of cancer disease, we would have to wait for many years," he admitted. Rather than secure an immediate and complete victory, the IACI pursued a new path. On this new path, the organization "will by all means and by our present work try to alleviate the torments and pain of cancerous patients as far as possible."[38]

That profound admission denigrated cancer laboratory researchers, reducing them to pie-in-the-sky dreamers. The real cancer work appreciated by the IACI was now to be diagnosis and surgery, although various remedies and palliatives would be applied. The only national organization of cancer researchers still affiliated with the IACI could not abide the international agency's revamped ambitions. Angered by German high-handedness, intransigence, and incompetence, as well as abandonment of the IACI's prime directive, the American Association for Cancer Research called a meeting several months after the Brussels debacle to discuss its future in the IACI. Researchers at this meeting recounted several grievances. The AACR maintained that the IACI's late and limited agenda prevented them from meaningful participation in the Brussels gathering. The IACI compounded this mistake with a powerful affront. It accepted as the official American delegation persons not appointed by the AACR. The IACI required subsidiary organizations to pay high dues, while the IACI provided no accounting of its finances. These injustices—a lack of respect and appreciation—caused the AACR to express its "strong feelings of dissatisfaction." The group concluded it had "not benefited" from IACI affiliation. The IACI's new agenda had deserted and rejected cancer laboratories. It made it abundantly clear "that the functions of the American Society for the Control of Cancer are more in accord with the purposes of the International Association." Consequently, the organization notified both the IACI and the ASCC of its decision to resign from the international body. To provide a home for cancer laboratory research, the AACR pledged to found and support its own journal, devoted entirely to the areas that the IACI had forsaken.[39]

The war in Europe impeded international cancer efforts. The moribund IACI officially became a war casualty. Its monthly periodical ceased publication in 1914. The planned Copenhagen meeting never happened. In fact, the IACI never held another international meeting. Physicians and surgeons throughout England and the continent mobilized to treat the wounded or to serve in other ways. Cancer research in Europe became almost an afterthought. Generations of mice used for cancer experiments were shipped to the United States to avoid becoming military casualties.[40]

In a number of other ways, 1915 was a watershed year in the cancer war. Bashford, intimately tied to the British cancer research effort and one of the longest standing research directors, resigned his post at the Imperial Cancer Research Fund. His spirit and health broken by the libel case and his failure to conquer cancer, Bashford was succeeded by James Alexander Murphy. Bashford's assistant for a decade, Murray lacked Bashford's fire and nose for controversy, preferring to engage in behind-the-scenes research.[41] Beebe, who had labored long to determine the chemistry of tumors and who had been a pillar of the AACR, allegedly began an affair with his graduate student, welched on a loan from his wife's sister, and began to hawk a vegetable extract as a cancer cure. He was soon dismissed from his post at Columbia and in the Crocker for cause.[42] Ehrlich and Wassermann both died, and their chemotherapeutic efforts collapsed.[43] With the military co-opting physicians, the great statistical army was not free to compile and record the fate of cancer patients. Leyden was long dead, and Czerny forced out of his Heidelberg perch. He died before the end of the year.[44] In the United States, the American Society for the Control of Cancer was in its ascendancy. Even though he was director of the Crocker, Wood found himself devoting considerable time to its efforts.[45] In 1915, the Pennsylvania Medical Society unveiled an ambitious program. It called on all medical journals to devote an issue to methods to increase public awareness about cancer detection. Some seventy-odd journals complied.[46]

Several investigators took the occasion of the dramatic moment to compile the cancer research of the previous decades. In a world of science, compilation, followed by systematization, was an important step to knowledge. Gathering what had been done in one format and then attempting to order it, or to allow the natural order to disclose itself, held the promise of enlightenment; it revealed patterns hidden to the otherwise unfocused eye. Such a project was not unique to the 1910s. Scientists had long undertaken literature reviews—articles that were little more than encyclopedic surveys of some aspects of cancer research—de rigueur. In 1907, and again in 1910, this practice created two huge compendiums that set out all the cancer research from the ancients through the past several decades. Jacob Wolff's *Die Lehre Von Der Krebskrankheit Von Den Ältesten Zeitsen Bis Zur Gegenwart* and John Thomas's *Le Cancer* both aimed to collect the universe of cancer knowledge less as a place from which to proceed than as a place from which to reason. The act of accumulation was tantamount to discovery, as the sum total of what had been done was subjected to the rational mind. Patterns were inevitably uncovered, and insight was the natural consequence.[47]

Insight did not materialize from these heavy volumes. Failure did not discredit the technique. A great quantity of cancer research was published in the years immediately before World War I, and two Americans tried to harness the new material. William H. Woglom published his *Studies in Experimental Cancer: A Review* as a way of drawing a base line for Columbia's new Crocker cancer effort. William Seaman Bainbridge, longtime gynecologist/surgeon at the New York Skin and Cancer Hospital, published his *The Cancer Problem* a year later, in 1914.

These magnificent tomes were testament to the Tower of Babel that had come to characterize cancer research. Contradictory research, disputes, and seemingly unrelated criteria puzzled the researchers as they tried to make sense out of the cacophony that constituted cancer research for the past forty-five years. These books were to help accomplish that. In a manifest Aristotelian way, the various activities, observations, and results were shoehorned into established, long-standing categories. For instance, Woglom, who had worked in England with Bashford, divided his data into earlier observations on the transmissibility of cancer, transplanted tumors, resistance, hypersusceptibility, spontaneous tumors, and tumors of a nature still undefined. While each major division had a series of subsections, Woglom's opus merely reflected a priori assumptions. It mirrored the status quo.[48]

Bainbridge's magnificent collection was only marginally better, but was certainly far broader. Bainbridge attempted to gather in his book all knowledge of cancer, not just cancer research. As a consequence, it had entire sections on treatments, diagnosis, radiology, surgery, and campaigns to have the public and physicians understand the important of early diagnosis and surgery. His cancer research part was more conventional. Although not a laboratory researcher, Bainbridge had attended the initial international cancer meeting in Heidelberg in 1906 and was a student of cancer investigation. This part of the work centered on causality. Statistical considerations, etiology, predisposing causes, histopathology, and immunity reactions each was received its own treatment.[49]

These beautiful compendiums were monuments to what had preceded them. Just as surely as if they had been built in concrete and stone, they were elaborate, man-made structures, the consequence of ideas. In this case, they memorialized the death of a dream, the dream of a quick victory over cancer, the dream that laboratory science held the key, the dream that the bacteriological vision and analogies among what was known and what was unknown would provide access to cancer's inner workings. The two tomes were fitting tributes to that vision.

These majestically constructed intellectual tombs housed many truths, of course, but their compilers remained oblivious. Surveying the causality literature, Bainbridge maintained that "the whole trend of investigation points not to a single cause" of cancer, "but to a number of causes." That nod to the then-current notion that each case of cancer required an irritating agency or agent, as well as the actual disease-causing entity, was followed up by another intriguing proposition. Despite the work of the previous decades, Bainbridge still believed that the term cancer masked several other distinct maladies. He noted that "syphilis, tuberculosis, actinomycosis, blastomycetes, and even leprosy . . . were formerly confused with cancer." All were "now known to be separate entities, each with its specific cause. Who can tell to what further extent this process of differentiation and isolation may lead," he concluded.[50]

Bainbridge interpreted the phenomena that he had recorded within the broad consensus of those who had generated it. Each earlier investigator had searched to pinpoint cancer's cause and each had presented their data. When researchers offered discordant results, efforts then revolved around two simple propositions. Either the results required homogenization or one was correct and the other in error. Analogies to previous experience—taking what was known and applying it as precedent to what was unknown to make it known—provided the measure upon which to decide most matters.

Things were rarely that clear. Persons could make different analogies about the very same situation or condition; by their very virtue of being like something but not necessarily exactly that something, analogies were never deterministic. Only opinions were deterministic. Analogies served as forum and focus for contentiousness. In this case, Bainbridge followed in well trodden footsteps. He forced the data to fit his preconceived notions of how disease operated.

In 1915, two prominent researchers did something very different. They shunned established models and offered a radically different explanation for cancer's cause. Their methods were, at first glance, strikingly similar to those that had preceded them. They laid out the evidence that investigators had uncovered during the past several decades and placed it in categories.

But rather than attempt to square the circle—to find the best analogy for often contradictory evidence—they disaggregated it. Rather than an Aristotelian approach, they attempted something more akin to Lord Bacon and decided that new categories of analysis were required.

Surprisingly, the peripatetic Gaylord was the inaugural voice of this conceptual shift. In a piece published in early 1915, Gaylord began in what, for him, was a characteristic way. He launched first into a defense of the parasitic theory of cancer. In Gaylord's archeology, his own trout research, along with Rous's and Fibiger's experiments, were central. This research proved that a parasitic agent operated in cancer. Once he declared victory for his long-held theory, he then moved on to the new idea. He disentangled cancer. He pulled out various research results, and the threads with them, and took them at face value. Again, Rous, Fibiger, and Gaylord himself were at the heart of the new notion. Each offered a different cancer pathway and mechanism. Rather than a single disease, Gaylord now concluded that cancer was a category of diseases, a collective noun. Cancer, in Gaylord's formulation, defined a class of diseases, each of which has a similar series of symptoms, clinical manifestations, and cellular pathology, but which also remained distinctive entities. As distinctive entities, each cancer could have its own agent. Searching for *the* cause of cancer was, therefore, nonsensical. Cancers had many causes, although Gaylord deemed different filterable viruses a major culprit for many of these diseases. What exactly a filterable virus was, Gaylord remained unsure. He recognized what he called inclusions within many tumors, and within diseases, produced by filterable viruses generally, and wondered if they constituted a chemical or living agency. In the end, however, it did not matter. Filterable viruses were but one cause for cancers.

Gaylord summed up his new view in clear terms. "Cancer," he argued, "represents a great group of pathological changes having many points of similarity which have led us to classify them under one head, cancer." In "this group there must be a great range of agents," he reasoned, "probably a number of specific viruses which we have yet to discover and to study." The "cancer problem"—the subject around which Gaylord and other cancer laboratory researchers had repeatedly framed their results and arguments—"will be broken up into a great field" of distinctive causalities. To nail down these numerous cancer-causing agents "will require many years of patient and extensive work of many investigators."[51]

Gaylord's work was illustrative. It was not based on a new discovery. Everything he cited had been in the public domain for some time and had been known to cancer researchers far longer. What marked Gaylord's theory as different was that it was conceived from a different premise, a premise at odds with the ideas that had guided research for nearly a half century. It took the inability to find the cause of cancer as a failure, not of people and performance, but of thought. Rather than accept a model used for decades, Gaylord advocated what was an essentially pluralistic theory. It rendered cancer a composite rather than a single disease.

Ewing offered a similar view at the end of 1915. Unlike Gaylord, he had no specific ax to grind. In his years affiliated with Cornell, he had weighed in on the cancer conquest battle from many sides. In that sense, Ewing was an agnostic, not wedded as a partisan to any view except the dominant view—cancer was a disease with a specific cause. His early work with canines and the transmission of cancer through genital transplant during coitus marked him as a careful researcher. In was no wonder, then, that two relatively recent works of great care captivated Ewing. He took particular note of Rous's work with chicken sarcoma, especially his demonstration that three distinct agents seemed to account for three different kinds of tumors. He also admired Fibiger's exquisite work with a specific type of cockroach and a certain kind of gastric carcinoma in rats. The work of both of these men had detractors. Several argued that the cancer they uncovered was not cancer at all, but a type of benign tumor, a theory that helped explain why such conscientious researchers got the profoundly interesting results that they had.

Ewing was having none of that. Rous's and Fibiger's great skill and care as investigators meant to Ewing that both men were correct in their observations. And, for that to be the case, the assumption that had challenged them must be wrong. Rather than a single entity with one cause, cancer was surely a mass of diseases. Rous's and Fibiger's contributions, Ewing argued, "seem to me to point to the necessity of regarding all forms of neoplasms as specific diseases." These diseases were "connected only by the fact that they are neoplastic in greater or less degree, but differing in their etiology, clinical course and therapeutic possibilities." He then offered his own analogy about how drastic his reconceptualization of cancer was: "Tuberculosis and bubonic plague are infectious diseases of inflammatory nature." In Ewing's mind, those two diseases were "quite as closely related as Fibiger's gastric carcinoma of rats and pipe smokers' cancer of the lip." We must "abandon" the "habit of regarding cancer as a protean disease of uniform significance." The "interests of progress" demanded it. "When cancer research properly occupies itself in the study of the distinctive features of different cases of malignant disease, especially when it abandons the idea of a universal cure for cancer, it will be in accord with sound pathological sense."[52]

Ewing's and Gaylord's new approach to cancer did nothing to undermine the public information awareness campaign. Indeed, it provided a potent explanation for why it was critical. Since cancer was a composite disease, comprised of numerous neoplastic disorders, each with its own etiology, pathology, and prognosis, prevailing on medical men and the public to recognize the specific malady at its earliest state was the sole recourse. Therapists and laboratory scientists might develop a means to fight one of the several cancers, but the others would persist. Early diagnosis, which now must include differentiation by cancer type, was the only sustainable approach.

The two New Yorkers' theory of cancer was the final nail in the coffin for the idea that cancer would be susceptible to a swift resolution. Control was now all that mattered in the battle, because it was all that could be achieved in the foreseeable future. At the same time, however, the multivariate view of cancer resurrected the cancer laboratory. Rather than one disease to conquer, they now needed to learn the intricacies of many similar but different neoplastic diseases, as well as how to differentiate among them. The immediate pressure to find a sudden strike to end the human plague of cancer had been transformed into a more deliberate, even systematic, investigation into the minutiae of each of the now seemingly separable neoplastic maladies.

The pluralist cancer model also reduced the making something so conundrum to human proportions. Results and observations no longer were true or false, black or white. Truth was relative, something in a particular context. Context became essential. Many investigators reporting on similar phenomena could be right once it was recognized that the measurements and data they published referred to different neoplastic diseases, diseases that could be differentiated by type of cell, tissue and organ attacked, the type of tumor produced, and mechanisms that generated them. This model was far more complicated than that which had engendered turn-of-the-century cancer laboratories. Yet its articulation helped resolve one of the fundamental tensions that had made cancer laboratories critical. The new cancer definition could make things so, simply by defining away everything else. It could not conquer cancer. It could only redefine cancer into something manageable. And it provided medical men and others with a new analogy to apply.

Epilogue

And the Band Plays On

In 1915, Frederick L. Hoffman, statistician for the Prudential Insurance Company of America, published his magnum opus, *The Mortality From Cancer Throughout the World*.[1] Two hundred pages of text followed by six hundred pages of statistical tables, the tome argued that, despite the lack of any sort of statistical consistency or comparability, the numbers showed that cancer in the world was increasing everywhere and at rates heretofore unanticipated. That menacing fact held important implications, and Hoffman set out to list some of the various behaviors, traits, and activities that made certain groups of citizens more liable to the disease than others. He also devoted himself to what he called life insurance medicine. His figuring demonstrated that individuals with cancer life insurance had significantly higher incidences of cancer than general populations, an important revelation for his employers and their trade association.

Hoffman's fundamental argument was that more and better statistics were necessary, because they would help pinpoint exactly which behaviors were risky behaviors. They would indicate levels of risk—something necessary to factor into insurance premiums—and alert well-designing men and women to exactly which behaviors they should work to get the great mass of humanity to cease.

There was more than an element of morality in the work, and Hoffman framed almost the entire book without discussion of cancer's cause. The book was nothing less than a call to immediate action. Hoffman sought to galvanize publics to move swiftly and decisively. He wanted people to act—to change before they got cancer. He wanted cancer rates greatly reduced, and he believed statistics held the key.

Despite Hoffman's confidence in statistics' inevitable mitigation of cancer rates, he had not constructed his book simply with statisticians in mind. His dedication told the story. It was "dedicated to the American Society for the Control of Cancer and the American Association for Cancer Research." These two representative organizations reflected the twin pillars of the world's first war against cancer—a cadre of professionals undertaking specialized research of a certain stripe to discover cancer's cause and perennial campaigns by those professionals dispossessed, or at least marginalized, by that new elite to get people to seek a surgeon at the first sign of cancer or a presumed precursor. The latter thrust targeted the here and now, the former aimed at an ultimate victory. Together they had become the cancer establishment. They were the permanent institutions through which the world would wage the cancer battle.

These and other similar institutions in Europe and elsewhere had become the cancer establishment without resolving the central question that motivated their creation. In all cancer research matters, they could not make things so. To be sure, the overwhelming majority of the new establishmentarians hewed to what I have called a bacteriological or Germ Theory perspective. They understood cancer to be a single disease and to have one causative agent. But beyond that agreement, precious little had been settled, despite the impressive institutional edifices that they had formed. Even things as relatively straightforward as whether cancer rates were truly increasing remained up in the air. Nowhere did the methods and procedures thought to make things so—science—unambiguously achieve that result. That remained true no matter if the science was that of the laboratory, the clinician, the statistician, the nomenclaturist, or the pathological anatomist.

Rarely did this profound impotence disrupt newly established programs and procedures or negate institutional cachet. Each group succeeded in securing a prime position in the cancer research nexus, even as its members had failed abjectly to determine cancer's cause. Their genius, their essential contribution, was quite basic. They got others to acknowledge them as a legitimate, perhaps even an essential, element of the cancer research nexus.

Clearly, that occurrence did not rely on facts or evidence. It began with a boldfaced contention. These individuals all claimed to possess special skills or knowledge, which they asserted was instrumental to finding the cause of cancer. Their authority ultimately derived from their declaration as cancer research experts. That pronouncement proved both critical and ironic; the men and women comprising these groups lacked the various areas of expertise that their claims had averred. In effect, each group's collective identification of cancer researchers—their self-definition—predated the acquisition of the special skills that they professed had made them indispensible.

Their initial inability to make things so was direct testament to their inadequate skill set for their newly constructed task. Their subsequent capacity to forge their cohort into an entity that ultimately demonstrated a modicum of consistency and talent, and to do so in real time, solidified their recognition as critical to the cancer quest. Put more simply, they consolidated authority by working to achieve those very cancer research attributes that they originally claimed to possess. That did not enhance their ability to make things so, but it provided them a fundamentally similar platform upon which to base their case. Rather than make things so, they made themselves so, gaining credibility and gravitas.

At its heart, the making things so question was virtually irresolvable. It proved nearly impossible to rule situations out absolutely. Microbes and other living things presented an almost uncountable number of variations. Fractions of a degree of temperature, sunlight, slight variations in media or microbial strain, and duration of investigation all might cause differential results. Control was not possible. But that difficulty paled when compared to the problem of establishing initial constants upon which to run experiments. Each constant circumscribed options for that experiment. But a different constant would produce a different set of options and, therefore, data. The possibilities were virtually limitless.

Researchers becoming increasingly adept at running these experiments, and increasingly similar in preparation and training with which to run them, standardized results somewhat. But standardization restrained possibilities, eliminating everything outside the standard. It severely reduced the number of distinct tests to run. It limited vision and approach to that which had been standardized and institutionalized. It was the death knell to creativity. It was not that one perspective was privileged and all other possibilities took a back seat. In the case of science, privileging that specific approach necessarily eliminated everything else. The perspective of those who became the standard is all that remains.

None of this troubled the great mass of late nineteenth and early twentieth century people. Their initial concerns were more immediate. They were desperate, scared, confronted with an onslaught of cancer. The various groups of newly identified professional cancer researchers promised quick amelioration, just as had the quacks, which the scientists abhorred. As significant, the various groups of scientists that would eventually constitute the cancer research establishment prescribed a remedy consistent with cultural norms. Expertise of a certain type—a type apparently successful in analogous endeavors—would eradicate cancer. When that failed to occur, another scientific cohort seized on cancer control to manage the disease.

Managing the disease while others sought a cure was certainly a heady notion in 1915, but now, from the perspective of one hundred years on, it seems quaint, naïve, even hackneyed. Certainly none of the partisans involved in the initial war would have thought that those oncological institutions would still need to exist today. The ultimate deconstruction of the idea of a single cancer cause and its replacement with a pluralistic vision have done little to change the equation. The institutions erected during the world's first war against cancer have clearly failed. Cancer continues to plague humankind, and at an alarming rate. How is that so? Why and how do these hundred-year-old relics persist? Does the character of the institutions—government-supported, immense, professional bureaucracies dedicated above all to the preservation of a particular method and tightly circumscribed point of view—make them too big to fail? What rests at the heart of the matter? Is it simply inconceivable to face the truth, to admit that these banal dinosaurs have not remotely achieved their goals over the past century and show no signs of doing so anytime soon? Are we now powerless to admit abject failure? If that is the case, then we have created a diabolical trap for ourselves. We have invested our hopes, dreams, expectations into a single project that may not ever fulfill even its initial promise and from which we cannot emotionally extract or detach ourselves. We have gambled and gambled wrongly. We now must continue to feed the behemoth or abandon the patina of hope. That remains the ultimate tyranny of science and of professionalism.

NOTES

Introduction

1. Siddhartha Mukherjee, *The Emperor of All Maladies. A Biography of Cancer* (New York: Scribner's, 2010) is what its subtitle purports to be—cancer's biography. Often overlooked but influential histories of cancer are James T. Patterson, *The Dread Disease. Cancer and Modern American Culture* (Cambridge, MA: Harvard University Press, 1987); Sigismund Peller, *Cancer Research Since 1900* (New York: Philosophical Library, 1979); and Michael B. Shimkin, *Contrary to Nature* (Washington, DC: GPO, 1977). For other studies of cancer, see, for instance, David Cantor, "Cancer," *Companion Encyclopedia for the History of Medicine* (London: Routledge, 1997), 537–61; Jean-Paul Gaudilliere, "Cancer," in *The Cambridge History of Science*, vol. 6, *The Modern Biological and Earth Sciences*, ed. Peter Bowler and John Pickstone (Cambridge, UK: Cambridge University Press, 2009), 487–503; and Patrice Pinell, "Cancer," in *Medicine in the Twentieth Century*, ed. Roger Cooter and John V. Pickstone (Amsterdam: Harwood Academic, 2000), 671–86. James S. Olson compiled a bibliography of prominent cancer-related papers. See his *The History of Cancer. An Annotated Bibliography* (Westport: Greenwood Press, 1989). Wolfgang U. Eckart led a series of practitioners and others in an edited volume on cancer research. See his *100 Years of Organized Cancer Research* (Stuttgart: Georg Thieme, 2000).

2. Jean-Paul Gaudilliere, a leading scholar of cancer's past, put the matter simply: "We know little about the development of cancer histological diagnosis in the decades before 1920." He ironically concludes it likely was "a by-product of the laboratory revolution in medicine." See his "Cancer," *Cambridge History of Science*, vol. 6, especially p. 488. Several Athens, Greece–based physicians have put together a Francocentric compilation of bacteriological era theories of cancer. See G. Tsoucalas, K. Laios, M. Karamanou, V. Gennimata, and G. Androutsos, "The Fascinating Germ Theories on Cancer Parthogenesis," *JBUON* 19 (2014): 319–23.

3. See, for instance, F. Marchand, "Ueber Gewebswucherung und Geschwulstbildung mit Rücksicht auf die parasitäre Aetiologie der Carcinome," *Deutsche Medicinische Wolfenschrift* (hereafter *DMW*) 28 (1902): 693–96, 721–24; Dr. Olshausen, "Impfmetastasen der Carcinome," *DMW* 28 (1902): 750–51; L. Brieger, "Impfmetastasen der Carcinome," *DMW* 28 (1902): 840–41.

4. The classic, detailed discussion of cancer theories is Jacob Wolff, *The Science of Cancerous Disease from Earliest Times to the Present*, a translation of the 1907 edition of Wolff's *Die Lehre von der Krebskrankheit von den altesten Zeiten Bis Zur Gegenwart* by Barbara Ayoub (Canton, MA: Science History Publications, 1987), 93–271. Also of utility are L. J. Rather, Patricia Rather, and John B. Frerichs, *Johannes Muller and the Nineteenth-Century Origins of Tumor Cell Theory* (Canton, MA: Science History Publications, 1986); James S. Olson, comp., *The History of*

Cancer. An Annotated Bibliography (New York: Greenwood Press, 1989), 138–47; L. P. Bignold, Brian L. D. Coghlan, and Hubertus P. A. Jersmann, *David Paul Von Hansemann: Contributions to Oncology* (Basel: Birkhauser Verlag, 2007), 45–60; and Russell Maulitz, "Rudolf Virchow, Julius Cohnheim and the Program of Pathology," *Bulletin of the History of Medicine* 52, 2 (1978): 162–82. Iwona Mitrus, Ewa Bryndza, Aleksander Sochanik, and Stanislaw Szala, "Evolving Models of Tumor Origin and Progression," *Tumor Biology* 33 (2012): 911–17, is a fine practitioner history. A good contemporary summary is Joseph Janvier Woodward, *On the Structure of Cancerous Tumors and the Mode in Which Adjacent Parts Are Invaded* (Washington, DC: Smithsonian Institution, 1873). Creating a usable past implies a continuity that did not, in fact, exist. See Victor A. Triolo, "Nineteenth Century Foundation of Cancer Research. Advances in Tumor Pathology, Nomenclature, and Theories of Oncogenesis," *Cancer Research* 25 (1965): 75–106, for how that has been handled for cancer research.

5. A thoughtful, intriguing discussion of nineteenth-century disease theories and the rise of the Germ Theory in its several guises is K. Codell Carter, *The Rise of Causal Concepts of Disease: Case Histories* (Burlington, VT.: Ashgate Publishing, 2003). Carter is especially interested in the rise of epidemiological thinking, the project by which universal causes comes to define diseases.

6. For bacteriology and the Germ Theory of Disease, see, for example, Michael Worboys, *Spreading Germs: Disease Theories and Medical Practice in Britain, 1865–1900* (Cambridge, UK: Cambridge University Press, 2000), especially pp.193–277; Christoph Gradmann, *Laboratory Disease. Robert Koch's Medical Bacteriology*, trans. Elborg Foster (Baltimore: Johns Hopkins University Press, 2009); Nancy Tomes, *The Gospel of Germs. Men, Women, and the Microbe in American Life* (Cambridge, MA: Harvard University Press, 1998); and W. E. Bynum, *Science and the Practice of Medicine in the Nineteenth Century* (Cambridge, UK: Cambridge University Press, 1994). I would be remiss if I did not cite William Bulloch, *A History of Bacteriology* (Oxford: Oxford University Press, 1938). An underappreciated volume that highlights bacteriology as medical template is Hubert A. Lechevalier and Morris Salotorovsky, *Three Centuries of Microbiology* (New York: McGraw-Hill, 1965). Claire Salomon-Bayet, ed., *Pasteur Et La Revolution Pastorienne* (Paris: Payot, 1986), argues specifically that bacteriology as the dominant medical approach changed the character of French, German, and English governance. Jack D. Ellis, *The Physician-Legislators of France: Medicine and Politics in the Early Third Republic, 1870–1914* (New York: Cambridge University Press, 1990), 175–206, provides copious examples of how French government incorporated bacteriology. For France alone, and especially the learned professions and their dalliance with the bacteriological idea, see Bruno LaTour, *The Pasteurization of France*, trans. Alan Sheridan and John Law (Cambridge: Harvard University Press, 1988).

7. Nancy J. Tomes and John Harley Warner, "Introduction to Special Issue on Rethinking the Reception of the Germ Theory of Disease: Comparative Perspectives," *Journal of the History of Medicine and Allied Sciences* 52 (1997): 7–16. The other work in the volume supports their critical contention.

8. Worboys maintains that the Germ Theory in its various incantations would "transform every aspect of medicine." See Worboys, *Spreading Germs*, 8.

9. Theodore M. Porter, *Trust in Numbers. The Pursuit of Objectivity in Science and Public Life* (Princeton: Princeton University Press, 1995), 217. Porter's volume is a continuation of his earlier work. See his *The Rise of Statistical Thinking, 1820–1900* (Princeton: Princeton University Press, 1986). Objectivity, especially as it pertained to science and observation, has gotten a broader treatment in Lorraine Daston and Peter Galison, eds., *Objectivity* (New York: Zone Books, 2010). Here, it is almost always described as the province of a group, a community that shared common approaches to their subject and sometimes common backgrounds and perspectives.

10. Some scholars might attribute this situation not to an inability to recreate the "experiment" but to a differences in geographic explorations.

11. The use of analogy in the sciences and medicine has generated a substantial literature. A convenient introduction is Fernand Hallyn, ed., *Metaphors and Analogies in the Sciences* (Amsterdam: Springer Netherlands, 2000).

12. Christoph Gradmann, "Spirit of Scientific Rigour: Koch's Postulates in Twentieth-Century Medicine," *Microbes and Infection* 16 (2014): 885–92.

13. Of interest on the early years of vitamins is Kenneth J. Carpenter, *Beriberi, White Rice, and Vitamin B: A Disease, A Cause, and A Cure* (Berkeley: University of California Press, 2000).

14. Philosophers of science would parse that situation as the necessary cause was not a sufficient cause. Other things would be required for a disease to eventuate, but those various things would be plural by definition. If there had only been one auxiliary factor, it would not be auxiliary at all but a second necessary cause.

15. Although concerned with post-1945 history of cancer, David Cantor recognizes that at the heart of cancer research rested a "power struggle," generally although not exclusively about "scientific knowledge and expertise." See his "Cancer," in *Companion Encyclopedia of the History of Medicine*, vol. 1, ed. W. F. Bynum and Roy Porter (London: Routledge, 1993), 537–61.

16. For a good exposition about the "geographical" thinking and what it entailed when it came to critical inquiry, see the introduction and essays in David N. Livingstone and Charles W. J. Withers, eds., *Geographies of Nineteenth-Century Science* (Chicago: University of Chicago Press, 2011). Also of use are Jeremy Vetter's articles, "Introduction: Lay Participation in the History of Scientific Observation," *Science in Context* 24 (2011): 259–80; "Introduction," *Knowing Global Environments: New Historical Perspectives on the Field Sciences* (New Brunswick: Rutgers University Press, 2010), 1–16; and "Labs in the Field? Rocky Mountain Biological Stations in the Early Twentieth Century," *Journal of the History of Biology* 45 (2012): 587–611. For an attempt to reduce geographies of exploration to the functionalist sociological categories of "sites, regions, territories and borders," see Dairmid A. Finnegan, "The Spatial Turn: Geographic Approaches in the History of Science," *Journal of the History of Biology* 41(2008): 369–88. Also of utility is Robert E. Kohler, "Practice and Place in Twentieth-Century Field Biology: A Comment," *Journal of the History of Biology*, 45 (2012): 579–86.

17. Gradmann sees in the work of Koch and others the continual use of the metaphor of war. In the conclusion to *Laboratory Disease*, he speculates about

bacteriology generally being cast in terms of battles, as a war against opposition forces. See especially pp. 230–33.

18. See, for example, Bruno Latour and Steve Woolgar, *Laboratory Life: The Construction of Scientific Facts*, 2nd ed. (1979; Princeton: Princeton University Press, 1986); Ludwik Fleck, *Genesis and Development of a Scientific Fact*, trans. Thaddeus J. Trenn and Robert K. Merton (Chicago: University of Chicago, 1979); Barbara Clow, *Negotiating Disease: Power and Cancer Care, 1900–1950* (Montreal: McGill-Queens University Press, 2001); Harry M. Marks, *The Progress of Experiment: Science and Therapeutic Reform in the United States, 1900–1990* (Cambridge, UK: Cambridge University Press, 1997); Bruno Latour, *Science in Action* (Cambridge, MA: Harvard University Press, 1987); Deborah Bruton, ed., *Medicine Transformed: Health, Disease and Society in Europe, 1800–1930* (Manchester: Bath Press, 2004), 92–118; and Daston and Galison, *Objectivity*. Attempts to provide a universal template for the manufacture of certainty has become a major historical piece. Useful on the ethos and science as ideational bond is Peter Dear, "Science is Dead; Long Live Science," *Osiris* 27 (2012): 37–55. Also of note is Georges Canguilhem, "What is Scientific Ideology," in his *Ideology and Rationality in the History of the Life Sciences*, trans. Arthur Goldhammer (Cambridge, MA: MIT Press, 1990), 27–41.

19. Most of the studies of scientific communities either concentrate on the seventeenth and eighteenth centuries, when few barriers beyond station existed, or on the extremely streamlined emergence of new or redrafted professional groups in the nineteenth and twentieth centuries, when the newly configured groups could stake out scientific-social space in scientific areas uninhabited or not well populated. The latter is thought to be space-driven, a response to social, geographical, or cultural circumstance. That is reversed. Self-identification preceded those events. John V. Pickstone, "Sketching Together the Modern Histories of Science, Technology, and Medicine," *Isis* 102 (2011): 122–33, comes at the problem from a different angle. Philosophers of science have devoted attention to the questions of the durability of the application of research programs. See, for instance, Imre Lakatos, "Falsification and the Methodology of Science Research Programmes," in *Criticism and the Growth of Knowledge*, ed. Imre Lakatos and Alan Musgrove (Cambridge, UK: Cambridge University Press), 91–196; and Imre Lakatos and Paul Feyerabend, *For and Against Method, Including Lakatos's Lectures on Scientific Method and the Lakatos-Feyerabend Correspondence*, ed. Matteo Motterlini (Chicago: University of Chicago Press, 1999).

20. Clifford Geertz, *The Interpretation of Cultures: Selected Essays* (New York: Basic Books, 1973); and Michel Foucault, *The Archaeology of Knowledge and the Discourse on Language* (New York: Vintage, 1982).

21. In the case of cancer researchers, self-identification preceded knowledge, technical competence, and skill. I have written about this rethinking of the nature of the professionalization process in a few other venues. See my "Professional Revolution and Reform in the Progressive Era: Cincinnati Physicians and the Elections of 1897 and 1900," *Journal of Urban History* 5 (1979): 183–207; *Agricultural Science and the Quest for Legitimacy: Farmers, Agricultural Colleges and Experiment Stations, 1870–1890* (Ames: Iowa State University Press, 1986); and "Setting the Standard: Fertilizers, State Chemists and Early National Commercial

Regulation, 1880–1887," *Agricultural History* 61 (1987): 47–73. See also my "When Numbers Failed: Social Scientists, Modernity and the New Cities of the 1920s and 1930s," in *Great Depression: People and Perspectives*, ed. Hamilton Cravens (Santa Barbara: ABC-CLIO, 2009), 165–84, for the brief and vain attempt in social science professions to shun the "objectivity" of statistics for attempts to describe through words the intricacies characterizing the new cities of the period. They ultimately returned to statistical analyses—an analysis they knew was flawed and incomplete—because it provided them legitimacy within government and among their cohorts.

22. A nice summary of the results/state of the art of laboratory historical sociology can be found in Robert E. Kohler, "Lab History: Reflections," *Isis* 99 (2008): 761–68. Also of interest is the fine collection by Andrew Cunningham and Perry Williams, eds., *The Laboratory Revolution in Medicine* (Cambridge, UK: Cambridge University Press, 1992).

23. Some hospitals, in the course of attending to impoverished cancer victims, performed experiments upon them and even engaged in some laboratory experiments, but those activities were but a minor facet of their affairs.

24. Caroline C. S. Murphy, "From Friedenheim to Hospice: A Century of Cancer Hospitals," in *The Hospital in History*, Lindsay Granshaw and Roy Porter (London: Routledge, 1989), 221–42.

25. A good, not quite contemporaneous discussion of the origins of the cancer control movement throughout the western world is *Cancer Control: Report of an International Symposium Held Under the Auspices of the American Society for the Control of Cancer* (Chicago: Surgical Publishing Company, 1927). Of use are Kirsten E. Gardner, *Early Detection: Women, Cancer, and Awareness Campaigns in the Twentieth-Century United States* (Chapel Hill: University of North Carolina, 2006); Walter Sanford Ross, *Crusade: The Official History of the American Cancer Society* (New York: Arbor House, 1987); and Donald F. Shaughnessy, "The Story of the American Cancer Society" (PhD diss., Columbia University, 1957).

Chapter 1

1. Robert T. Morris, MD, "Recent Views Respecting Cancer," *Popular Science Monthly* 32 (1887): 534; and "Cancer," *Science* 12 (1888): 67.

2. Lorraine Daston and Peter Galison, *Objectivity* (New York: Zone Books, 2010); Theodore M. Porter, *Trust in Numbers: The Pursuit of Objectivity in Science and Public Life* (Princeton: Princeton University Press, 1995).

3. For the work of the sanitarians, see, for instance, R. A. Lewis, *Edwin Chadwick and the Sanitary Movement, 1832–1854* (London: Longmans, Green and Co., 1952); Christopher Hamlin, "Providence and Putrefaction: Victorian Sanitarians and the Natural Theology of Health and Disease," *Victorian Studies* 28 (1985): 381–411; John Griscom, *The Sanitary Condition of the Laboring Population of the New York* (New York: Harper and Brothers, 1845); and Sandra Hempel, *The Strange Case of the Broad Street Pump: John Snow and the Mysteries of Cholera* (Berkeley: University of California Press, 2007).

4. For the contributions of the new bacteriologists, see, for instance, Edwin Ackerknecht, *Rudolf Virchow: Doctor, Statesman, Anthropologist* (Madison:

University of Wisconsin, 1953); Victor Robinson, *The Life of Jacob Henle* (New York: Medical Life Company, 1921); K. Codell Carter, "Edwin Kleb's Grundversuche," *Bulletin of the History of Medicine* 75 (2001): 771–81; and Thomas D. Brock, *Robert Koch: A Life in Medicine and Bacteriology* (Raleigh, NC: Science Tech Publishing, 1988).

5. For analogies made between the cancer microbe and either tuberculosis or syphilis, see, for instance, Henry T. Butlin, "An Address on the Investigation of the Causes of Cancer," *British Medical Journal* (hereafter *BMJ*) 2 (1885): 51–53; "The Parasitic Origin of Cancer," *Cincinnati Lancet and Clinic* 14 (1885): 541–42; Dr. Doutrelepont, "Syphilis und Carcinom," *DMW* (November 1887): 1016–18; "Glasgow Pathological and Clinical Society, January 27, 1886," *BMJ* 2 (1886): 494–501; Dr. Ziemassen, "Lungen-Tuberculose-Syphilis oder- Carcinom," *Berliner Klinische Wochenschrift* (hereafter *BKW*) (March 1887): 219–21; "Microscopic Characters of Cancer," reprinted from the Indiana Medical Journal, *Cincinnati Medical News* 18 (1885): 837–39; "The Bacillus of Cancer," *Science* 11 (1888): 44–45; Lester Curtis, trans., "Studies in the Etiology of Carcinoma," trans. from *BKW*, no. 10, *Chicago Medical Journal and Examiner* 56 (1888): 284–92; and "The Study of Cancer and Tuberculosis," *BMJ* 1 (1898): 1474–75. For some other efforts in Leyden's laboratory, see Dr. Scheurlen, "Die Aetiologie des Cancinoms," *DMW* (1887): 1033–34.

6. The one cause, one disease matrix so infused late nineteenth-century medical thought that it was exceedingly difficult, perhaps almost impossible, to devise a rational alternative. In that sense, two books deserve mention here: Lucien Febvre, *The Problem of Unbelief in the 16th Century: The Religion of Rabelais* (Cambridge, MA: Harvard University Press, 1985); and James Turner, *Without God, Without Creed: The Origins of Unbelief in America* (Baltimore: Johns Hopkins University Press, 1986) both discuss thought and action in terms of cognition—in terms of what was conceivable, tenable.

7. What Hansemann lacked in numbers, he made up in persistence. See, for instance, David Hansemann, "Ueber den primären Krebs der Leber," *BKW* (April 1890): 353–56; Dr. Hansemann, "Die Carcinomliteratur im Jahre 1889 vom pathologischeanatomischen Standpunkte," *BKW* (1890): 519–21, 543–44; David Hansemann, *Studien Uber Die Spezifictat, Den Altruismus Und Die Anaplasie Der Zellen: Mit Besonderer Berucksichtigung Der Geschwulste* (Berlin: A. Hirschwald, 1893); E. Ziegler, "Bemerkungen," *BKW* (January 1894): 102; Hugo Ribbert, "Ueber Die Parasitare Natur Des Carconoms," *DMW* 27 (1901): 811–13; Dr. Alexander-Katz, "Zur Parasitaren Aetiologie Des Carcinoms," *DMW* 27 (1901): 876–77; D. V. Hansemann, "Ueber die Parasitäre Natur des Carcinoms," *DMW* (1902): 44–45; Prof. Hansemann, "Was wissen Wir über die Ursache der Bösartigen Geschwülste?," *BKW* (1905): 313–18; Hugo Ribbert, "Beiträge Zur Entstehung der Geschwülste. Eine Kritische Besprechung von. D. Hansemann," *Zeitschrift Für Krebsforschung* (hereafter *ZFK*) 5 (1907): 522–28; and D. V. Hansemann, "Zur Bezeichnung der Bosartigen epithelialen Neubildungen," *ZFK* 7 (1908): 1–2.

8. The idea of predisposition—acting in such a way as to increase one's likelihood to cancer—never truly vanished. See, for instance, James Sawyer,

"Note on the Causation of Cancer," *Lancet* 1 (1900): 848–49; John Haddon, "The Connexion Between Feeding and Cancer," *Lancet* 1 (1900): 965; C. N. Saldanha, "The Social Factor in the Genesis of Cancer," *Lancet* 1 (1900): 1246–47; and "The Pathogenesis and Therapeutics of Cancer," *Cincinnati Lancet-Clinic* 57 (1906): 408. For a rather circumspect article about medical research, see Frederick C. Shattuck, "How Progress Comes in Medicine," *Cincinnati Lancet-Clinic* 56 (1906): 665–70.

9. See, for example, John Francis Churchill, *A Letter to the Registrar-General on the Increase of Cancer in England and Its Cause* (London: D. Stott, 1887); "The Increase of Cancer," *Boston Medical and Surgical Journal* (hereafter *BMSJ*), 128 (1893): 270; "Increase in Cancer in Prussia," *Medical News* 74 (1899): 461; "Increase of Mortality By Cancer," *Journal of the American Medical Association* (hereafter cited as *JAMA*) 28 (1897): 603–4; and R. Romme, "La Frequence Croissante Du Cancer," *Revue Des Maladies Cancereuses*," 5 (1900): 104–6.

10. For irritation and specialized cancers, see James Earle, *The Chirurgical Work of Percivall Pott, F.R.S.*, vol. 3 (London: Wood and Innes, 1808); Newton M. Shaffer, *Pott's Disease* (New York: George Putnam and Sons, 1879); Herbert L. Snow, *Clinical Notes On Cancer: Its Etiology and Treatment* (London: J. & A. Churchill, 1883); "Inflammation Masking Cancer," *American Practitioner* 5 (1888): 255; and John V. Shoemaker, "Clinical Studies in Carcinoma," *Medical Bulletin* 11 (1889): 224–26. Also see, for instance, "The Origin of Cancer," *Cincinnati Lancet-Clinic* 16 (1886): 720–21; Dr. Schill, "Ueber Den Regelmässigen Befund Von Doppelpunktstäbchen im carinomatösen und sarcomatösen Gewebe," *DMW* (1887): 1034–35; F. Hirschfeld, "Eine Bemerkung zu Herrn Dr. Klemperer's Arbeit: Ueber den Stoffwechsel und das Coma der Krebskranken," *BKW* (November 1889): 979–80; "The Pathology of Inflammation," *BMSJ* 123 (1890): 67–68, 377–79; G. Winter, "Ueber die Frühdiagnose des Uteruskrebes," *BKW* (August 1891): 809–13; D'Arcy Power, "Some Effects of Chronic Irritation Upon Living Tissue, Being the First Steps in a Rational Study of Cancer," *BMJ* 2 (1893): 830–34; J. Meplaux, "Nature Inflammatoire Du Sarcome," *Revue Des Maladies Cancereuses* 2 (1897): 191; and "Trauma in the Etiology of Malignant Disease," *Medical News* 74 (1899): 559. For discussion of the seed-soil metaphor in some detail, see Worboys, *Spreading Germs*, 235–37 and passim.

11. Joseph Coats, "An Address on Certain Considerations in Regard to the Infective Nature of Cancer," *BMJ* 2 (1893): 53–57. Also of interest are Herr Scheurlen, "Zur Aetiologie des Carcinoms," *DMW* (1887): 1069; and Jules Felix, "L'Etiologie Des Affections Cancereuses," *Revue Des Maladies Cancereuses* 1 (1896): 146–57.

12. G. Sims Woodhead, "The Morton Lecture on Cancer and Cancerous Diseases," *BMJ* 1 (1892): 954–60. Also see E. Calmette, "De L'Etiologie Coccidienne Du Cancer," *Revue Des Maladies Cancereuses* 2 (1897): 185–86; and A. Borrell, "Dans La Derniere Séance, M. Wlaeff a Lu a La Societe Une Note Intitulee: Contribution a L'Étude Du Traitment Des Tumeurs Malignes Et Des Parasites De Cette Affection," *Comptes Rendus Hebdomadaires Des Seances Et Memoires De La Societe De Biologie* 53 (1901): 108–9.

13. Samuel G. Shattuck, "The Morton Lecture on Cancer and Cancerous Diseases," *BMJ* 2 (1894): 1065–67. Of interest is Herbert Snow, *Twenty-Two Years' Experience in the Treatment of Cancerous and Other Tumors* (London: Bailliere, Tindall and Cox, 1898), 34–49.

14. William Russell, "An Address on a Characteristic Organism of Cancer," *BMJ* 2 (1890): 1356–60. For similar sentiments, see, for instance, Ludwig Makara, "Untersuchungen über Die Aetiologie Des Carcinoms," *DMW* (1888): 634–35; Jules Felix, "De L'Etiologie Des Affections Cancereuses," *Revue Des Maladies Cancereuses* 1 (1896): 209–24; and E. Camelot, "Le Cancer Est-il De Nature Parasitaire," *Journal Des Sciences Medicales De Lille* (February 1896): 194–228; F.-J. Bosc, "Recherches Su La Nature (Parasitaire) De Formations Intracellulaires Dans Un Cancer Du Sein," *Comptes Rendus Hebdomadaires Des Seances Et Memoires De La Societe De Biologie* 51 (1899): 444–46; G. Lemeire, "Le Parasitisme Dans Le Cancer," *Revue Des Maladies Cancereuses* 5 (1900): 81–93, 123–41, 165–83, 213–25, and 6 (1901): 77–80. Many of the ever disagreeing Britishers were charter members of the Pathological Society of Great Britain and Ireland. Not all investigators uncovered convincing evidence of the cancer microbe. See, for instance, Emil Senger, "Studien Zur Aetiologie Des Carcinoms," *BKW* (March 1888): 185–89; Simon Duplay and Maurice Cazin, "De Greffes Cancereuses," *Le Semaine Medicale* (1892): 61–62; Guiseppe Von Pianese, *Beitrag Zur Histologie Und Aetiologie Des Carcinoms, aus dem Italienischen Ubersetzt von R. Teauscher* (Jena: G. Fischer, 1896); Maurice Cazin, "La Theorie Psorospermique Du Cancer," *Revue Des Maladies Cancereuses* 1 (1896): 3–7; and M. F. Curtias, "A Propos Des Parasites Du Cancer," *Comptes Rendus Hebdomadaires Des Seances Et Memoires De La Societe De Biologie* 51 (1899): 191–93.

15. For Pasteur, see Rene J. Dubos, *Louis Pasteur: Freelance of Science* (Boston: Little, Brown, and Company, 1950); and Gerald Geison, *The Private Science of Louis Pasteur* (Princeton: Princeton University Press, 1995). Several scholars have explored how, in real time, Koch's postulates have been applied. See, for instance, Alfred S. Evans, *Causation and Disease: A Chronological Journey* (New York: Plenum Medical, 1993); Victoria A. Harden, "Koch's Postulates and the Etiology of Rickettsial Diseases," *Journal of the History of Medicine and Allied Sciences* 42 (1987): 277–95; and K. Codell Carter, "Koch's Postulates in Relation to the Work of Jacob Henle and Edwin Klebs," *Medical History* 29 (1985): 353–74.

16. Useful on this point is Christoph Gradmann, *Laboratory Disease: Robert Koch's Medical Bacteriology*, trans. Elborg Forster (Baltimore: Johns Hopkins University Press, 2009), especially 70–76, 122, 221.

17. A. P. Ohlmacher, "A Critique of the Sporozoan Theory of Malignant Neoplasms from a Micro-Technical Standpoint," *JAMA* 22 (1894): 973–76.

18. H. G. Plimmer, "A Preliminary Note Upon Certain Organisms Isolated From Cancer and Their Pathogenic Effects Upon Animals," *Lancet* 1 (1899): 826–27. For similar events, see F. J. Bosc, "Les Parasites Du Cancer Et Du Sarcome (Morphologie, Repartition)," *Revue Des Maladies Cancereuses* 3 (1899): 207–9; M. Bra, "D'un Champignon Parasite Du Cancer," *Compte Rendue Societie Biologie* (1898): 1050–53; M. Bra, "Le Champignon Parasite Du Cancer," *Le Presse Medicale* (February 1899): 87–91; and M. Jurgens, "Les Protozoaires Du Cancer," *Le Semaine Medicale* 18 (1898): 455.

19. See, for example, N. Senn, "The Present Status of the Carcinoma Questions," *JAMA* (1901): 804–15; R. B. Greenough, "On the Presence of the So-Called 'Plimmer's Bodies' in Carcinoma," *BMSJ* (1901): 59–62; and E. R. LeCount, "The Analogies Between Plimmer's Bodies and Certain Structures Found Normally in the Cytoplasm," *Journal of Medical Research* (hereafter *JMR*) 7 (1902): 383–93. Plimmer's work remained controversial years later. See, for instance, Apolant and G. Emden, "Ueber Die Entstehung Plimmer'scher Körperchen Aus Kerndegenerationen," *ZFK* 3 (1905): 579–83; and D. V. Hansemann, "Ueber die Funktion der Geschwulstzellen," *ZFK* 4 (1906): 565–77.

20. H. G. Plimmer, "Rhapalocephalus Carcinomatoeus," *Journal of Pathology and Bacteriology* 2 (1893): 486–92.

21. A good, extended debate over the local vs. constitutional origins of cancer can be found in P. S. Connor, "Cancer: Has It a Constitutional or Local Origin?" *Cincinnati Lancet and Clinic* 2 (1879): 381–82, 385–86; and G. A. Fackler, "Dicussion on Cancer," *Cincinnati Lancet-Clinic* 20 (1888): 491–500. Also see "Infectiveness of Cancer," *Compendium of Medical Science* 5 (1888): 313–14; "Origin of Cancer," *Popular Science* 29 (1886): 569; "The Microbe of Cancer," *Cincinnati Medical News* 20 (1887): 744–46; "The Inoculation of Carcinoma," *Cincinnati Lancet-Clinic* 21 (1888): 423; "The Question of the Nature and Meaning of Malignant New Growths," *Lancet* 2 (1888): 29–30; Henry Campbell, "In What does Cancer Consist?" *Lancet* 2 (1888): 444–45; "The Cause of Cancer Infectivity," *Cincinnati Lancet-Clinic* 21 (1888): 398; George Thomas Beatson, "On the Etiology of Cancer, With a Note of Some Experiments," *BMJ* 1 (1899): 399–400; and J. T. Roberts, "Medical Society of London, Infectivity of Malignant Growths," *BMJ* 2 (1899): 1195–96.

22. See Alan I Marcus "From Individual Practitioner to Regular Physician: Cincinnati Medical Societies and the Problem of Definition among Mid-Nineteenth Century Americans," in *Technical Knowledge in American Culture: Science, Technology, and Medicine in America Since the Early 1800s*, ed. Hamilton Cravens, Alan I Marcus, and David M. Katzman (Birmingham: University of Alabama Press, 1996), 55–70. Also of interest is "Cancer Craze," *American Practitioner* 5 (1888): 255; and James P. Warbasse, "Are the Parasitic Theories of the Etiology of Carcinoma Tenable?" *Brooklyn Medical Journal* (1894): 145–54.

23. For success as the basis for reputation, see, for instance, Alan I Marcus, *Plague of Strangers: Social Groups and the Origins of Municipal Services, Cincinnati, 1819–1870* (Columbus: Ohio State University Press, 1991); and "Setting the Standard: Fertilizers, State Chemists and Early National Commercial Regulation, 1880–1887," *Agricultural History* 61 (1987): 47–73.

24. For Koch and tuberculin, see Thomas D. Brock, *Robert Koch: A Life in Bacteriology and Medicine* (New York: ASM Press, 1999); and Gradmann, *Laboratory Disease*, 95–134.

25. Warbasse, "Are the Parasitic Theories," 145–54, provides article citations for over eighty-five separate cancer germs identified before 1894. For other lists of citations to specific germs as cancer agents, see, for example, M. Armand Ruffer and J. Herbert Walker, "On Some Parasitic Protozoa found in Cancerous Tumours," *Journal of Pathology and Bacteriology* 1 (1893): 198–215; and "Micro-Organisms in Tumors," *JAMA* 34 (1900): 692–93.

26. Woods Hutchinson, *The Cancer Problem: Or, Treason in the Republic of the Body* (New York: Tucker Publishing Co., 1900). Also see, for instance, Mayet, "De L'Inoculation Du Cancer," *Revue Des Maladies Cancereuses* 1 (1896): 64.

27. See, for example, Theodore M. Porter, *The Rise of Statistical Thinking 1820–1900* (Princeton: Princeton University Press, 1986); and Mary Poovey, *A History of the Modern Fact: Problems of Knowledge in the Sciences of Wealth and Society* (Chicago: University of Chicago, 1998).

28. H. Percy Dunn, "English Experience With Cancer," *Popular Science Monthly* 26 (1885): 688–90; "The Alleged Increase of Cancer," *Lancet* 2 (1888): 1192; "Pathological Studies of Cancer," *Medical Bulletin* 11 (1889): 226–27; Spencer Wells, "The Morton Lecture on Cancer and Cancerous Diseases," *BMJ* 2 (1888): 1201–6; "Microbe of Cancer," *Indiana Medical Journal* 9 (1890): 42; Alfred Haviland, "Increase of Cancer: Its Probable Cause," *Lancet* 2 (1890): 316–18; D'Arcy Power, "An Experimental Investigation in Causation of Cancer," *BMJ* 2 (1894): 636–38; "The Victims of Cancer Houses," *BMSJ* 131 (1894): 149–50; "Cancer Houses," *BMJ* 2 (1897): 1760; "Cancer Houses and Cancer Areas," *JAMA* 28 (1897): 232–33; "Cancer in Relation to the Dwelling," *BMJ* 2 (1898): 1571–72; W. Roger Williams, "Note on Multiple Family Cancer," *BMJ* 2 (1898): 1612–13; Edmund Andrews, "Supposed Increase of Cancer," *JAMA* 32 (1899): 1406–9; "The Cancer Problem," *Medical News* 75 (1899): 181–82; and "Cancer Mortality Among the Jews," *Science* 12 (1890): 331.

29. See, for instance, Herbert L. Snow, *The Proclivity of Women to Cancerous Diseases and to Certain Benign Tumours* (London: Churchill, 1891); "Climate and Cancer," *BMJ* 2 (1895): 1333; J. Rebulet, "Influence De L'Heredite Sur La Frequence Du Cancer En Normandie," *Revue Des Maladies Cancereuses* 2 (1897): 19–25; Leon Noel, "Sur La Topographie Et La Contagion Du Cancer," *Revue Des Maladies Cancereuses* 2 (1897): 137–45, 201–13; Edward Noel Nason, "The Influence of Locality on the Prevalence of Malignant Disease," *BMJ* 1 (1898): 679–81; Roswell Park, "An Inquiry into the Etiology of Cancer with Some Reference to the Latest Investigations of the Italian Pathologists," *Medical News* 72 (1898): 603–5; "The Influence of Locality on the Prevalence of Cancer," *BMJ* 1 (1899): 812–13; E. Lloyd Jones, "The Topical Distribution of Cancer," *BMJ* 1 (1899): 813–16; Gilbert Barling, "An Address Entitled A Modern View of Cancer," *BMJ* 2 (1899):1461–65; "Geographic and Statistic Methods as Auxiliary Factors in the Study of Carcinoma," *JAMA* 33 (1899): 1047–48; "The Etiology of Cancer," *Lancet* 2 (1900): 753; and Irving Phillips Lyon, "Cancer Distribution and Statistics in Buffalo for the Period 1880–1899, With Special Reference to the Parasitic Disease," *American Journal of the Medical Sciences* 121 (1901): 629–92.

30. The literature is voluminous. See, for instance, "Increase of Cancer in Prussia," *Medical News* 74 (1899): 461; "Increase of Mortality By Cancer," *JAMA* 28 (1897): 603–4; and Joseph Frank Payne, "Increase of Cancer," *JAMA* 33 (1899): 1066. *The Practitioner*, a London-based medical periodical, devoted an entire monthly issue to cancer surveys. See Arthur Newsholme, "The Statistics of Cancer," *Practitioner* 62 (1899): 371–84; Alfred Haviland, "The Medical Geography of Cancer in England and Wales," *Practitioner* 62 (1899): 400–17; and D'Arcy Power, "The Local Distribution of Cancer and Cancer Houses," *Practitioner* 62 (1899): 418–29.

31. For the use of colonies and sports of nature, see, for instance, Antonello Gerbi,*The Dispute of the New World: The History of a Polemic, 1750–1900*, trans. Jeremy Moyle (Pittsburgh: University of Pittsburgh Press, 1973); and Murphy D. Smith, *A Museum: The History of the Cabinet of Curiosities of the American Philosophical Society* (Philadelphia: American Philosophical Society, 1996).

32. Charles Fiessinger, "La Pathologenie Du Cancer," *Revue De Medecine* (1893): 13–34; and Fiessinger, "Nouvelles Recherches Sur L'Etiologie Du Cancer," *Revue De Medecine* (1893); 706–20.

33. M. Bosc, "JHistogenese, Etiologie, Prophylaxie Et Inoculabilite Du Cancer et Du Sarcome," *La Semaine Medicale* (1898): 166; E. Lloyd Jones, "The Topical Distribution of Cancer," *BMJ* 1 (1899): 813–17; Marie Bra, "Physiologie Pathologique," *Comptes Rendus Academie Des Sciences* 129 (1899): 118–21; Marie Bra, *La Cancer Et Son Parasite (Action Therapeutique Des Produits Solubles Du Champignon* (Paris: Societe D'Editions Scientifiques, 1900); O. Govaerts, "Cancereux Soignes En 1897 Et 1898, Habitant Le Voisinage De La Sambre," *Revue Des Maladies Cancereuses* 5 (1900–1901): 106–8; and J Chevalier, "Le Cancer: Maladie Parasitaire," *Revue Des Maladies Cancereuses* 6 (1901–1902): 30. The Germans took note in 1900, 1901, and 1902, but they did not try to join environmental conditions to the disease. Rather, they recognized a potent analogy between human cancer and various tumor-like plant growths. See *Verhandlungen des Comite fur Krebsforschung, 1900–1902* (Berlin: The Comite, 1902), 19–22 , 76–78; and Robert Behla, "Ueber 'Cancer á Deux' und Infektion des Krebses," *DMW* 27 (1901): 427–31.

34. Roswell Park, "A Further Study Into the Frequency and Nature of Cancer," *Medical News* 74 (1899): 385–91; "Cancer Among Fish," *Washington Post*, May 25, 1909, 6; "Searching in Fish for the Germ of Cancer," *Washington Post*, September 4, 1910, MT4; and "Want Bureau to Study Fish Cancer," *Trenton Evening Times*, February 16, 1912, 4. Also of interest is "The Relation of Trees to Cancer," *Cincinnati Lancet-Clinic* 48 (1902): 674–75. For yellow fever, bubonic plague, and their vectors, see, for instance, George M. Sternberg, "Transmission of Yellow Fever by Mosquitoes," *Annual Report of the Smithsonian Institution for 1900* (Washington, DC: GPO, 1901); and Marilyn Chase, *The Barbary Plague: The Black Death in Victorian San Francisco* (New York: Random House, 2004), 28–104.

35. "Study of Fish Diseases," *Report of the Commissioner of Fisheries for the Fiscal Year 1910* (Washington, DC: GPO, 1911), 17–18, 39; George M. Bowers, "Fishery Experiment Station and Laboratory," *Report of the Commissioner of Fisheries for the Fiscal Year 1911* (Washington, DC: GPO, 1913), 67–68; and Hugh M. Smith, "Diseases of Fishes," *Report of the Commissioner of Fisheries for the Fiscal Year of 1913* (Washington, DC: GPO, 1914), 32.

36. "Is Cancer of a Poisonous Nature?" *Cincinnati Lancet-Clinic* 26 (1891): 204; "The Cancer Antitoxin," *Lancet* 2 (1895): 127–28; "The Toxin Therapy and Malignant Disease, *Medical News* 73 (1898): 264; and "The Treatment of Cancer By Its Own Toxins," *JAMA* 33 (1899): 1657. For a history of the diphtheria antitoxin, see Derek S. Linton, *Emil Von Behring: Infectious Disease, Immunology, Serum Therapy* (Philadelphia: American Philosophical Society, 2005).

37. William B. Coley, "The Treatment of Malignant Tumors By Repeated Inoculations of Erysipelas: With A Report of Ten Original Cases," *American Journal*

of the Medical Sciences 105 (1893): 487–510; "Erysipelas Toxins in the Treatment of Malignant Tumors," *JAMA* 23 (1894): 650–51; N. Senn, "The Treatment of Malignant Tumors by the Toxins of the Streptococcus of Erysipelas," *JAMA* 25 (1895): 131–34; "Coley Macht," *BKW* (1895): 512; Charles Richet, "Effets Toxiques Des Injections Veineuses De Tumeurs Cancereuses Ulcerees," *Comptes Rendus Hebdomadaires De La Societe De Biologie* 47 (1895): 601–2; V. Czerny, "Serotherapie Du Cancer Et Du Sarcome," *Revue Des Maladies Cancereuses* 1 (1896): 127–28; M. Kopfstein, "Action Du Serum De L'erysipele Sur Le Carcinome Et Les Autres Tumeurs Cancereuses," *Revue Des Maladies Cancereuses* 1 (1896): 131–33; "An Antitoxin for Carcinoma," *Lancet* 2 (1895): 1154; R. Emmerich and M. Zimmermann, "Quelques Cas De Cancere Et De Sarcome Traites Par Le Serum Anti Cancereux," *Revue Des Maladies Cancereuses,"* 1 (1896): 186–87; D. Boinet, "Toxine Cancereuse," *Comptes Rendue De La Societie de Biologie* 22 (1895): 476; E. Opitz, "Ueber die Veränderungen des Carcinomgewebes bei Injectionen mit 'Krebsserum' (Emmerich) Und Alkohol," *BKW* (August 1896): 754–56; "Traitment Des Cancers Inoperables," *La Semaine Medicale* (1900): 138–39; "The High-Frequency Treatment of Cancer," *Cincinnati Lancet-Clinic* 48 (1902): 673; Dr. Wlaeff, "Contribution A L'Étude Du Traitment Des Tumeurs Malignes Par Le Serum Anticellulaire," *Revue Des Maladies Cancereuses* 5 (1901): 65–78; "Value of the X-Ray in Cancer," *Cincinnati Lancet-Clinic* 51 (1903): 391–92; J.- B. Charcot, "Quelques Faits Relatifs A Des Recherches Sur La Serotherapie Du Cancer," *Comptes Rendus Hebdomadaires De La Societe De Biologie* 54 (1902): 15–16; and "The Treatment of Cancer With Radium," *Nature* 71 (1905): 588. At least one German investigator tried to kill cancer by restoring cellular chemistry and making it difficult for the invader to survive. See Karl Scherk, "Ein Vorschlag zur erforschung der Aetiologie des Carcinoms," *ZFK* 1 (1903): 239–42.

38. For emphasis on collective experience, see Francis Bacon, *Novum Organum* (1620; Indianapolis: Bobbs-Merrill, 1960); and Henry D. Shapiro, "Daniel Drake's 'Sensorium Commune' and the Organization of the Second American Enlightenment," *Cincinnati Historical Society Bulletin* 27 (1969): 42–62. Also see James E. McClellan III, *Science Reorganized: Scientific Societies in the Eighteenth Century* (New York: Columbia University Press, 1985); Roger Hahn, *The Anatomy of a Scientific Institution: The Paris Academy of Sciences, 1666–1803* (Berkeley: University of California, 1971): Michael Hunter, *Establishing the New Science: The Experience of the Early Royal Society* (Woodbridge, UK: Boydell Press, 1989); and Henry E. Lowood, *Patriotism, Profit, and the Promotion of Science in the German Enlightenment: The Economic and Scientific Societies, 1760–1815* (New York; Garland, 1991).

39. Harry M. Marks, "'Until the Sun of Science . . . the True Apollo of Medicine has Risen'': Collective Investigation in Britain and America, 1880–1910," *Medical History* 50 (2006): 147–66, is a fine overview of the collective movement. Also see R .M. S. McConaghey, "The BMA and Collective Investigation," *BMJ* (1956): 2666–71.

40. See, for example, George Murray Humphry, "President's Address," *BMJ* (1880): 241–44; "The Cancer-Inquiry of the Collective Investigation Committee," *Cincinnati Lancet and Clinic* 14 (1885): 384–85; "The Collective Investigation of Cancer," *Lancet* 1 (1890): 377, 887; Theodore A. McGraw, "Our Present Knowledge

of Tumors and Cancers," *JAMA* 25 (1895): 387–95; and "An Inquiry as to the Increase and Infectiousness of Cancer," *BMSJ* 141 (1899): 641.

41. S. Duplay, "Introduction," *Revue Des Maladies Cancereuses* 1 (1896): 1–2.

Chapter 2

1. "The Government Researches in Pathology and Medicine," *Nature* 12 (1875): 470–72.

2. Much of this story and many of the original documents were printed in Edwin A. Mirand, *Legacy and History of Roswell Park Cancer Institute, 1898–1998* (Virginia Beach, VA: Donning, 1998). Also see Roswell Park, "An Inquiry into the Etiology of Cancer with Some Reference to the Latest Investigations of the Italian Pathologists," *American Journal of the Medical Sciences* 115 (1898): 503–19. Park retrospectively discussed the formation of the laboratory in "Again the Question of Cancer," *Medical News* 76 (1900): 324–31. Also see "Medical College and Hospital Notes," *Buffalo Medical Journal* 38(1898–99): 146. A more positivistic statement was Victor A. Triolo, "Nineteenth Century Foundations of Cancer Research. Origins of Experimental Research," *Cancer Research* 24 (1964): 4–27.

3. Mirand, *Legacy and History*; "Editorial," *Buffalo Medical Journal* 38(1898–1899): 454; "Alumni Reunion," *Buffalo Medical Journal* 38(1898–1899): 609; and Roswell Park, "A Further Study Into the Frequency and Nature of Cancer," *Medical News* 74 (1899): 384–91.

4. "Cancer Research," *Lancet* 2 (1902): 682–83; George H. Simmons, "Etiology of Malignant Tumors," *JAMA* 34 (1900): 691–92; "Living Things in Cancers," *New York Times* (hereafter *NYT*), September 20, 1896, 9; "A Week's Paris Gossip," *NYT*, April 24, 1899, 7; "What Interests Berlin," *NYT*, May 6, 1900, 7; J. Riddle Goffe, "The Increase of Cancer," *Medical News* 74 (1899): 399–400; "New York Academy of Medicine," *Medical News* 76 (1900): 59–60; and "Cell Inclusions In Carcinoma Interpreted As Blastomycetes," *JAMA* 32 (1899): 1181–82.

5. "Cancer," *JAMA* 33 (1899): 433; "Etiology of Cancer, American Public Health Association Annual Meeting," *JAMA* 33 (1899): 1291; "Our London Letter," *Medical News* 75 (1899): 151; "The Increase of Cancer," *Lancet* 2 (1899): 191; "The Buffalo State Pathological Laboratory," *Buffalo Medical Journal* 39 (1899–1900): 65; and "The Increase of Cancer Real Not Apparent," *Medical News* 75 (1899): 530.

6. "The Middlesex Hospital," *Hackney Express and Shoreditch Observer*, July 15, 1899, 4; "A Step Forward in Research," *The Charity Record*, September 7, 1899, 100; "Scheme to Combat Cancer," *London Daily Mail*, December 2, 1899, 3; "The Middlesex Hospital-Research Laboratories For the Investigation of the Cause of Cancer," *London Daily Mail* December 12, 1899, 1; "The Middlesex Hospital," *Echo*, December 12, 1899, 1; and "The Middlesex Hospital," *The Charity Record*, September 20, 1900, 864, and October 18, 1900, 892.

7. Thomas Wakely, "The Investigation of Cancer," *Lancet* 2 (1899): 224–25; and "The Etiology of Cancer," *Lancet* 1 (1900): 1085–86.

8. George B. Shattuck, "Cancer and Modern Research," *BMSJ* 140 (1899): 457–58; and "Dr. H. R. Gaylord," *Buffalo Medical Journal* 38 (1898–1899): 901.

9. "The Study of Cancer and Tuberculosis," *BMJ* 1 (1898): 1474–75; "An Inquiry As To the Increase and Infectiousness of Cancer," *BMSJ* 141 (1899): 641;

"$100,000 to Study Cancer," *Medical News* 76 (1900): 30; "Berlin," *Lancet* (1900): 660; "Proposed Legislation," *NYT*, February 1, 1899, 1; "C. P. Huntington Dead," *NYT*, August 15, 1900, 1; J. Collins Warren, "Introduction," *Journal of the Boston Society of Medical Sciences* 5 (1900): 31–32; "Great Gifts Last Year," *NYT*, February 1, 1902, BR1; "Money Gifts to Harvard," *NYT*, March 14, 1902, 1; "Mrs. C. P. Huntington's Gift," *NYT*, May 24, 1902, 7; and Frontispiece and Introduction, *Reports of the Collis P. Huntington Fund for Cancer Research*, vol. 1 (New York City, 1905).

10. See, for example, "Increase in Cancers," *JAMA* 35 (1900): 768; "Cancer Mortality in Essex," *BMJ* 2 (1900): 242; E. N. Nason, "Some Remarks Upon An Analysis of 5,000 Cases of Death From Malignant Disease," *BMJ* (1901) 1: 1199–1201; "Carcinoma in Sweden," *JAMA* 36 (1901): 521; "Cancer in South Australia," *BMJ* 1 (1902): 162; "Cancer in Holland," *BMJ* 1 (1902): 852; "Cancer in Egypt and the Causation of Cancer," *BMJ* 2 (1902): 917; "The Distribution of Cancer in Scotland," *BMJ* 2 (1902): 1590; "Cancer in the German Empire," *JAMA* 38(1902): 851; "Cancer in Italy," *American Medicine* 4(1902): 766; "Cancer in Germany," *Medical News* 81 (1902): 949; Charles Templeman, "A Contribution to the Study of Cancer Mortality," *BMJ* 1 (1903): 356–59; "Cancer in Ireland," *BMJ* 1 (1903): 370–71; W. J. Barclay, "Tuberculosis and Cancer in New Zealand," *Lancet* 2 (1903): 822–24; "Cancer in Hungary," *Medical News* 83 (1903): 316; "Cancer in Norway," *American Medicine* 5 (1903): 515–16; "Empire Review," *Nature* 69 (1904): 541; "Cancer in Spain," *BMJ* 1 (1904): 99; "Cancer Research in Portugal," *BMJ* 1 (1904): 428; "Paris," *BMJ* 2 (1904): 39–40; and "Cancer Research in Greece," *JAMA* 42 (1904): 779.

11. "Cancer Among the Jews," *BMJ* 2 (1901): 1023, 1 (1902):681–82, 747–48; and "Cancer," *Lancet* 1 (1902): 261. Also see Irving Phillips Lyon, "Cancer Distribution and Statistics in Buffalo for the Period 1880–1899, With Special Reference to the Parasite Theory," *American Journal of Medical Sciences* 71 (1901): 629–51; Dr. Wutzdorff, "Ueber Die Verbreitung der Krebskrankheit in Deutschen Reiche," *DMW* (1902): 161–66; and Algernon T. Bristow, "The Hypothesis of Cohnheim Concerning Carcinoma," *Brooklyn Medical Journal* (1903): 444–51.

12. "Cancer in Tropical Countries," *BMJ* 2 (1902): 273, 730; "Cancer Among Hindoos," *Lancet* 1 (1902): 57; "Cancer in India and China," *Lancet* 1 (1902): 192–93, 921; "Carcinoma and Malaria," *JAMA* 38 (1902): 622; and "Cancer and Meat-Eating," *BMJ* 1 (1902): 1120.

13. "A Comparative Statistical Study of Cancer Mortality," *BMJ* 1 (1903): 929–32, 989–91, 1051–52, 1110–11, and 1154–56; and "Cancer Mortality," *BMJ* 2 (1904): 77–78. For the Galton Institute and Pearson, see Theodore M. Porter, *Karl Pearson: The Scientific Life in a Statistical Age* (Princeton: Princeton University Press, 2005).

14. "Cancer Distribution and Statistics," *JAMA* 36 (1901): 1740; "Cancer in Buffalo," *BMJ* 2 (1901): 827–28; "Cancer Among Sailors," *Medical News* 80 (1902): 89; Arthur Newsholme, "The Possible Association of the Consumption of Alcohol with Excessive Mortality from Cancer," *BMJ* 2 (1903): 1529–30; and "Cancer Mortality of the Thames Valley," *JAMA* 42 (1904): 1187.

15. *Verhandlungen des Comite fur Krebsforschung, 1900–1902* (Berlin: The Comite, 1902), iii–v, 1–4; and "Verhandlugen Des Comites für Krebsforschung,"

DMW 27 (1901): 301–5. For the social context in which the Comite began its work, see Peter Baldwin, *Contagion and the State in Europe, 1830–1930* (Cambridge: Cambridge University Press, 1999).

16. *Verhandlungen*, 5–8; and "Verhandlungen Des Comites Für Krebsforschung," *DMW* 27 (1901): 305–8.

17. "Collective Investigations of Cancer in Germany," *BMJ* 1 (1900): 532; *Verhandlungen*, 48; "Collective Investigation of Cancer," *BMJ* 2 (1900): 1209; "Study of Carcinoma in Germany," *Medical News* 77 (1900): 620; "Cancer in Germany," *BMJ* 1 (1901): 171; "Work of Cancer Investigating Committee," *JAMA* 36 (1901): 1670; and "Zur Krebsstatistik," *DMW* 27 (1901): 92 and 28 (1902): 348.

18. *Verhandlungen*, 9–12.

19. "Cancer Research," *Lancet* 2 (1902): 682–83.

20. E. E. Von Leyden, "Eröffnung der Abteilung für Krebsforschung an der I. Medizinischen Klinik Der Kgl. Charité zu Berlin," *ZFK* 1 (1903): 73–78; and "Oeffentliches Sanitätswesen. Die neue Abteilung für Krebsforschung der I. medizinischen Klinik in der Königlichen Charité Zu Berlin," *DMW* 29 (1903): 434–35. Also see E. V. Leyden, "Weitere Untersuchungen Zur Frage Der Krebsparasiten," *ZFK* 1 (1903): 393–414. Leyden was also interested in testing reported cures at his cancer hospital. See E. V. Leyden and F. Blumenthal, "Vorlaufige Mittheilungen Uber Einge Ergebnisse der Krebsforschung auf der Medizinischen Klinik," *DMW* 28 (1902): 637–38.

21. "Special Correspondence," *BMJ* 2 (1901): 1438; "Cancer Study in Germany," *Medical News* 79 (1901): 831; "War on Cancer," *American Medicine* 3 (1902): 623; and *Verhandlungen*, 35–37, 66–68.

22. "The Causation of Cancer," *BMJ* 1 (1901): 1281–82; *Verhandlungen*, 84–91; "Inhaltsverzeichniss Der Sitzungsprotokolle," vom 21 Marz 1902 bis 28 Februar 1903, *Verhandlungen*, 14, 25–38; "Cancer Inquiries in Germany and Russia," *BMJ* 1 (1901): 1103; L. L. Levschine, "Concerning Collective Investigations on Cancer," *New York Medical Journal* (hereafter *NYMJ*) 73 (1901): 434; "Zeitschrift f. Krebsforschung, Jena," *JAMA* 41 (1903): 941; "A Record of Cancer Investigations," *Medical Record* 64 (1903): 223; Drs. Weinberg and Gastpar, "Die bösartigen Neubildungen in Stuttgart von 1873 bis 1902," *ZFK* 2 (1904): 195–200; Dr. Foucault, "Sur Une Etude Statistique Sur La Mortalite Cancereuse," *Bulletin De L'Academie De Medecine* 1 (1904): 449–55; Sousa Junior, "O Cancro No Porto," *ZFK* 2 (1904): 373–75; and Jozsef Barabas, "Beiträge zur Statistik und Lokalisation des Krebses," *ZFK* 3 (1905): 158. For an organizational history of the various German cancer efforts through World War II, see Gustav Wagner and Andrea Mauerberger, *Krebsforschung in Deutschland. Vorgeschichte Und Geschichte Des Deutschen Krebsforschungszentrums* (Berlin: Springer-Verlag, 1989), 3–45.

23. "Zur Einführung," *ZFK* 1 (1904): 1–3.

24. *London Daily Mail*, January 19, 1901, 1, 63. "The Endowment of Research on Cancer," *BMJ* 1 (1902): 158; and Sandhurst, "Middlesex Hospital," *Charity Record and Hospital Times* (1902): 357. For donations to the Middlesex effort in 1902 and 1903, see *The Cancer Charity of The Middlesex Hospital: Report of the Year 1903* (London: Mitchell, Hughes, and Clarke, 1904), 13, 38–42, 86, 90.

25. "The Endowment of Research on Cancer," *BMJ* 1 (1902): 158; Cuthbert E.

Dukes, "The Origin and Early History of the Imperial Cancer Research Fund," *Annals of the Royal College of Surgeons* 36 (1965): 325–38; and "Sir Henry Morris," *BMJ* 1 (1926): 1066–67.

26. "A Scheme of Organized Research on Cancer," *BMJ* 1 (1902): 228–29; and Thomas Wakely, "The Investigation of Cancer," *Lancet* 1 (1902): 246–47.

27. "A Scheme of Organized Research on Cancer," 228–29; and "Krebsforschung In England," *DMW* 28 (1902): 528.

28. Wakely, "The Investigation of Cancer" and "A Scheme of Organized Research on Cancer," 228–29. The English effort drew the attention of the Americans and Germans. See "London Letter," *JAMA* 38 (1902): 1171; and "Krebsforschung in England," *DMW* 28 (1902): 528.

29. "Researches on Cancer," *Lancet* 1 (1902): 343–44.

30. "The Proposed Cancer Investigation," *BMJ* 1 (1902): 480; and Dawson Williams, "Cancer Research—The Scheme of the Royal Colleges," *BMJ* 1 (1902): 921–22.

31. Thomas Wakely, "Cancer Research," *Lancet* 1 (1902): 1121–22.

32. "The Royal Colleges and the Investigation of Cancer," *Lancet* 1 (1902): 1131–32. See also "Our London Letter," *Medical News* 80 (1902): 222.

33. "Cancer Research," 922. The BMSJ commented on the plan to organize researchers worldwide. See "Organized Cancer Research," *BMSJ* 146 (1902): 476.

34. F. W. Tunnicliffe, "Proposed Organised Research on Cancer," *Nature* 65 (1902): 467–69. Also of interest is L. Aschoff, "Notizen Uber Den Gegenwartigen Stand Der Krebsforschung in London Und Paris," *ZFK* 1 (1903): 112–24.

35. "British Fiscal Campaign Is Already in Full Swing," *NYT*, August 2, 1903, 4; "Cancer Research," *BMJ* 1 (1902): 1051–52; "Cancer Research," *BMJ* 1 (1902): 1109; "Royal College of Surgeons of England," *Lancet* 2 (1902): 101–2, 178–79. Also see Joan Ausoker, *A History of the Imperial Cancer Fund, 1902–1986* (Oxford: Oxford University Press, 1988).

36. "Cancer Research," *BMJ* 2 (1902): 409; "Cancer Research Fund," *Lancet* 2 (1902): 452–53, 1342; "Cancer Research Fund," *JAMA* 39 (1902): 1470; "The British Cancer Research Fund," *BMJ* 2 (1902): 1555; "British Fiscal Campaign Is Already in Full Swing; The Third Annual Meeting," *Nature* 105 (1904): 253; "Cancer Research," *Nature* 106 (1904): 279–80; and "A Cure for Cancer May Have Been Found," *NYT*, July 9, 1904, 7.

37. "Cancer Research in America," *BMJ* 1 (1902): 731; Roswell Park, "New York State Department of Health—Cancer Laboratory, University of Buffalo," *Buffalo Medical Journal* 57 (1902): 569–78; "An International Commission for the Study of Cancer," *BMJ* 1 (1902): 916; and *Fourth Annual Report of the Work of the Cancer Laboratory of the New York State Board of Health For the Year 1902–3* (Albany, NY: Evening Union Company, 1903), 5–19.

38. "Cancer Research," *BMJ* 2 (1902): 336–37; "Cancer Research in London," *Medical News* 81 (1902): 516; "Liverpool," *Lancet* 1 (1903): 268; and "The Liverpool Cancer Research Fund in Connexion with University College and the Royal Infirmary," *Lancet* 1 (1903): 556.

39. *First Annual Report of the Liverpool Cancer Research-The Mrs. Sutton Timmis Memorial Fund* (Liverpool: University Press of Liverpool, 1904), 3–7.

40. For the search for the germ of cancer outside of Europe and North America,

see, for instance, "Cancer Research in Australia," *Empire Review* 38 (1904): 117–21; and Carlos de Menezes and Antunes Lemos, "Eliologia Do Cancro," *ZFK* 2 (1904): 368.

41. "Natural History of Cancer," *JAMA* 44 (1905): 1155; and "Syphilis and Cancer," *JAMA* 44 (1905): 1407. Also see Robert Reyburn, "Causes of Cancer," *Medical Record* 62 (1902): 171–73.

42. "Cancer Research Fund," *BMJ* 2 (1903): 317–18; "Liverpool," *Lancet* 1 (1904): 1383.

43. W. T. Councilman, "The Modern Conceptions and Methods of Medical Science," *BMSJ* 151(1904): 425–33. Among the clearest contemporary statement is Jacques Loeb, *The Mechanistic Conception of Life* (Chicago: University of Chicago Press, 1912). Historians have considered the late nineteenth and early twentieth centuries in this light. See, for instance, the much overlooked Garland Allen, *Life Science in the Twentieth Century* (New York: Wiley, 1975), 73–111. Not all animals were deemed appropriate for laboratory service. See A. M. Trotter, "Six Cases of Carcinoma of the Ox," *Journal of Comparative Pathology and Therapeutics* 16 (1903): 244–52. Some veterinarians disputed whether cancer was a common animal disease. See C. Cunningham, "Cancer Cases," *Journal of Comparative Pathology and Therapeutics* 16 (1903): 163–69.

44. "A Gleam of Hope in Cancer," *Medical News* 87 (1905): 848–49.

45. "Cancer Research," *Lancet* 2 (1903): 413–14.

Chapter 3

1. Harvey Gaylord, "The Protozoon of Cancer," *American Journal of the Medical Sciences* 71(1901): 503–39; Harvey R. Gaylord, "Remarks on the Work of the Buffalo Laboratory on the Investigation of Cancer," *Buffalo Medical Journal* 39 (1901): 549–53; "Cancer Parasite Discovered," *NYT*, March 30, 1901, 6; "Finds Cause of Cancer," *Daily Mail*, (Hagerstown, MD), May 3, 1901, 1; "The Germ of Cancer," *The Gleaner* (Kingston, Jamaica), May 25, 1901, 1; "The Cause of Cancer," *Traverse City Evening Record*, May 6, 1901, 2; and "The Protozoon of Cancer," *JAMA* 36 (1901): 1324–25.

2. "The New Cancer Parasite," *American Medicine* 1 (1901): 100–1; "The Protozoon of Cancer," *Medical News* 78 (1901): 707–9; "Johns Hopkins Hospital Medical Society," *JAMA* 36 (1901): 1420; George B. Shattuck, "Another Alleged Cause of Cancer," *BMSJ* 144 (1901): 480–82; and "The Nature of the Cancerous Process," *NYMJ* 74 (1901): 560.

3. "American Surgical Association," *Medical News* 78 (1901): 754; "Nature of the Cancerous Process," *BMSJ* 145 (1901): 16–18; and Roswell Park, "The Nature of the Cancerous Process," *JAMA* 37 (1901): 671–74.

4. "The Recent Buffalo Investigations Regarding the Nature of Cancer," *NYMJ* 73 (1901): 909; Edward N. Liell, "The Present Status of Cancer: Its Etiology and Pathology—the Value of Laboratory Research," *Medical News* 81 (1902): 545–48; Leo Loeb, "Cell Implantation in the Production of Tumors," *JAMA* 40 (1903): 974–77; Alexander Theodore Brand, "The Etiology of Cancer," *BMJ* 2 (1902): 238–42; and "Biological Aspect of Carcinoma," *Medical News* 87 (1905): 1004–5. For contemporary insect vectors, see "The Study of Ticks and the Diseases Caused By Them," *NYMJ* 71 (1900): 735–36.

5. "The Buffalo Campaign Against Cancer," *NYMJ* 81 (1905): 130; "Cancer Serums," *BMJ* 1 (1905): 542; "The Immunization of Mice to Cancer," *Medical News* 86 (1905): 477–78; "Some Recent American Studies of Cancer," *NYMJ* 81 (1905): 601–2; "New Studies in Cancer," *Cincinnati Lancet-Clinic* 55 (1905): 554–55; "Serum for Cancer," *Medical News* 87 (1905): 910; and G. H. A. Clowes and F. W. Baeslack, "Further Evidence of Immunity Against Cancer in Mice After Spontaneous Recovery," *Medical News* 87 (1905): 968–71.

6. "Deductions from the Experimentations Tending to Determine the Cause of Cancer," *Medical News* 87 (1905): 713–14; "Recent Results in Cancer Research Which Bear on the Parasitic Theory," *JAMA* 45 (1905): 1351; and "Cancer and Parasites," *Medical News* 87 (1905): 950.

7. "Cancer Bacillus Discovered?" *NYT*, April 27, 1900, 7; "What Interests Berlin," *NYT*, May 6, 1900, 7; "The Micro-Organism of Malignant Growths," *NYMJ* 71 (1901): 735; "The Parasites of Cancer Again Discovered," *JAMA* 36 (1901): 1784–85; "Etiology of Cancer," *JAMA* 37 (1901): 481; "Cause of Malignant Tumors," *Medical News* 79 (1901): 499–500; "Malignancy," *JAMA* 37 (1901): 864; "Professor Max Schuller's Views on Malignancy," *NYMJ* 74 (1901): 487–493; Dr. M. Schuller, "Das Wesen Der Schuller'schen Krebsparasiten," *DMW* 27 (1901): 623–24; and Max Schuller, "Die Parasiten Im Krebs Und Sarkom Des Menachen," *BKW* (1902): 16.

8. "Schuller's Cancer Parasite," *American Medicine* 2 (1901): 514; Friedrich Volcker, "The Character of Schuller's Carcinoma Parasites," *DMW* 27 (1901): 322–24; A. Rose, "Parasites of Cancer and Sarcoma," *American Medicine* 2 (1901): 726–27; "A Tale of Cancer and Cures," *Medical News* 79 (1901): 1033–34; and "Our Berlin Letter," *Medical News* 80 (1902): 618.

9. "XX Congress For Internal Medicine," *American Medicine* 3 (1902): 811–12; "Pathological Anatomy and Cancer Investigation," *BMJ* 1 (1903): 269; "Meeting of the Cancer Research Committee," *JAMA* 38 (1902): 1546; "Origin of Cancer," *NYMJ* 81 (1905): 973; "Vienna," *BMJ* 1 (1905): 1297; Georg Kelling, "Zur Entscheidung der Frage über die Ursache des Krebses," *ZFK* 3 (1905): 258–64; Herr V. Leyden, "Ueber die parasitäre Theorie in der Aetiologie der Krebse," *Centralblatt Fur Bakteriologie, Parasitenkunde Und Infektionskrankheiten* 36 (1905): 458–62; E. V. Leyden, "Ueber die parasitären Theorie in der Aetiologie der Krebse," *BKW* (1905): 345–50; and "Berliner medizinische Gesellschaft, Sitzung Vom 15 März 1905," *BKW* (1905): 373–79, 404–9, and "22 März 1905," 442–44. For variola, see, for example, "American Association of Pathologists and Bacteriologists," *Medical News* 82 (1903): 959; R. L. Thompson, "The Bacteriolytic Complement Content of the Blood Serum in Variola," *JMR* 10 (1903): 71–88; and "The Cancer and Variola Parasites," *Medical News* 82 (1903): 1183.

10. "Malaria as a Cure for Cancer," *NYT*, April 7, 1902, 8; "The Cancer Mystery," *NYT*, September 23, 1902, 8; "Cancer Research," *JAMA* 41 (1903): 343; "New Treatment of Cancer," *The Standard* (Ogden, UT), November 6, 1903, 4.

11. "Oeffentliches Sanitatswesen—Die Nene Abtheilung Fur Krebsforschung Der I. Medizinischen Klinik In Der Koniglichen Charite Zu Berlin," *DMW* 29 (1903): 434–35.

12. "Special Correspondence—Berlin," *BMJ* 2 (1904): 150; and "Cancer

Research Committee," *JAMA* 43 (1904): 1909–10. Cancer inspection stations were also on Leyden's agenda.

13. "Cancer Research in Germany," *BMJ* 1 (1905): 319; "Cancer Statistics in Stuttgart," *BMJ* 1 (1905): 1159; Hans Leyden, "Die Krebssterblichkeit in Montevideo," *ZFK* 3 (1905): 308–11; and "Die Bösartigen Neubildungen in Stuttgart 1873–1902," *ZFK* 4 (1906): 30–44.

14. "The Parasitic Theory of Cancer," *BMJ* 1 (1905): 1056.

15. "Malignant Mouse Tumors," *NYMJ* 82 (1903): 453; "Transplantation of Tumors," *JAMA* 43 (1904): 1872–73; and "Experimental Cancer and Immunity," *American Medicine* 12 (1906): 290.

16. "Cancer Investigation," *JAMA* 35 (1900): 1562; Harvard Medical School, *The Caroline Brewer Croft Fund Cancer Commission* (Boston: Harvard, 1907), reports 1 and 2; Edward H. Nichols, "First Annual Report of Work on the Etiology of Cancer," *Boston Society of Medical Science* 5 (1900): 57–58; David Riesman and A. O. J. Kelly, "Clinical Medicine," *American Medicine* 3 (1902): 923; and "Cancer Research in the United States," *Lancet* 1 (1902): 1845–46;

17. "Cancer Research Reports," *Medical News*, 86 (1905): 88.

18. *The Caroline Brewer Croft Fund Cancer Commission*, report 3; "The Third Annual Report of the Harvard Cancer Commission," *Medical News* 85 (1904): 889–90; "The Present Status of Cancer Investigation," *BMSJ* 152 (1905): 352–53; "Recent Cancer Research," *American Medicine* 9 (1905): 543; and "The American Cancer Commission," *BMJ* 1 (1905): 106.

19. Leo Loeb, "Further Investigations in Transplantation of Tumors," *JMR* 8 (1902): 44–75; "The Transmissibility of Cancer," *JAMA* 43 (1904): 127–28; and "The Energy of Tumor Growth," *NYMJ* 82 (1905): 406.

20. *Reports of the Collis P. Huntington Fund for Cancer Research* (New York: n.p., 1905), vol. 1; B. H. Buxton and Phillip Shaffer, "Enzymes in Tumors," *JMR* 13 (1905): 543–54; and "Pathological Chemistry of Tumors," *Medical News* 86 (1905): 427.

21. "The Imperial Cancer Research Fund," *BMJ* 2 (1904): 146–49.

22. "Cancer Research at the Middlesex Hospital," *BMJ* 1 (1903): 35–36; Alexander G. R. Foulerton, ed., *Archives of the Middlesex Hospital*, vol. 2, *Second Report From the Cancer Research Laboratories* (London: Macmillan and Co., 1904); W. S. Lazarus-Barlow, ed., *Archives of the Middlesex Hospital, Vol. 3, Third Report From the Cancer Research Laboratories* (London: Macmillan and Co., 1904); and "The Middlesex Hospital Cancer Research Laboratories," *BMJ* 2 (1904): 845–46.

23. Karl Pearson, "Report on Certain Cancer Statistics of Messrs. W. T. Hillier and I. Tritsch, of the Cancer Research Laboratories, Middlesex Hospital," in *Archives of the Middlesex Hospital*, vol. 2, 127–37; "Cancer Research at Middlesex Hospital," *BMJ* 1 (1904): 1271; and "The Influence of Heredity in Cancer," *JAMA* 42 (1904): 1626–27. Others saw the existence of cancer in tuberculosis patients not as causal but as a matter of predisposition to both. See E. Boinet, "Cancer Et Tuberculese," *Bulletin De L'Academie De Medecine* 53 (1907): 228–30.

24. E. F. Bashford, "The Problems of Cancer," *BMJ* 2 (1903): 127–29; and "Cancer Research," *BMJ* 2 (1903): 373–74.

25. Henry Morris, "The Bradford Lecture on Cancer and Its Origin," *BMJ* 2

(1903): 1505–11; and "The Bradshaw Lecture," *Nature* 69 (1903): 157. For Connheim, see, for example, Russell C. Maulitz, "Rudolf Virchow, Julius Cohnheim and the Program of Pathology," *Bulletin of the History of Medicine* 52 (1978): 162–82; and "Julius Cohnheim (20 July 1839–15 August 1884) and His Work. Papers from a Festschrift," *Zentralblatt für allgemeine Pathologie und pathologische Anatomie* 130 (1985): 281–347.

26. H. G. Plimmer, "The Parasitic Theory of Cancer," *BMJ* 2 (1903): 1511–15.

27. See, for example, "Cancer," *NYMJ* 79 (1904): 36–38; and Herbert Tempest Dufton, "Cancer and Its Origin," *BMJ* 1 (1904): 105–6.

28. J. Bretland Farmer, J. E. S. Moore, and C. E. Walker, "On the Resemblances Exhibited Between the Cells of Malignant Growths in Man and Those of Normal Reproductive Tissues," *Proceedings of the Royal Society of London* 72 (1903–1904): 499–504. Also see "The Resemblances Between the Cells of Malignant Growths in Man and Those of Normal Reproductive Tissues," *Lancet* 2 (1903): 1830–31; "Royal Society," *Nature* 102 (1904): 285.

29. E. F. Bashford and J. A. Murray, "The Significance of the Zoological Distribution, the Nature of the Mitoses, and the Transmissibility of Cancer," *Proceedings of the Royal Society of London* 73 (1904): 66–76. The piece was reprinted in *BMJ* 1 (1904): 269–71, and *Lancet* 1 (1904): 413–16.

30. See, for instance on these points, "Cancer and Its Origin," *BMJ* 1 (1904): 51, 162, 218, 402; "Recent Cancer Research," *BMJ* 1 (1904): 259; "Cancer and Parthenogenesis," *Nature* 103 (1904): 392; H. J. W, "The Cancer Problem," *Cincinnati Lancet-Clinic* 52 (1904): 86; "Cancer," *NYMJ* 79 (1904): 469–70; "Scotland," *BMJ* 1 (1904): 800; Robert Bell, "The Biological Significance of Malignant Growths," *BMJ* 1 (1904): 865; H. J. Campbell, "Note on the Causation of Cancer," *BMJ* 1 (1904): 1004–5; "The Biology of Cancer," *JAMA* 42 (1904): 650–51; "The Nature and Etiology of Cancer," *Lancet* 2 (1904): 467–68; Albert S. Grunbaum, "The Germ Cell Theory of Cancer," *BMJ* 2 (1904): 1634; and "Cancer," *NYMJ* 81 (1905): 46. The Farmer group recanted its epic research a year later, when it acknowledged that, while some cancer cells divided like reproductive cells, others divided in a more conventional manner. See, for example, J. Bretland Farmer, J. E. S. Moore and C. E. Walker, "On the Cytology of Malignant Growths," *Proceedings of the Royal Society of London*, Series B, 518 (1906): 336–53; and J. E. S. Moore and C. E. Walker, *The Maiotic Process in Mammalia* (London: Williams & Norgate, 1906).

31. *Scientific Reports on the Investigations of the Cancer Research Fund, No. 1* (London: Taylor and Francis, 1904); "The Biological and Comparative Aspects of Cancer," *Lancet* 1 (1904): 448–49; and "George H. Simmons, "Recent Developments in the Study of Cancer Etiology," *JAMA* 43 (1904): 125–26.

32. "Cancer Research," *BMJ* 2 (1903): 1558–60; "The Cancer Research Fund," *BMJ* 1 (1904): 1027; "Report of the English Cancer Research Fund," *Medical News* 84 (1904): 1088–89; "Cancer Research," *Medical News* 85 (1904): 131, 227–28; "British Cancer Research Fund," *Medical News* 84 (1904): 38–39; "Cancer Research," *JAMA* 43 (1904): 133; and "Recent Studies of Disease Organisms," *Nature* 70 (1904): 519–20.

33. E. F. Bashford, "An Address on the Growth of Cancer," *Lancet* 1 (1905): 837–41; "Imperial Cancer Research Fund," *BMJ* 2 (1905): 96–99; "Scientific Report of the Imperial Cancer Research Fund," *Lancet* 2 (1905): 246–48; and "The

Statistical Investigation of Cancer," *BMJ* 2 (1905): 590–91.

34. "The Age Incidence of Cancer," *Lancet* 1 (1905): 1031–32; "Cancer," *NYMJ* 81 (1905): 825–26; "The Growth of Cancer," *American Medicine* 9 (1905): 839; "The Age of Cancer," *BMJ* 2 (1905): 594–95; F. W. Forbes-Ross, "Observations on Certain Features Exhibited By Cells in Their Relation to Cancer," *BMJ* 2 (1905): 1101–2.

35. "Visit of French Physicians and Surgeons to London, October, 1904," *Lancet* 164 (1904): 1111–16.

36. French investigators heavily favored a microbial explanation for cancer. See M. Jaboulay, "Le Parasite Du Cancer Epitheliale (premiere note)," *ZFK* 3 (1905): 156; Charles Ladame, "Le Corpuscule De Feinberg," *ZFK* 3 (1905): 156–57. So too did many of their German counterparts. See, for instance, Dr. Feinberg, "Zur Lehre Des Gewebes Und Der Ursache Der Krebsgeschwulste," *DMW* 28 (1902): 185–87; and Ludwig Feinberg, "Ueber Die Verhutung De Infektion Mit Der Erregern Der Krebsgeschwulate," *BKW* (1906): 172.

37. Best for the French medical profession is George Weisz, *The Medical Mandarins: The French Academy of Medicine in the Nineteenth and Early Twentieth Centuries* (Oxford: Oxford University Press, 1995). Also of use is Gerald L. Geison, *Professions and the French State, 1700–1900* (Philadelphia: University of Pennsylvania Press, 1984).

38. "Dr. Doyen and the Microbe of Cancer," *Lancet* 1 (1902): 126–27; "The Etiology and Treatment of Cancer," *Lancet* 1 (1902): 322–23; "The Toxin Treatment of Cancer," *BMJ* 1 (1904): 507; "M. Doyen's Cancer Serum," *BMJ* 2 (1904): 1181–82; "Radium Fails in Cancer," *Chicago Tribune*, February 28, 1904, 13; Eugene Louis Doyen, *Etiologie et Traitement Du Cancer* (Paris: A. Maloine, 1904); "Doyen's Cancer Serum," *JAMA* 44 (1905): 145; "The New Treatment of Cancer," *NYMJ* 81 (1905): 259; "M. Doyen's Researches on Cancer," *BMJ* 1 (1905): 729–30; "The 'Microbe Doyen,'" *Lancet* 1 (1905): 955–56; "Cancer," *New York Journal of Medicine* 82 (1905): 768; and "Cancer Serums," *BMJ* 1 (1905): 542–43.

39. "The Mode of the Origin of Neoplasms," *Lancet* 2 (1905): 100. For Doyen's career generally, see Jacques HM Cohen, "The Scandalous Dr. Doyen, or the Solitary Tragedy of a Prodigy," trans. by Karine Debbasch, http://www.bium.univ-paris5.fr/histmed/medica/doyen_eng.htm.

40. Initiation of *Revues Des Maladies Cancereuses* in 1893 reflected a desire for cancer researchers to share information, but that desire had not generated an institutional structure outside of the periodical. In 1902, then-editor of the *Revues*, E. Ozenne, chided his French colleagues for not imitating the Germans, Russians, and English and establishing something formal and substantive. With cancer rates apparently skyrocketing, he attributed the lack of action in France to his nation's medical men "continuing to remain deaf to the voice of pity." See E. H. Ozenne, "Societies Contre Le Cancer," *Revue Des Maladies Cancereuses* 6 (1902): 11.

41. Johannes Orth, "On the Morphology of Carcinoma and the Parasitic Theory of its Etiology," *Annals of Surgery* 40 (1904): 773–81. Also see W. L. Rodman, "Cancer," *JAMA* 45 (1905): 371–78. For a positivistic summary of the "contributions" of the cancer research institutes taken from the perspective of the second half of the twentieth century, see Victor A. Triolo, "Nineteenth Century foundations of Cancer Research: Origins of Experimental Research," *Cancer Research* 24 (1964): 4–27. The eleventh edition of the *Encyclopedia Britannica* was

so taken by the creation of cancer laboratories and the world's war on cancer that it traced the development of these institutions. See *Encyclopedia Britannica*, 11th ed., vol. 5 (1911), 176–77.

42. E. F. Bashford, "Are the Problems of Cancer Insoluble," *Lancet* 2 (1905): 1670–74.

Chapter 4

1. See, for example, R. T. Hewlett, "The Present Position of the Cancer Problem," *Nature* (1905): 295–97; "Contributions to the Cancer Problem," *American Medicine* 10 (1905): 416; Wilhelm Alex Freund, "Zur Naturgeschichte der Krebskrankheit nach klinischen Erfahrungen," *ZFK* 3 (1905): 1–33; "The Present Position of the Cancer Problem," *Current Opinion* 40 (1906): 296–97; "The Cancer Problem," *BMJ* 2 (1906): 1733; J. Bland-Sutton, "A Lecture on the Cancer Problem," *Lancet* 1 (1907): 1339–45; Charles Gordon Mackay, "Case That Seems to Suggest a Cure to the Possible Solution of the Cancer Problem," *BMJ* 2 (1907): 138–40; F. B. Skerrett, "The Cancer Problem—A Suggestion," *BMJ* 2 (1907): 1206–7; and "The Cancer Problem," *JAMA* 49 (1907): 1877.

2. "The Imperial Cancer Research Fund," *Lancet* 1 (1906): 243; "The Imperial Cancer Research Fund," *Lancet* 2 (1906): 305–6; E. F. Bashford, "Advance in Knowledge of Cancer," *Nature* 79 (1908): 261–64; "The Imperial Cancer Research Fund,"NYMJ 81 (1909): 86–87; and "Imperial Cancer Research Fund," *Lancet* 2 (1910): 265–69.

3. E. F. Bashford, "Are the Problems of Cancer Insoluble," *Lancet* 2 (1905): 1670–74; and J. Jackson Clarke, "The Problem of Cancer," *BMJ* 2 (1905): 1679.

4. E. F. Bashford, "The Application of Experiment to the Study of Cancer," *Scientific Progress in the Twentieth Century* 2 (1907): 1–29. Bashford believed that animal experiments were critical to understanding human cancer. See his "The Growth of Cancer," *Transactions of the Medical Society of London* 28 (1905): 210–29; and "The Comparative Study of Cancer," *Journal of the Royal Sanitary Institute* 25 (1904): 852–56.

5. Nicholas Senn, "A Plea for the International Study of Carcinoma," *JAMA* 46 (1906): 1254–58; and "The Fifteenth International Medical Congress," *NYMJ* 83 (1906): 466. For self and human experimentation, see Susan E. Lederer, *Subjected to Science: Human Experimentation in America Before the Second World War* (Baltimore: Johns Hopkins University Press, 1995), 11 and passim.

6. Dawson Williams, "The Problems of Cancer Research," *BMJ* 1 (1906): 1242–43. For Williams's career generally, see "Obituary-Sir Dawson Williams, C.B.E., M.D," *BMJ* 1 (1928): 414–25.

7. Accentuation of the concept of basic or pure research and its various and political uses was a later nineteenth and early twentieth century ploy. Historians have often noted its successes. See, for example, Leonard S. Reich, *The Making of American Industrial Research: Science and Business at GE and Bell, 1876–1926* (London: Cambridge University Press, 1985); and Daniel J. Kevles, *The Physicists: The History of a Scientific Community in Modern America*, (New York: Vintage, 1979), 45–59.

8. Etienne Burnet, "La Lutte Contre Le Cancer," *Revue De Paris* (January–

February 1906): 149–68; R. Ledous-Lebard, "La Lutte Contre Le Cancer," *These Pour Le Doctorat En Medecine* (Paris: Masson Et Cie, 1906); and M. E. Roux, "Sur Un Travail De M. Le Dr. A. Borrel, Intitule: Tumeurs Cancereuses Et Helminthes," *Bulletin De L'Academie De Medecine* 2 (1906): 141–44.

9. "Cancer Research in Germany," *BMJ* 1 (1906): 753; "An International Conference," *BMJ* 1 (1906): 1534; "Berlin," *Lancet* 1 (1906): 1862; "An International Conference on Cancer," *BMJ* 2 (1906): 656. Gaylord's call was mentioned retrospectively in "Vorwort," *ZFK* 5 (1907): 17–18. About the institute at Heidelberg, see Vinzenz Czerny, *Das Heidelberger Institut für experimentelle Krebsforschung* (Tübingen: Verlag Der H. Laupp'schen Buchhandlung, 1912), 1–14; and "Vermischtes," *ZFK* 1 (1903): 496. An international conference to consider cancer had the precedent of an international tuberculosis conference. That analogous conference met in Berlin in 1899.

10. Walther Poppelmann, "Krebs und Wasser?" *ZFK* 4 (1906): 39–44; Hans Leyden, ed., "Bericht über die am I. September 1902 in Spanien veranstaltete Krebssammelforschung," *ZFK* 1 (1903): 47–72; Dr. Weinberg, "Kritische Bemerkungen zu Der Breslauer Statistik des Krebses beider Ehegatten und der Frage des Krebses der Ehegatten überhaupt," *ZFK* 4 (1906): 83–90; and "Krebsforschung in Hamburg," *DMW* (1907): 2163.

11. "A Cancer Institute at Heidelberg," *BMJ* 1 (1906): 219; "International Cancer Conference," *BMJ* 2 (1906): 725–26, 884, 957–58. For the pomp, see "Internationale Konferenz Fur Krebsforchung 1906," *ZFK* 5 (1907): 18–42. For the pathological anatomists, see Hugo Ribbert, *Die Entstehung Des Carcinoms* (Bonn: 1905); and O. Israel, "Die biogenetische Theorie der Geschwülste und die Aetiologie des Carcinoms," *BKW* (1905): 350–53.

12. "Verhandlungen der Internationalen Konferenz für Krebsforschung Vom 25. Bis 27. September 1906 zu Heidelberg Und Frankfurt a.M.," *ZFK* 5 (1907): 3–19.

13. "Verhandlungen," 20–22. Bashford published similar sentiments about comparative and biological studies of cancer in *Third Scientific Report of the Investigations of the Imperial Cancer Research Fund* (London: Taylor and Francis, 1908), 1–60.

14. "Verhandlungen," 24–26.

15. Francis Carter Wood, "A Review of the Advances in Our Knowledge and Treatment of Cancer in the Last Thirty Years," *Medical Record* 88 (1915): 1–4.

16. "Verhandlungen," passim; "International Cancer Conference," 957–58; "Die I. Internationale Konferenz für Krebsforschung, Heidelberg-Frankfurt a. M. 25–27 September 1906," *DMW* (1906): 1682–86, 1727–28; and "The Cancer Conference," *BMJ* 2 (1906): 962. Also see C. O. Jensen, "Experimentelle Untersuchungen über Krebs bei Mäusen," *ZFK* 1 (1903): 134–38; C. O. Jensen, "Ueber einige Probleme der experimentellen Krebsforschung," *ZFK* 7 (1908): 279–85; "Cancer on Mice," *JAMA* 47 (1906): 468; "The Experimental Analysis of the Growth of Cancer," *NYMJ* 84 (1906): 1093–94; F. R. Skerrett, "The Cancer Problem—A Suggestion," *BMJ* 2 (1907): 1206–7; E. E. Tyzzer, "The Inoculable Tumors of Mice," *JMR* 17 (1907): 137–53. For an early German report on the Jensen mouse, see E. V. Leyden and F. Blumenthal, "Vorläufige Mittheilungen über einige

Ergebnisse der Krebsforschung auf der I. Medizinischen Klinik," *DMW* 28 (1902): 637–38. Newspapers carried the important news that mice speeded the cancer quest. See, for instance, Maynard Evans, "On a Vast Army of Mice Rests Hope of Finding a Cancer Cure," *Atlanta Constitution*, Nov. 18, 1906, 3; and "Cancer 'Cures' Rejected," *Washington Post*, July 11, 1909, 8. For a history of the laboratory mouse in America, see Karen Rader, *Making Mice: Standardizing Animals for American Biomedical Research, 1900–1955* (Princeton: Princeton University Press, 2004), 25–58. Rats have their own history. See Mark A. Suckow, Steven H. Weisbroth, and Craig L. Franklin, *The Laboratory Rat* (Waltham, MS: Academic Press, 2005), 17–31.

17. "Verhandlungen," 258–59. For a more extensive argument, see E. V. Leyden, "Ueber den Krebs der Mäuse," *ZFK* 4 (1906): 1–13. For another paean to the mouse, see, for instance, A. Borrel and M. Haaland, "Tumeurs De La Souris," *CRSB* (1905): 14–15.

18. Henry T. Butlin, "Carcinoma is a Parasitic Disease," *BMJ* 2 (1905): 1565–71; and "The First International Conference on Cancer," *JAMA* 47 (1906): 1312.

19. Verhandlungen," passim.

20. "The International Conference on Cancer," *Lancet* 2 (1906): 1098–99, 1171–73; and "International Cancer Conference, 1906," *BMJ* 1 (1907): 1487. Conference proceedings were printed as a special issue of *Zeitschrift für Krebsforschung*. Others articulated a finer justification for eschewing theory when searching for prevention and cure. They accentuated empiricism. See "Hypothesis and Treatment in Relation to Cancer," *BMJ* 2 (1908): 1509–10. In Britain, Middlesex Hospital moved decisively into treatment, especially examining claims of curative substances. See "The New Cancer Research Laboratories at the Middlesex Hospital," *Lancet* 2 (1905): 1149 and *BMJ* 2 (1905): 1069; and "Organization of Cancer Research," *BMJ* 1 (1906): 1227–28. See also "Cancer Research in Dundee," *BMJ* 1 (1908): 474. In the United States, the Croft group inaugurated clinical experiments to test cures. See "The Clinical Study of Cancer," *NYMJ* 87 (1908): 72–73; "Cancer Research," *BMJ* 1 (1908): 475; and "The Harvard Cancer Commission," *BMJ* 1 (1910): 1505.

21. "Verhandlungen," 64–65, 249–50; "International Cancer," 958; and "Verhandlungen Des Deutschen Zentralkomitees für Krebsforschung," *ZFK* 6(1908): 429–33. The conference was hardly alone in making the transition to prevention. See, for example, Charles P. Childe, "The Educational Aspects of the Cancer Question," *BMJ* 2 (1907): 135–38; Henry Trentham Butlin, "The Contagion of Cancer in Human Beings: Auto-Inoculation," *Lancet* 2 (1907): 279–83; and Azevedo Neves, "Die Portugiesische Kommission für Krebsforschung," *ZFK* 7 (1908): 180–83. For a state of the art statement on German cancer research on the eve of creation of the IACI, see L. Michaelis, "Weitere experimentelle Untersuchungen über Tierkrebs," *DMW* (1907): 826–28.

22. P. Juliusburger, "7081 Todesfälle an Krebs von 1885–1899 bei der 'Friedrich Wilhelm' Preussischen Lebens-und Garantie-Versicherungs-Aktien-Gesellsch. in Berlin," *ZFK* 3 (1905): 106–31; and "Bericht über die von der Schwedischen Aerztegesellschaft veranstaltete Sammelforschung über die Krebskrankheit in Schweden während der Zeit vom 1. Dezember 1905 Bis 28. Februar 1906," *ZFK* 7 (1908): 3–44.

23. "Imperial Cancer Research Fund," *BMJ* 2 (1907): 26–29.

24. The story of the AACR is recounted in Victor A. Triolo and Ilse L. Riegel, "The AACR, 1907–1940: Historical Review," *Cancer Research* 21 (1961): 137–42. Also see G. H. A. Clowes, "Cancer Research Fifty Years Ago and Now," *Cancer Research* 16 (1956): 1–4. For the AACR's early efforts, see "American Association for Cancer Research," *JAMA* 50 (1908): 63–67; and *JAMA* 51 (1908): 158–59, 251–54. For the founding of International Association of Cancer Investigation, see "International Conference on Cancer," *Lancet* 1 (1908): 1661–62; and "Internationale Vereinigung Fur Krebsforschung, Berlin, 23, Mai 1908," *DMW* 34 (1908): 1039–41. For early efforts, see Pierre Delbet and R. Ledoux-Lebard, *Travaux De La Deuxieme Conference Internationale Pour L'Étude Du Cancer Tenue A Paris Du 1st Au 5 Octobre 1910* (Paris: Librairie Felix Alcan, 1911). For the Rockefeller Institute, see E. Richard Brown, *Rockefeller Medicine Men: Medicine and Capitalism in America* (Berkeley: University of California Press, 1979); Darwin H. Stapleton, ed., *Creating a Tradition of Biomedical Research: Contributions to the History of the Rockefeller University* (New York: Rockefeller University Press, 2004); and Karen Deane Ross, "Making Medicine Scientific: Simon Flexner and Experimental Medicine at the Rockefeller Institute for Medical Research, 1901–1945 (PhD diss., University of Minnesota, 2006). Also see "Rockefeller Plans for Vast Institute," *NYT*, February 22, 1903, 1; "Rockefeller Gives $2,600,000 Outright," *NYT*, November 24, 1907, 1; and "Institutes for Medical Research," *BMSJ* 156 (1907): 196. For attempts to develop laws of tumor transplantation through understanding the biology and chemistry of tumors, see, for instance, W. Ford Robertson and M. C. W. Young, "Further Researches Into the Etiology of Carcinoma: Note Upon Certain Histological Features of Carcinomatous Tumours Revealed By An Improved Ammonio-Silver Process," *Lancet* 2 (1907): 358–61; "The Cancer Problem," *NYMJ* 91 (1910): 187–88. For an example of an organization spawned by the forming of the IACI, see Azevedo Neves, "Die Portugiesische Kommission für Krebsforschung," *ZFK* 7 (1908): 180–83.

25. Etienne Burnet, "Le Cancer," *La Revue De Paris* (March 1908): 325–50; President Bouchard, "Séance Du Lundi 15 Juin 1908," *Bulletin De L'Association Française Pour L'Étude Du Cancer*(hereafter cited as *L'Étude*) 1 (1908): 15; Philippe Jeanteur and Paul Cappelaere,"Bientot Centenaire," *Bulletin Du Cancer* 93 (2006): 3–4; J.-F. Bernaudin, "IL y a 100 ANS: 1908, l'annee 01 du Bulletin du Cancer," *Bulletin Du Cancer* 95 (2008): 791–95; Jean-Francoise Bernaudin, "*Le Bulletin De L'Association Française Pour L'Étude Du Cancer* De 1909 A 1914: *Le Bulletin Du Cancer* Dans Sa Premiere Periode," *Bulletin Du Cancer* 100 (2013): 1251–59; and Patrice Pinell, *The Fight Against Cancer: France 1890–1940*, trans. David Madell (London: Routledge, 1992), 39–41.

26. L' Association Française Pour L'Étude Du Cancer, "Statuts," *L'Étude* 1 (1908): 1–11. For a good discussion of the concept of public utility, see Jann Passler, *Composing the Citizen: Music as Public Utility in Third Republic France* (Berkeley: University of California Press, 2009), 68–82 and passim. For physicians in French public service, see Jack D. Ellis, *The Physician-Legislators in the Early Third Republic, 1870–1914* (Cambridge, UK: Cambridge University Press, 1990).

27. The new organization's constitution was published in Triolo and

Riegel, "American Association," 165–166. For an early draft, see "Internationale Vereinigung Fur Krebsforschung, Berlin, 23. Mai 1908," *DMW* 34 (1908): 1039–40. Despite the specificity of the constitution, not all researchers knew exactly what the organization would do. Jensen called for it to initiate and co-ordinate hereditarian experiments. See C. O. Jensen, "Ueber einige Probleme der experimentellen Krebsforschung," *ZFK* 7 (1908): 279–85.

28. "Bericht der wissenschaftlichen Abteilung der russischen Gesellschaft zur Bekämpfung des Krebses," *ZFK* 9 (1910): 61–66; and K. Yamagiwa, ed., *Gann: Ergebnisse der Krebsforschung in Japan* (Tokyo: Handaya, 1907).

29. "Cancer Research," *BMJ* 1 (1908): 1149; "The Cancer Problem," *BMJ* 1 (1909): 51; and "Imperial Cancer Fund," *BMJ* 2 (1908): 162–64. Germany took the opportunity to redouble its cancer efforts by establishing a fund named after Leyden and paralleling the British effort. See "Ernst von Leyden Foundation for Cancer Research and the Campaign Against Cancer," *JAMA* 52 (1909): 146.

30. Pierre Delbet, "Rapport Annuel Du Secretary General," *L'Étude* 3 (1910): 53–55.

31. "Imperial Cancer Research Fund," *BMJ* 2 (1909): 151–54; "International Cancer Research Union," *BMJ* 1 (1909): 1085; "A Special General Meeting," *BMJ* 1 (1910): 283; "The Second International Congress," *BMJ* 1 (1910): 565; and "Our London Letter," *Medical Record* 76 (1909): 238–39.

32. "International Conference for the Study of Cancer," *Lancet* 1 (1910): 1443; and "The Second International Conference," *BMJ* 1 (1910): 643.

33. "Imperial Cancer Research Fund," *Lancet* 2 (1910): 265–69; "Imperial Cancer Research Fund," *BMJ* 2 (1910): 205–9; and "The Progress of Cancer Research," *Nature* 84 (1910): 126–28.

34. "Conference on Cancer," *Lancet* 2 (1910): 1108, 1175; "The International Cancer Conference," *BMJ* 2 (1910): 1266–68; "Paris Letter," *JAMA* 55 (1910): 1567–68; Reid Hunt, "Second International Conference for the Study of Cancer (Paris, October 1–5, 1910) and Ninth International Antituberculosis Conference (Brussels, October 5–8, 1910)," *Public Health Reports* 25 (1910): 1624–25; "The International Cancer Conference At Paris," *Nature* 84 (1910): 545–46; "Cancer Research," *BMJ* 1 (1911): 1008–9; and "The International Conference on Cancer Research," *Lancet* 1 (1911): 1091–92.

35. Pierre Delbet, P. Manetrier, and A. Herrenschmidt, "Essai De Nomenclature Des Cancers Pour L'usage International," *Travaux De La Deuxieme Conference Internationale*, 252–90. For a sense of the diversity of statistical measurement that the IACI hoped to overcome, see Dr. Abramowski, "Zur Frage des endemischen Vorkommens von Krebs," *ZFK* 6 (1908): 404–11; A. Hvuslef, "Ueber das Auftreten von Krebs in den Landbezirken von Norwegen," *ZFK* 7 (1908): 184–89; S.A. Gavalas, "Die Verbreitung der Krebskrankheit in Griechenland," *ZFK* 7 (1908): 605–15; and M. Guillot, "Le Probleme De L'Heredite Cancereuse En Normandie," *L'Étude* 1 (1908): 112–21.

36. Each of the following is in *Travaux De La Deuxieme Conference Internationale*. They included R. Ledoux-Lebard, "La Statistique Du Cancer," 449–67; Professor J. Dollinger, Ergebnisse der Krebsstatistiken "469–512; Prof George Meyer, "Methoden Der Statistik (Internationaler Fragebogen)," 513–24;

"Sketch for a Question Form for an International Cancer Statistic," 567–68, 572; and "Discussion on Statistics and Nomenclature," 650–64. For some examples of the types of taxonomic issues the IACI hoped to correct, see J. Orth, "Ueber Heilungsvorgange An Epitheliomen Nebst Allgemeinen Bemerkungen Uber Epitheliome," *ZFK* 1 (1903): 413–44.

37. "Conference on Cancer," *Lancet* 2 (1910): 1108, 1175; "The International Cancer Conference," *BMJ* 2 (1910): 1266–68; "Paris Letter," *JAMA* 55 (1910): 1567–68; "Cancer Research," *BMJ* 1 (1911): 1008–9; and "The International Conference on Cancer Research," *Lancet* 1 (1911): 1091–92. The physical confrontation was remembered in Pierre Delbet, *L'Emprise Allemande* (Paris: Felix Alcan, 1915), 29–30. Any number of international organizations for human good contributed to the cancer debate. See "A Cancer Exhibition," *BMJ* 2 (1907): 541; and Vere G. Webb, "Do Fleas Spread Cancer?" *Lancet* 1 (1908): 853–54.

38. In Britain, Middlesex Hospital moved decisively into treatment, especially examining claims of curative substances. See "The New Cancer Research Laboratories at the Middlesex Hospital," *Lancet* 2 (1905): 1149 and *BMJ* 2 (1905): 1069; "Organization of Cancer Research," *BMJ* 1 (1906): 1227–28; "Cancer Hospital," *Charity Record and Hospital Times*, 1907, 99; and W. S. Lazarus-Barlow, ed., "Sixth Report From the Cancer Research Laboratories," in *Archives of the Middlesex Hospital*, vol. viii (London: Macmillan and Co., 1907); see also "Cancer Research in Dundee," *BMJ* 1 (1908): 474.

39. "Medical News," *BMJ* 2 (1908): 213; and "French Cancer Research Association," *JAMA* 51 (1908): 514. Some argued that the restricted nature of L'Association undercut its utility. See, for example, Auguste A. Housquains, "Paris Letter. The Fight Against Cancer," *Interstate Medical Journal* (1911): 1057–59.

40. A. Borrel, "Le Problem Etiologique Du Cancer," *Bulletin de L'Association Franc, Aise Pour L'Étude Du Cancer* 1 (1908): 15–25. Germans beyond the pathological anatomists also celebrated the mice. See, for instance, Carl Lewin, "Experimentelle Beiträge zur Morphologie und Biologie Bösartiger Geschwulste bei Ratten und Mäusen," *ZFK* 6 (1908): 267–314. Since the pathological anatomists concerned themselves with cellular changes, they characteristically had no use for experimental animals. A typical argument was J. Orth, "Die Morphologie der Krebse und die parasitäre Theorie," *BKW* (1905): 281–83, 326–30.

41. "Rockefeller Gives Another $500,000," *NYT*, May 31, 1908, 1; "Rockefeller Gives More Land to Son," *NYT*, July 17, 1909, 1; and "More Rockefeller Millions to Science," *NYT*, October 18, 1910, 3

42. "Legislature Asked for Vivisection Law," *NYT*, March 26, 1908, 2; "Vivisection's Part in the Battle With Disease," *NYT*, October 18, 1908, SM2; and "Medical Men Defend Tests on Animals," *NYT*, November 24, 1909, 18.

43. James Ewing, "Animal Experimentation and Cancer," *JAMA* 54 (1910): 267–69; James A. Ewing, "Experiments in Cancer," *NYT*, February 28, 1909, SM10; and "Blood Cures Cancer," *Washington Post*, January 13, 1910, 11.

44. "Wealth and Science Joining Hands For the Conquest of Cancer," *NYT*, December 19, 1909, SM10. The article was simultaneously published in the *Washington Post* with small alterations. See "All the World is Battling With

Cancer," *Washington Post*, December 19, 1909, SM1; and "Medical Research and Cancer," *JAMA* 55 (1910): 1477–78.

45. "Vivisection's Part."

46. Leo Loeb, "Recent Progress and Present Status of Experimental Research in Cancer," *JAMA* 55 (1910): 1530–32.

47. "Cancer Research," *BMJ* 1 (1908): 475; "The Clinical Study of Cancer," *NYMJ* 87 (1908): 72–73; Cancer Commission of Harvard University, *A Course of Lectures on Tumors* (Boston: Medical School of Harvard University, 1909), 5–18, 47–64, 65–82; "The Harvard Cancer Commission," *BMJ* 1 (1910): 1505; *The Fifth Report of the Cancer Commission of Harvard University* (Boston: Medical School of Harvard University, 1909); E. E. Tyzzer and Thomas Ordway, "The Huntington Hospital and the Scope of its Work," *BMSJ* 166 (1912): 887–89; "Cancer Hospital Opened," *JAMA* 58 (1912): 1124; and *First Annual Report of the Collis P. Huntington Memorial Hospital for Cancer Research, 1912–1913* (Boston: Cancer Commission of Harvard University, 1913).

48. "Report of Cancer Laboratory, New York State Department of Health," *BMSJ* 161 (1909): 128–29; "For the State Cancer Laboratory," *Buffalo Medical Journal* 66 (1910–11): 397–98; "The State Cancer Laboratory," *Buffalo Medical Journal* 66 (1910–11): 443–45; "New York State Institute for the Study of Malignant Disease," *Buffalo Medical Journal* 66 (1910–11): 581–88; and Harvey R. Gaylord, "New York State Institute for the Study of Malignant Disease," *Buffalo Medical Journal* 66 (1910–11): 623–24.

49. W. B. C., "Cancer Research," *Science* 35 (1912): 979–80; "Geo. F. Baker Aids New York Hospital," *NYT*, November 15, 1912, 1; "May Give Radium to Many Hospitals," *NYT*, October 25, 1913, 8; "and $1 Million Dollars Pledged to Cancer Hospital," *NYT*, May 2, 1914, 6.

50. For the bequest and the new institution, see "The George Crocker Special Research Fund," *Science* 30 (1909): 870–71; "Columbia Prepares Report on Cancer," *NYT*, January 13, 1910, 5; "The Mystery of Cancer," *Los Angeles Times*, October 30, 1910, V13; "Funds," *Science* 37 (1913): 409; "The Crocker Research Laboratories," *JAMA* 62 (1914): 466; and Francis Carter Wood, "Report of the Director of the George Crocker Special Research Fund for the Academic Year Ending June 30, 1914," in *Annual Reports of the President and Treasurer of Columbia University to the Trustees With Accompanying Documents for the Year Ending June 30, 1914* (New York: Columbia, 1914), 205–12. For Crocker's suit against Doyen, see "Crocker Sues Dr. Doyen," *NYT*, January 13, 1907, 6.

Chapter 5

1. George H. Simmons, "The Parasitic Origin of Malignant Neoplasms," *JAMA* 46 (1906): 657. For Schmidt's work, see, for example, "The Etiology of Cancer," *NYMJ* 83 (1906): 1312; and "Says He Has a Cancer Cure," *NYT*, September 2, 1906, 4.

2. "Dr. Borrel on Cancerous Tumours and Helminthes," *BMJ* 2 (1906): 392; "Cancerous Tumours and Helminthes," *JAMA* 47 (1906): 812; Emile Roux, "Sur Un Travail De M. le Dr. A. Borrel, Intitile: Tumeurs Cancereuses Et Helminthes," *Bulletin De L'Academie De Medecine* 56 (1906): 141–44; A. Borrel, "Acariens

Et Cancer Du Systeme Pilaire," *CRSB* 65 (1908): 486–88; A. Borrel, "Acariens Et Cancer," *L'Étude* 1 (1909): 29–53; and A. Borrel, "Parasitisme Et Tumeurs," *Travaux De La Deuxieme*, 193–205. Borrel also noted similarity between cancer families and those families whose members suffered leprosy. He thought a mite was the vector. A. Borrel, "Demodex Et Infections Cutanees," *CRSB* 65 (1908): 596–97. Later earthworms were substituted for nematodes by Hiram Dana Walker, a Buffalo physician who had long worked with earthworm-borne parasites causing disease in chickens. See "Earthworms and Cancer," *Lancet* 2 (1910): 417; as well as H. D. Walker, *The Gape Worm of Fowls: The Earthworm Its Intermediate Host* (Franklinville, NY: Walker and Bickwell, 1897); H. D. Walker, *Cancer and Sarcoma* (Buffalo, NY: Self-published, 1909); and "Carcinoma and Sarcoma: The Earthworm Their Original Host," *Lancet-Clinic* 105 (1911): 479–80.

3. H. G. Gaylord, "Evidences that Infected Cages Are the Source of Spontaneous Cancer Developing Among Small Caged Animals," *BMJ* 2 (1906): 1555–58; and H. G. Gaylord and G. H. A. Clowes, "Evidences that Infected Cages Are the Source of Spontaneous Cancer Developing Among Small Caged Animals," *JAMA* 48 (1907): 15–21; and "American Association for Cancer Research," *JAMA* 50 (1908): 63–64 and 52 (1909): 409. This thesis was adopted elsewhere. See, for example, E. E. Tyzzer, "A Series of Twenty Spontaneous Tumors in Mice with the Accompanying Pathological Changes and the Results of the Inoculation of Certain of These Tumors into Normal Mice," *JMR* 17 (1907/08): 155–95; and P. Ehrlich and H. Apolant, "Ueber Spontane Mischtumoren der Maus," *BKW* (1907): 1399–1401. Others pointed to instances of mouse-human cancer contagion. See, for example, W. Ford Robertson, "Experimental Evidence of the Infective Origin of Carcinoma," *Lancet* 1 (1909): 1591–93. Bashford denied that cancer epidemics among mice existed and attributed these occurrences to old age. See "Cancer Problems," *BMJ* 1 (1907): 217–18; and "Epidemiological Society," *Lancet* 1 (1907): 227.

4. "A Carcinoma Parasite," *BMSJ* 156 (1907): 185–86; and Gary N. Calkins, "A Spirochete in Mouse Cancer, Spirochaeta Microgyrata (Lowenthal) Var. Gaylordi," *Journal of Infectious Diseases* 4 (1907): 171–74. Also see "An Interesting Sunday Times," *NYT*, February 4, 1907, 8. For reports from the buffalo lab about spirochetes and epidemic cancer among mice, see Harvey R. Gaylord, "Report of the Cancer Laboratory," *Documents of the Senate of the State of New York, 1909* (Albany: J. B. Lyon, 1909), 579–91.

5. Harvey R. Gaylord, "Parasitism and Cancer," *New York State Journal of Medicine* 7 (1907): 189–90; and "American Association for Cancer Research," *JAMA* 52 (1909): 410–11. Gaylord had made a similar argument about smallpox and cancer parasites. See H. R. Gaylord, "On the Analogy Between Smallpox and Cancer," *Medical Review of Reviews* 10 (1904): 900–906. For the contemporary excitement about the spirochetes, see H. B. Fantham, "The Spirochetes: A Review of Some Border-line Organisms Between Animals and Plants," *Science Progress in the Twentieth Century* 3 (1908–1909): 148–62. For their alleged relations to trypanosomes, see G. D. Parker, "Sleeping Sickness," *Science Progress in the Twentieth Century* 3 (1908–1909): 657–66.

6. Harvey R. Gaylord, "A Spirochete in Primary and Transplanted Carcinoma of the Breast in Mice," *Journal of Infectious Diseases* 4 (1907): 155–70; and "Cancer

Research," *JAMA* 50 (1908): 1196–97. Also see "Discussion—Sur La Curabilite Du Cancer En General Et Le Traitment Du Cancer De La Langue En Particulier," *Bulletin De L'Academie De Medecine*, 51 (1906): 464–79; Simon Flexner, "Spirochaeta (Treponema) Pallida and Syphilis," *Journal of Experimental Medicine* (hereafter *JEM*) (1907): 464–72; "Spirochetes in Mouse Cancer," *BMSJ* 156 (1907): 548; Drs. Boutie and Minouflet, "Presentations D'Ouvrages Manuscrits Et Imprimes," *Bulletin De L'Academie De Medecine* 52 (1907): 317; F. B. Mallory, "The Results of the Application of Special Histological Methods to the Study of Tumors," *JEM* 10 (1908): 575–91; and Richard Weil, "The Biochemical Investigation of Malignant Tumors and Its Diagnostic applications," *JAMA* 55 (1910): 1532–35.

7. "The Cause of Cancer Probably Discovered; Its Cure Possible," *NYT*, February 3, 1907, SM3; and "An Interesting Sunday Times," *NYT*, February 4, 1907, 8. Calkins circumspection was justified. At the late May 1907 meeting of the Association of Pathologists and Bacteriologists—the very same meeting where the group formed the AACR—Gaylord presented his work as several other researchers provided contrary results. See "Spirochetes and Cancer," *BMSJ* 156 (1907): 679.

8. The *NYT* juxtaposed the work of Beard and the Buffalo group. See "The Two Theories of Cancer Origin," *NYT*, February 18, 1907, 16.

9. The situation was recounted in Ralph W. Moss, "The Life and Times of John Beard, DSc (1858–1924)," *Integrative Cancer Therapies* 7 (2008): 229–51. Calkins's statements were symptomatic of organized medicine's point of view. See also William Seaman Bainbridge, "Transmissibility and Curability of Cancer," *BMSJ* 156 (1907): 835–42.

10. For Beard's reasoning, see J. Beard, "The Cancer Problem," *Lancet* 1 (1905): 281–83; J. Beard, "The Cancer Problem and Research," *Lancet* 1 (1905): 385–86; John A. Shaw-Mackenzie, "The Etiology and Treatment of Cancer," *BMJ* 1 (1905): 1183; and "Cancer Research," *JAMA* 46 (1906): 728–29. Farmer and his coworkers continued to delve into the similarities of gamete and cancer cell division. See, for instance, "A Recent Advance in the Knowledge of Cancer," *Nature* 75 (1907): 587–89; J. Bland-Sutton, "A Lecture on the Cancer Problem," *Lancet* 1 (1907): 1339–45; and "The Cytological Investigation of Cancer," *Lancet* 1 (1908): 1495–96.

11. "Berlin—Researches on Cancer," *Lancet* 1 (1907): 122; and J. Beard, "The Recent Discussion on Cancer in Berlin," *Lancet* 1 (1905): 1160–61. Leyden's laboratory had been long interested in the chemistry of cancer cells. See Hans Wolff, "Ein Beitrag Zur Chemie des Carcinoms," *ZFK* 2 (1905): 95–105.

12. J. Beard, "The Action of Trypsin Upon the Living Cells of Jensen's Mouse-Tumour," *BMJ* 1 (1906): 140–41; and "The Action of Trypsin Upon the Living Cells of Jensen's Mouse-Tumour," *BMJ* 1 (1906): 360.

13. A. Howard Pirie, "The Experimental Evidence," *BMJ* 1 (1906): 318. Also see "Trypsin and Amylopsin in Malignant Growths," *JAMA* 47 (1906): 445.

14. W. A. Pusey, "Trypsin in Malignant Growths," *JAMA* 46 (1906): 1763.

15. For C. W. Saleeby's forays into the muckraking magazines, see, for example, his "The Coming Conquest of Cancer," *Harpers Weekly* 50 (1906): 301, 311; "Cancer-Can It Be Cured," *McClures* 47 (1906): 438–45; "Has Science Conquered Cancer," *Harpers Weekly* 50 (1906): 1237–38; and "Trypsin and Some Positive Cancer Cures,"

Harper's Weekly 51 (1907): 84, 88–91. His magnum opus was published as *The Conquest of Cancer: A Plan of Campaign* (New York: Frederick A. Stokes, 1907). Saleeby was especially adept at translating detailed medical concepts into laymen's terms.

16. The *NYT* was a particularly attentive trypsin denizen. See, for instance, "An Authoritative Assurance," *NYT*, March 4, 1906, 8; "Hope for Cancer Cure From New Discoveries," *NYT*, July 26, 1906, 7; "Claimed too Much too Quickly," *NYT*, August 15, 1906, 6; "Cancer Cured By Trypsin," *NYT*, December 16, 1906, 6; "Demands Fair Trial For Trypsin in Britain," *NYT*, December 17, 1906, 3; "Cancer Patients Cured By Trypsin Injections," *NYT*, December 23, 1906, 5; "Scolded, But Not Squelched," *NYT*, December 31, 1906; "Medical News for Laymen," *NYT*, January 1, 1907, 8; "Favors Reports of Cures," *NYT*, January 3, 1907, 8; "The Cause of Cancer Probably Discovered; Its Cure Possible," *NYT*, February 3, 1907, SM3; and "Medical Secretions," *NYT*, February 10, 1907, 6. An interesting reflection of anxiety over cancer was Dr. Römer, "Ueber Krebsangst," *ZFK* 4 (1906): 75–82.

17. "The 'Coming Conquest of Cancer,'" *JAMA* 46 (1906): 729; "The 'Conquest' of Cancer," *BMJ* 2 (1906): 1830; "The Treatment of Cancer," *Nature* 75 (1906): 177–78; "The Beard Treatment of Cancer," *JAMA* 49 (1907): 1779; "Another 'Cancer' Boom," *BMJ* 1 (1907): 1446–47; and "The Trypsin Treatment of Cancer," *Lancet* 2 (1908): 1231–32.

18. "Trypsin in Treatment of Cancer," *JAMA* 47 (1906): 644; "A Resume of Cancer Research," *Racine [WI] Daily Journal*, October 10, 1906, 4; "The Treatment of Cancer," *Nature* 75 (1907): 247; "The Trypsin Treatment of Cancer," *BMJ* 1 (1907): 158–59; "Report on the Trypsin Treatment of Cancer," *BMSJ* 156 (1907): 129–31; "Westminster Hospital," *Lancet* 1 (1907): 360–61; "The Interlude of Cancer," *NYMJ* 85 (1907): 277; " "Conquest of Cancer," *JAMA* 48 (1907): 832; "The Trypsin Treatment of Cancer," *BMJ* 1 (1907): 519–20; William Seaman Bainbridge, "Trypsin in Cancer: A Preliminary Statement," *BMJ* (1907): 486–89; William J. Morton, "A Case of Cancer Treated By Trypsin," *NYMJ* 85 (1907): 443–44; Winfield S. Hall, "Treatment of Cancer with Trypsin," *Surgery, Gynecology and Obstetrics* 4 (1907): 641–43; "Cancer Treated With Trypsin," *JAMA* 52 (1909): 1714; Stephen Rushmore, "The Effect of Trypsin on Cancer and on the Germ Cells in Mice," *JMR* 21 (1909): 591–96; and William Seaman Bainbridge, "The Enzyme Treatment for Cancer—Final Report," *Medical Record* 76 (1909): 85–92. Note Beard's defense in 1912. See J. Beard, "A Biological View of the Cancer Cell," *BMJ* 1 (1912): 162–63.

19. "The 'Conquest' of Cancer," *BMJ* 1 (1908): 96–99, 232–35; "Ferments, Antiferments, and Cancer," *BMJ* 2 (1908): 347–48; German trypsin successes were regularly reported in the *NYT*. See, for instance, "Cancer Expert on Trypsin," *NYT*, May 29, 1907, 4; "The Search for A Cancer Cure," *NYT*, June 16, 1907, 6; and "John Beard on Trypsin," *NYT*, October 31, 1907, 8.

20. "The Annual Meeting," *Nature* 76 (1907): 226–27; "Imperial Cancer Research Fund," *BMJ* 2 (1907): 26–29; "Trypsin and Amlopsin in the Treatment of Cancer," *BMJ* (1908): 522–23; "The Enzyme Treatment of Cancer," *BMJ* 2 (1909): 218–20; "The Enzyme Treatment of Cancer," *Lancet* 2 (1909): 1079–80; and "American Association for Cancer Research," *JAMA* 54 (1910): 226–27. For

Beard, see Ralph W. Moss, "The Life and Times of John Beard, DSc (1858–1924)," *Integrative Cancer Therapies* 7 (2008): 229–51.

21. Clarence Edward Skinner, "Roentgenization in the Treatment of Cancer," *JAMA* 47 (1906): 1541–44; Robert Reyborn, "Causes and Cure of Cancer and Some of the Causes of Failure in Treating Malignant Growths By X Rays and Electric Currents," *New York Journal of Medicine* 83 (1906): 538–40; "New Cancer 'Cure' Fails," *NYT*, June 16, 1907, C4; W. S. Lazarus-Barlow, ed., "Sixth Report From the Cancer Research Laboratories," in *Archives of the Middlesex Hospital*, vol. viii (London: Macmillan and Co., 1907); "Imperial Cancer Fund," *BMJ* 2 (1907): 26–29 and 2 (1908): 162–64; Leopold Freund-Wien, *Die Elektrische Funkenbehandlung (Fulguration) Der Carcinome* (Stuttgart, 1908); "Electricity in Treatment of Cancer," *JAMA* 50 (1908): 1001; "'Fulguration' Treatment of Cancer," *BMJ* 2 (1908): 426–27; Georg Arndt and August Laqueur, "Experimentelle Untersuchungen Uber die Fulguration An Lebenswichtigen Organen," *BKW* (1908): 1440–44; "Cancer Fulguration," *BMSJ* 161 (1909): 35–37; "The Therapeutic Application of Radium," *BMJ* 1 (1909): 1250–51, 1557; Walter Valentin Keating-Hart, "Traitment Du Cancer Par La Fulguration," *L'Étude* 1 (1909): 1–24; "Radium and Cancer," *Nature* 14 (1909): 219–20; and Charles G. Barkla, "the Treatment of Cancer By X Rays," *BMJ* 2 (1910): 1532–33. By 1909, x-rays were thought also to contribute to cancer. H. Coenen, "Das Rontgencarcinom," *BKW* (1909): 292–94.

22. See, for instance, C. Jacobs and Victor Geets, "On the Treatment of Cancer By Therapeutic Inoculations of a Bacterial Vaccine," *Lancet* 1 (1906): 964–66; "Methylene Blue in the Treatment of Cancer," *JAMA* 48 (1907): 1626; William B. Coley, "The Treatment of Sarcoma with the Mixed Toxins of Erysipelas and Bacillus Prodigiosus," *BMSJ* 158 (1908): 175–82; "Principles of Antiferment Treatment of Cancer," *JAMA* 51 (1908): 797–98; "Treatment of Cancer," *BMJ* 2 (1908): 1719–20; George W. Gay, "The Medical Treatment of Malignant Disease," *BMSJ* 160 (1909): 297–302; "The Far Eastern Association of Tropical Medicine," *Lancet* 1 (1910): 1228; "Cancer," *Lancet-Clinic* 103 (1910): 580–81; and Harry A. Duncan, "Bacterial Treatment of Malignant Disease," *NYMJ* 91 (1910): 1055–56.

23. Harvey R. Gaylord and George H. A. Clowes, "On Spontaneous Cure of Cancer," *Surgery, Gynecology and Obstetrics* 2 (1906): 633–56. Gaylord was not alone. Also see "Spontaneous Tumors in Mice," *NYMJ* 87 (1908): 173; L. Negre, "Quelques Recherches Sur Le Cancer Spontane Et Le Cancer Experimental Des Souris," *Annals De L'Institut Pasteur* 24 (1910): 125–42; and "American Association for Cancer Research," *JAMA* 55 (1910): 340. Also see Anton Sticker, "Die Immunität und die spontane Heilung der Krebskrankheit nach fen Ergebnissen der modernen experimentellen Forschung," *ZFK* 7 (1908): 55–68. Spontaneous "cure" of cancer seemed so important that newspapers covered the matter. See, for example, "Editorial," *NYT*, April 16, 1906, 8; and "British Medical Association," *Lloyd's Weekly News*, August 26, 1906, 6.

24. W. Roger Williams, "The Nature of Jensen's Mouse Tumor," *Transactions of the Pathological Society of London* 58 (1906–1907): 38–42; W. Roger Williams, *The Natural History of Cancer, with Special Reference to Its Causation and Prevention* (London: W. Heinemann, 1908); "Have We Been Aiding the Quacks?" *NYT*, January 2, 1907, 6; and William Seaman Bainbridge, "Transmissibility and

Curability of Cancer," *BMSJ* 156 (1907): 835–42. For a rejoinder, see J. Beard, "The Scientific Criterion of a Malignant Tumor and the Nature of Jensen's Mouse-Tumor," *Medical Record* 71 (1907): 403–4.

25. G. H. A. Clowes and F. W. Baeslack, "On the Influence Exerted on the Virulence of Carcinoma in Mice By Subjecting the Tumor Materials to Incubation Previous to Inoculation," *JEM* 8+(1906): 481–503; Waldemar Loewenthal, "Tierversuche mit Plasmodiophora brassicae und synchytrium taraxaci nebst Beiträgen zur Kenntnis des letzteren," *ZFK* 3 (1905): 46–60; E. F. Bashford, "Illustrations of Propagated Cancer," *BMJ* 1 (1906): 1211–14; "Experimental Research in Connection With the Transplantation of Carcinoma in Mice," *NYMJ* 85 (1907): 331; Guthrie McConnell, "Sudan Oil in the Transplantation of Tumors," *JMR* 18 (1908): 381–82; Carl Lewin, "Experimentelle Krebsforschung Und Infektionstheorie," *DMW* 35 (1909): 710–14; Frederick P. Gay, "A Transmissible Cancer of the Rat Considered from the Standpoint of Immunity," *JMR* 20 (1909): 175–201; "Royal Society of Medicine," *Lancet* 2 (1909): 1588–89; and "American Association for Cancer Research," *JAMA* 54 (1910): 310–12. Antivivisectionists railed against animal experimentation. In Britain, researchers mobilized to counter the threat. "The Research Defence Society," *Lancet* 1 (1908): 1863–64.

26. See, for instance, E. E. Tyzzer, "The Relation of Heredity to Cancer," *JAMA* 55 (1910): 1535–37; "American Association for Cancer Research," *JAMA* 51 (1908): 253, 52 (1909): 410, and 54 (1910): 311.

27. Simon Flexner and J. W. Jobling, "Restraint and Promotion of Tumor Growth," *Proceedings of the Society of Experimental Biology and Medicine* 5 (1907): 16–18; Simon Flexner and J. W. Jobling, "Metaplasia and Metastasis of a Rat Tumor," *Proceedings of the Society of Experimental Biology and Medicine* 5 (1907): 52–53; J. W. Jobling, "Multiple Tumors in Mice," *Proceedings of the Society for Experimental Biology and Medicine* 6 (1908–1909): 10; and Simon Flexner and Maud L. Menten, *Studies Upon a Transplantable Rat Tumor* (New York: Rockefeller Institute for Medical Research, 1910. The French characteristically saw the cancer parasite killing epithelial tissue, which led to a cancerous transference of the connective tissue. See, for instance, M. A. Adamkiewicz, "Transformatio Du Cancer En Tissu Conjonctif Sous L'Influence De La Cancroine," *Bulletin De L' Academie De Medecine* 51 (1906): 290–92. The antivivisection movement was particularly intense in New York State. As head of the Rockefeller, Flexner acted as one of the leading proponents of the status quo. See, for example, "Vivisection's Part in the Battle With Disease," *NYT*, October 18, 1908, SM2; and "Medical Men Defend Tests on Animals," *NYT*, November 24, 1909, 18.

28. "American Association for Cancer Research," *JAMA* 50 (1908): 65–66; George W. Crile, "The Cancer Problem," *JAMA* 50 (1908): 1883–87; A. Brault and G. Faroy, "Sur L'Histogenese du Cancer," *Travaux De La Deuxieme*, 65–87; J. W. Vaughan, "Some Modern Ideas of Cancer, *JAMA* 54 (1910): 1510–14; and Charles H. Mayo, "The Prophylaxis of Cancer," *JAMA* 55 (1910): 1605–7.

29. S. P. Beebe and James Ewing, "A Study of the So-Called Infectious Lymophosarcoma of Dogs," *JMR* 15 (1906): 209–28; S. P. Beebe, "The Growth of Lymphosarcoma in Dogs," *JAMA* 49 (1907): 1492–93; "American Association for Cancer Research," *JAMA* 50 (1908): 64, and *JAMA* 51 (1908): 158, 251; and H.

Dominici, "Note Sur Les Lymphosarcomes," *L'Étude* 2 (1909): 120–40.

30. George W. Crile and S. P. Beebe, "Transfusion of Blood in the Transplantable Lymphosarcoma of Dogs," *JMR* 13 (1908): 385–405; and "American Association for Cancer Research," *JAMA* 52 (1909): 411.

31. An extensive exposition of Ehrlich's mouse research can be found at P. Ehrlich, *Arbeiten aus dem Königlichen Institut für Experimentelle Therapie Zu Frankfurt A. M., Heft I. Aus Der Abteilung für Krebsforschung* (Jena: Gustave Fischer, 1906).

32. Frederick P. Gay, "The Problem of Cancer Considered From the Standpoint of Immunity," *BMSJ* 161 (1909): 207–12; "Recent Work Upon the Cause of Cancer," *American Journal of Surgery* 21 (1907): 57–58; and J. A. Murray, "Die Beziehungen zwischen Geschwulstresistenz und histologischem Bau Transplantierter Mäusetumoren," *BKW* (1909): 1520–24.

33. I have written about the unity of Ehrlich's thought in almost the same words in "From Ehrlich to Waksman: Chemotherapy and the Seamed Web of the Past," in Elizabeth Garber, ed., *Beyond History of Science: Essays in Honor of Robert E. Schofield* (Bethlehem: Lehigh University Press, 1990), 266–83. Also see John Parascandola, "The Theoretical Basis of Paul Ehrlich's Chemotherapy," *Journal of the History of Medicine* 36 (1981): 19–43; and Ernst Baumler and Paul Ehrlich, *Scientists for Life*, trans. Grant Edwards (New York: Holmes & Meier, 1984). Some investigators claimed that cancer operated by producing poisonous substances that doomed nearby cells. See "The Poisons of Cancer, " *BMJ* 2 (1909): 1488–89.

34. For a fine list with texts of Ehrlich's publications, see http://www.pei.de/cln_092/nn_163900/EN/institute-en/paul-ehrlich-en/publications/paul-ehrlich-publications-en.html?__nnn=true. See especially "Professor Paul Ehrlich and His Collaborators," *Collected Studies in Immunity*, trans. Charles Bolduan (New York: John Wiley & Sons, 1906). For histories of immunology generally, see, for example, Arthur M. Silverstein, *Paul Ehrlich's Receptor Immunology: The Magnificent Obsession* (San Diego: Academic Press, 2002); and Pauline M. H. Mazumdar, *Species and Specificity: An Interpretation of the History of Immunology* (Cambridge, UK: Cambridge University Press, 1995).

35. "Effectual Vaccination of Mice Against Cancer," *JAMA* 46 (1906): 1715–16; Apolant, Ehlich, and Haaland, "Experimentelle Beitrage Zur Gescwulstlehre," *BKW* (1906): 37–42; "Herrn Geheimrat Ehrlichs Vortrag über Pathogenese des Krebses, gehalten im Kaiserin Friedrich-Hause am 9. März 1906, " *DMW* 32 (1906): 468–70; "Cancer Research at Frankfort," *BMJ* 2 (1906): 796; "The Recent Work," 57–58; "Immunization of Mice Against Cancer," *JAMA* 48 (1907): 558; "Berlin Letter," *JAMA* 51 (1908): 419–20; and Gay, "The Problem of Cancer Considered," 207–12. For similar efforts by others, see, for example, Isaac Levin, "The Reactive Cell Proliferation in the White Rat; And its Relation to the Genesis of Transplantable Tumors," *JEM* 10 (1908): 811–19; Isaac Levin, "Studies on Immunity in Cancers of the White Rat," *JEM* 12 (1910): 594–606; and William H. Woglom, "Resistance Produced in Mice Against Transplanted Cancer By Auto-Inoculation of the Spleen," *JEM* 12 (1910): 29–33.

36. "Cancer in Mice," *BMJ* 1 (1907): 1140–41; "American Association for Cancer Research," *JAMA* 50 (1908): 63–68; C. E. Walker, "The Action of Two

Sera Upon a Carcinoma Occurring in Mice," *Lancet* 2 (1908): 797–99; "Imperial Cancer Research Fund," BMJ 2 (1906): 207–9; "The Imperial Cancer Research Fund," *Lancet* 2 (1906): 314–15; E. J. Bashford, "The Investigations of the Imperial Cancer Research Fund," *BMJ* 2 (1906): 1554–55; E. F. Bashford, J. A. Murray, and M. Haaland, "Ergebnisse Der Experimentellen Krebsforschung," *BKW* (1907): 1194–97, 1238–43, 1433–45; "The Cancer Research Fund," *Lancet* 2 (1908): 177–78; "The Sixteenth International Congress of Medicine," *BMJ* 2 (1909): 797–98; "The Progress of Cancer Research," *Nature* 84 (1910): 126–28; "Imperial Cancer Research Fund," *BMJ* 2 (1910): 295–309; and E. F. Bashford and B. R. G. Russell, "Further Evidence on the Homogeneity of the Resistance to the Implantation of Malignant New Growths," *Proceedings of the Royal Society of London*, Series B, 82 (1910): 298–306.

37. Frederick P. Gay, "The Problem of Cancer Considered from the Standpoint of Immunity," *BMSJ* 161 (1909): 207–12; "Experimental Studies of Immunity in Cancer," *JAMA* 52 (1909): 474–75; and Max Koch, "Aus Den Verhandlungen der XII. Tagung der Deutschen Pathologischen Gesellschaft, gehalten zu Kiel vom 23–25 April 1908," *ZFK* 7 (1908): 495–512.

38. "The Marvels Wrought By Plastic Surgery," *NYT*, November 15, 1908, 6; "Tissues Live in Jars," *Washington Post*, October 19, 1910, 4; Alexis Carrel and Montrose T. Burrows, "Cultivation of Sarcoma Outside of the Body. A Second Note," *JAMA* 55 (1910): 1554; Alexis Carrel and Montrose T. Burrows, "Human Sarcoma Cultivated Outside of the Body. A Third Note," *JAMA* 55 (1910): 1732; Alexis Carrel and Montrose T. Burrows, "Cultivation of Tissues in Vitro and Its Technique," *JEM* 13 (1911): 387–96; Alexis Carrel and M. T. Burrows, "Cultivation in Vitro of the Thyroid Gland," *JEM* 13 (1911): 416–21; Alexis Carrel and Montrose T. Burrows, "On the Physiochemical Regulation of the Growth of Tissues," *JEM* 13 (1911): 562–73; and Alexis Carrel and Montrose T. Burrows, "An Addition to the Technique of the Cultivation of Tissues In Vitro," *JEM* 14 (1911): 244–47. Also see Leo Loeb, "On Some Conditions of Tissue Growth, Especially in Culture Media," *Science* 34 (1911): 414–15. For a good history of tissue culture research that paralleled Carrel's, see Jan A. Witkowski, "Experimental Pathology and the Origins of Tissue Culture: Leo Loeb's Contribution," *Medical History* 27 (1983): 269–88.

39. Robert A. Lambert and Frederic M. Hanes, "The Cultivation of Tissue in Plasma From Alien Species," *JEM* 14 (1911): 129–38; Robert A. Lambert and Frederic M. Hanes, "Characteristics of Growth of Sarcoma and Carcinoma Cultivated in Vitro," *JEM* 13(1911): 495–504; and Robert A. Lambert and Frederic M. Hanes, "A Study of Cancer Immunity By the Method of Cultivating Tissues Outside the Body," *JEM* 13 (1911): 505–10.

40. Gay, "The Problem of Cancer." Two other summaries of the state of art are V. Dungern, "Immunite," and Harvey R. Gaylord, "Immunity to Cancer," both in *Travaux De La Deuxieme*, 343–53 and 593–600, respectively. For more particularistic studies, see S. P. Beebe and James Ewing, "A Study of the Biology of Tumour Cells," *BMJ* 2 (1906): 1559–60; S. P. Beebe, "The Results of the Chemical Investigation of Tumors," *BMSJ* 156 (1907): 853–57; "Intermediate Host of Cancer," *JAMA* 46 (1906): 1244–45; "The Chemistry of Tumors," *JAMA* 46 (1906): 1615–16; Edmund Falk, "Injektionen Von Placentarblut Bei Carcinom,"

BKW (1908): 1394–96; George W. Crile and S. P. Beebe, "Transfusion of Blood in the Transplantable Lymphosarcoma of Dogs," *JMR* 18 (1908): 385–405; E. E. Tyzzer, "A Study of Inheritance in Mice With Reference to Their Susceptibility to Transplantable Tumors," *JMR* 21 (1909): 519–73; Alex M. Burgess, "The Nature of the Reaction of the Tissues of Susceptible and Non-Susceptible Mice to an Inoculable Tumor," *JMR* 21 (1909): 575–89; M. Haaland, "The Contrast in the Reactions to the Implantation of Cancer After the Inoculation of Living and Mechanically Disintegrated Cells," *Lancet* 1 (1910): 787–89; Peyton Rous, "An Experimental Comparison of Transplanted Tumor and a Transplanted Normal Tissue Capable of Growth," *JEM* 12 (1910): 344–65; and Peyton Rous, "Metastasis and Tumor Immunity," *JAMA* 55 (1910): 1895. For contagium vivum, see Robert Scanes-Spicer, "The Bradshaw Lecture on Cancer," *BMJ* 2 (1910): 2049–50; and M. R. Blanchard, "L'Origine Des Tumeurs," *Bulletin De L'Academie De Medecine* 63 (1910): 447–48. Investigators increasingly considered the tumor as if it were itself a parasitic agent. See, for example, W. H. Ransom, "A Critical Consideration of some Points in the Recent Bradshaw Lecturer on Carcinoma," *Lancet* 1 (1906): 849–52; "The Present State of Cancer Research," *JAMA* 48 (1907): 2000–2001; "Liverpool Medical Institution," *Lancet* 1 (1907): 430; J. W. Vaughn, "Sensitizations in Cancer," *NYMJ* 91 (1910): 1057–58; and "The Address in Surgery," *BMJ* 2 (1910): 274–75.

41. F. J. Bosc, "Essais De Serotherapie Anticancereuse," *CRSB* 2 (1906): 622–24, 701–4; "Bericht über die Tagung der Deutschen pathologischen Gesellschaft und der Gesellschaft Deutscher Aerzte und Naturforscher in Stuttgart 1906," *ZFK* 5 (1907): 516–22; Dr. Kelling, "Ueber Die Anwendung Und Die Deutung spezifischer serumreaktionen für die Carcinomforschung," *ZFK* 6 (1908): 315–60; Francesco Sanfelice, "Ueber Toxine und Antitoxine der Blastomyzeten in bezug auf die Aetiologie und Behandlung der bösartigen Geschwulste," *ZFK* 7 (1908): 564–604; "A Serum Treatment for Carcinoma in Mice," *Lancet* 2 (1908): 1474–75, 1772–73, 1846; "American Association for Cancer Research," *JAMA* 52 (1909): 407–10; Nicole Girard-Mangin, "Nature Des Poisons Cancereux," *CRSB* 67 (1909): 117–18; Isaac Levin, "Resistance to the Growth of Cancer Induced in Rats by Injection of Autolyzed Rat Tissue," *Proceedings of the Society for Experimental Biology and Medicine* 7 (1909–1910): 64–67; Isaac Levin, "Immunity to the Growth of Cancer Induced in Rats by Treatment With Mouse Tissue," *Proceedings of the Society for Experimental Biology and Medicine* 7 (1909–1910): 107–8; E. Vidal, "Recherches Sur Les Sensibilisatrices Contenues Dans Le Sang Des Animaux Traites Par Des Emulsions De Cancers Epitheliaux," *L'Étude* 3 (1910): 81–92; Maurice Guillet and M. Daufresue, "Examen Des Serums Cancereux Par La Methode De Deviation Du Complement," *L'Étude* 3 (1910): 34–39; Archibald Leitch, "Recent Cancer Research," *Lancet* 1 (1910): 1011–12; "The Treatment of Carcinoma With the Body Fluid of a Recovered Case," *BMSJ* 162 (1910): 363; and Ellen P. Corson White and Leo Loeb, "The Influence of an Inoculation With Tumor Material of Experimentally Decreased Virulence Upon the Result of a Second Inoculation With Tumor Material of Experimentally Decreased Virulence," *Proceedings of the Society for Experimental Biology and Medicine* 8 (1910–1911): 22–24. At least one investigator posited that an anaphylactic serum reaction weakened natural immunity and permitted tumors

to metastasize. This mechanism was explained in "Anaphylatic Seroreaction With Cancer," *JAMA* 53 (1909): 752. For the Wassermann test, see "The Present Status of the Wassermann Reaction as a Diagnostic Aid in Syphilis," *JAMA* 52 (1909): 638.

42. Ernest Fuld, "Ueber die Kelling'sche Serumreaktion bei Carinomatösen," *BKW* (1905): 535–38; Georg Kelling, "Ueber die Blutserumreaktion der Carinomatösen," *BKW* (1905): 905–11, 950–57; Charles E. Simon and Walter S. Thomas, "On Complement-Fixation in Malignant Disease," *JEM* 10 (1908): 673–89; Richard Weil, "The Hemolytic Reactions in Cases of Human Cancer," *JMR* 19 (1908): 281–93; "Hemolysis in Cancer," *JAMA* 51 (1908): 2162; Charles E. Simon, "Complement Fixation in Malignant Disease," *JAMA* 52 (1909): 1090–92; and E. C. Hort, "Diagnosis of Cancer By Examination of the Blood," *BMJ* 2 (1909): 966–70. For an extensive effort in one facility, see Freiherrn Von Dungern, "Ueber die Tätigkeit der biologisch-chemischen Abteilung des Instituts für Krebsforschung Von 1907–1911," *Heidelberger Institut,* 67–75. The German Cancer Committee even offered a prize for a successful diagnostic test for the disease. See "Prizes Offered by the German Central Committee for Cancer Research," *JAMA* 53 (1909): 1411.

43. E. F. Bashford, "An Address on Cancer in Man and Animals," *Lancet* 2 (1909): 691–701; "Cancer in Man and Animals," *JAMA* 53 (1909): 969–70; and "The Nature of Cancer," *Lancet* 1 (1910): 1557–58. Also of interest are "The Tumor Problem," *BMSJ* 160 (1909): 115; Alexander Theodore Brand, "The Specificity of Cancer and the General Principles of its Treatment and Prophylaxis," *Lancet* 1 (1910): 1471–72; S. P. Beebe, "The Chemistry of Cancer," *NYMJ* 92 (1910): 1058–60; and Max Borst, "Zelltheorie Des Carcinoms," and R. Paltauf, "Die Klinische Diagnostik des Krebses," both in *Travaux De La Deuxieme,* 601–13 and 614–36, respectively.

44. J. E. Salvin-Moore and C.E. Walker, "On The Relationship of Cancer Cells to the Development of Cancer," *Lancet* 1 (1908): 226–27; J. E. Salvin-Moore and J. O. Wakelin Barratt, "Note Upon the Effect of Liquid Air Upon the Graftable Cancer of Mice," *Lancet* 1 (1908): 227; "American Association for Cancer Research," *JAMA* 51 (1908): 252–53; and Harvey R. Gaylord, "The Resistance of Embryonic Epithelium, Transplantable Mouse Cancer, and Certain Organisms to Freezing with Liquid Air," *Journal of Infectious Diseases* 5 (1908): 443–48.

45. James Ewing, "Cancer Problems," *Archives of Internal Medicine* 1 (1908): 175–217; and E. E. Tyzzer, "The Hearing of the Experimental Investigation of Tumors on the Tumor Problem in General," *BMSJ* 161 (1909): 103–7.

46. Peyton Rous, "Parabiosis as a Test for Circulating Antibodies in Cancer," *JEM* 11 (1909): 809–14.

47. Peyton Rous, "An Experimental Comparison of Transplanted Tumor and a Transplanted Normal Tissue Capable of Growth," *JEM* 12 (1910): 344–66. Also see "American Association for Cancer Research," *JAMA* 51 (1909): 253.

48. Peyton Rous, "The Relations of Embryonic Tissue and Tumor Tissue," *JEM* 13 (1911): 239–47; Peyton Rous, "The Effect of Pregnancy on Implanted Embryonic Tissue," *JEM,* 13 (1911): 248–56; and "American Association for Cancer Research," *JAMA* 54 (1910): 311–12. For summaries of the ideas of irritation and

inflammation, see Leon Berard, "Traumatismes and Cancer," and C. Thiem, "Trauma Und Geschwulstbildung," both in *Travaux De La Deuxieme*, 355–69 and 401–27, respectively. Also see Dr. Herzfeld, "Tumor and Trauma," *ZFK* 3 (1905): 73–94; and M. Weinberg and Ugo Mello, "Recherches Sur Le Serum Des Cancereux," *CRSB* 67 (1909): 434–36, 441–43.

49. Peyton Rous, "Transmission of a Malignant New Growth By Means of a Cell-Free Filtrate," *JAMA* 56 (1911): 198; Peyton Rous, "A Transmittable Avian Neoplasm (Sarcoma of the Common Fowl)," *JEM* 12 (1910): 696–705; and "American Association for Cancer Research," *JAMA* 55 (1910): 342. For tumors and birds before Rous, see M. Ehrenreich and L. Michaelis, "Aus Dem Laboratorium der I. medizinischen Klinik [Abteilung für Krebsforschung] in Berlin," *ZFK* 4 (1906): 586–91; and V. Ellermann and O. Bang, "Experimentelle Leukämie bei Hühnern," *Centralblatt Fur Bakteriologie, Parasitenkunde Und Infektionskrankheiten* 46 (1908): 4–5, 595–604.

50. Peyton Rous, "A Sarcoma of the Fowl Transmissible By An Agent Separable from the Tumor Cells," *JEM* 13 (1911): 397–410. Also see "Report of Sections," *NYMJ* 95 (1912): 1219; and Moyer S. Fleisher, "Advances in Cancer Research," *Interstate Medical Journal* 18 (1911): 1039–45.

51. See, for instance, S. B. Wolbach, "The Filterable Viruses, A Summary," *JMR* 27 (1912): 1–25; and W. Ford Robertson and M. C. W. Young, "On the Protozoan Origin of Tumours," *BMJ* 2(1909): 868–73. The whole issue of viruses caused considerable consternation and confusion among researchers. It was outside their frame of reference and, as such, perplexed them. See, for instance, Sally Smith Hughes, *The Virus: A History of the Concept* (New York: Science History Publications, 1977); Alfred Grafe, *A History of Experimental Virology*, trans. Elvira Reckendorf (Berlin: Springer, 1991), especially 10–158; and Angela N. H. Creager, *The Life of A Virus: Tobacco Mosaic Virus as an Experimental Model, 1930–1965* (Chicago: University of Chicago Press, 2002), 17–35.

52. Rous's chicken sarcoma work became a template. A significant researcher had found cancer not from cells but from filtrate. This new model served as a platform from which to extend the analogy. If chicken sarcoma emerged from filtrate, then laboratory investigators might find filtrate-spawned cancer in other species. For a significant discussion of the tumult that sprang from this process, see, for example, "American Association for Cancer Research," *Zeitschrift für Krebsforschung* 11 (1912): 132–34. Even the most marginal theories were rejuvenated by Rous's study. See H. D. Walker, "The Production of Malignant Tumors From the Parasites of the Earthworm," *Medical Record* 82 (1912): 1167–68. For the problem of experiment generally, see, for instance, Leo Loeb, "Ueber einige Probleme der Experimentellen Tumorforschung," *ZFK* 5 (1907): 451–70; and A. Dietrich, "Der heutige Stand der Experimentellen Krebsforschung," *DMW* (1907): 495–99.

Chapter 6

1. E. F. Bashford and J. A. Murray, "The Significance of the Zoological Distribution, the Nature of the Mitoses, and the Transmissibility of Cancer," *BMJ* 1 (1904): 264–71; Marianne Plehn, "Die Shuppenträubung der Weißfische, verursacht durch das krebsbakterium," *Allgemeine Fischerei-Zeitung* 27 (1902): 40–44; Marianne Plehn ,"Bösartiger Kropf (Adeno-Carcinom der Thyreoidea) Bei

Salmoniden," *Allgemeine Fischerei-Zeitung* 27 (1902): 117–19; Ludwig Pick, "Ueber Einige bemerkenswerthe Tumorbildungen aus der Thierpatholoie, Insbesondere über gutartige und krebsige Neubildungen Bei Kaltblütern," *BKW* 40 (1903): 546–48; Ludwig Pick, "Der Schilddrüsenkrebs der Salmoniden, (Edelfische)," *BKW* 42 (1905): 1435–40, 1477–80, 1498–1502, and 1532–36; Marianne Plehn, "Koher Hammt Die Drehkrankheit Der Dalmoniden?" *Allgemeine Fischerei-Zeitung* 29 (1904): 151–53; Marianne Plehn, "Woher kommt die Krebskrankheit der Salmoniden?" *Allgemeine Fischerei-Zeitung* 29 (1904): 151–53; Marianne Plehn, "Ueber Geschwulste bei Kaltblütern," *ZFK* 4 (1906): 525–65; and "Endemic Cancer," *JAMA* 48 (1907): 165.

2. "American Association for Cancer Research," *JAMA* 52 (1909): 411.

3. "Cancer Among Fish," *Washington Post*, May 25, 1909, 6.

4. George M. Bowers, *Report of the Commissioner of Fisheries for the Fiscal Year 1909 and Special Papers* (Washington, DC: GPO, 1911), 15.

5. "American Association for Cancer Research," *JAMA* 54 (1910): 227–28.

6. "Fish Get Cancer," *Gettysburg Times*, February 14, 1910, 3; "Vaccination As Cure For Cancer," *Logansport Daily Reporter*, February 14, 1910, 4; "Cancer Cure," *Cedar Rapids Gazette*, February 18, 1910, 4; and "Sees Hope For Cancer," *Indianapolis Star*, February 20, 1910, 7.

7. "Mr. Taft Endorses A Health Bureau," *JAMA* 51 (1908): 414. See too Victor A. Triolo and Ilse L. Riegel, "The American Association for Cancer Research, 1907–1940: A Historical Review," *Cancer Research* 21 (1961): 143–44.

8. William Howard Taft, "Special Message," April 9, 1910. Online by Gerhard Peters and John T. Woolley, The American Presidency Project, http://www.presidency.ucsb.edu/ws/?pid=68499; "Editorial," *Buffalo Medical Journal* 65 (1910): 62; "Hope to Cure Cancer," *Washington Post*, February 14, 1910, 9; "Praises Ballinger," *Washington Post*, May 1 1910, 1; "We Learn," *BMJ* 1 (1910): 1062; and "Congress," *Science* n.s. 32 (1910): 54. Also see James T. Patterson, *The Dread Disease: Cancer and Modern American Culture* (Cambridge, MA: Harvard University Press, 1987), 59–60; and Richard Rettig, *Cancer Crusade: The Story of the National Cancer Act of 1971* (Princeton: Princeton University Press, 1977), 70–71.

9. "Cancer Research," *Washington Post*, April 12, 1910, 6; and "Cure for Cancer Sought Through Study of Fish," *NYT*, April 17, 1910, SM2. Also see "Taft Takes a Hand in Cancer Research," *Oakland Tribune*, April 21, 1910, 4.

10. "Cancer in Fishes," *JAMA* 54 (1910): 1380.

11. "International Cancer Conference," *BMJ* 2 (1910): 1267; and "Takes Issue With Taft," *Washington Post*, April 24, 1910, 6.

12. David Marine and C. H. Lenhart, "Observations and Experiments on the So-Called Thyroid Carcinoma of Brook Trout (Salvelinus Fontinalis) and Its Relation to Ordinary Goiter," *JEM* (1910): 311–37; "Thyroid Cancer of Brook Trout," *JAMA* 54 (1910): 1902.

13. Roswell Park, "Treatment of Cancer," *Buffalo Medical Journal* 66 (1910): 473.

14. "Searching for the Germ of Cancer," *Washington Post*, September 4, 1910, MT4; and "Cancer Test on Dogs," *Washington Post*, October 28, 1910, 4. The Bureau also experimented with dogs exclusively "drinking fishy water," water from hatcheries where cancer epidemics were known to exist. See "Cancer Test on

Dogs," *Indianapolis Star,* December 4, 1910, 38. Also see "To Use Dogs in Cancer Test," *Marshfield Times,* November 2, 1910, 4.

15. George M. Bowers, *Annual Report of the United States Commissioner of the Bureau of Fisheries for the Year 1910* (Washington, DC:, GPO, 1911), 17–18, 37–38.

16. David Marine and C. H. Lenhart, "Further Observations and Experiments on the So-Called Thyroid Carcinoma of the Brook Trout (Salvelinus Fontinalis) and its Relation to Endemic Goitre," *JEM* (1911): 455–75.

17. "Cancer in Fish," *JAMA* 56 (1911): 670.

18. George M. Bowers, *Report of the United States Commissioner of Fisheries for the Fiscal Year 1911* (Washington, DC: GPO, 1912), 67–68; "Want Bureau to Study Fish Cancer," *Trenton Times,* February 16, 1912, 4; and "Men May Catch Disease From Fish Says Bureau," *Evening Post* (Frederick, MD), March 14, 1912, 24. By 1912, investigations into the relationship between fish thyroid cancer and human cancer were winding down. The Buffalo group ended its involvement in Bureau activities that year. See George M. Bowers, *Report of the Commissioner of Fisheries for the Fiscal Year 1912 and Special Papers* (Washington, DC: GPO, 1914), 54; and *Report of the Commissioner of Fisheries for the Fiscal Year 1913 and Special Papers* (Washington, DC: GPO, 1914), 32.

19. Harvey R. Gaylord and Millard C. Marsh, "Carcinoma of the Thyroid in the Salmonoid Fishes," *Bulletin of the U. S. Bureau of Fisheries,* no. 32, 1912 (Washington, DC: GPO, 1914), 367–436, 441–57, 485–94. Gaylord earlier had announced the results of the chemotherapy experiments at the AACR's meeting in Philadelphia. See H. R. Gaylord, M. C. Marsh, and F. C. Bush, "Effect of Iodine, Mercury and Arsenic on Thyreoid Hyperglasias and Tumors in Fish," *ZFK* 12 (1913): 537–40.

20. Gaylord and Marsh, "Carcinoma," 463–84.

21. Gaylord and Marsh, "Carcinoma," 469, 498, 502–7. Also see "Tumours Produced by Viruses," *BMJ* 1 (1914): 389; and H. Ribbert, "Pathologische Anatomie," *DMW* 2 (1915): 507.

22. Van Bufren Thorne, "Laboratory Report Shows Germs Cause Fish Cancer," *NYT,* January 25, 1914, 47; David Marine, "Further Observations and Experiments On Goitre (So Called Thyroid Carcinoma) in Brook Trout (Salvelinus Fontinalis)," *JEM* 8 (1914): 70–88; David Marine, "The Rapidity of the Involution of Active Thyroid Hyperplasias of Brook Trout Following the Use of Fresh Sea Fish as Food," *JEM* 8 (1914): 376–82; and "Fish Cancer," *American Cancer* 20 (1914): 501. Also see "Goitre in Fishes," *BMJ* 2 (1915): 303; and A. T. Cameron and Swale Vincent, "Note on an Enlarged Thyroid Occurring in an Elasobranch Fish (Squalus Sucklii)," *JEM* 10 (1915): 251–56.

23. "Dr. Gaylord Unfair, Say Fish Experts," *NYT,* February 2, 1914, 4.

24. Harvey R. Gaylord, "Further Observations on So-Called Carcinoma of the Thyroid in Fish," *Journal of Cancer Research* 1(1916): 197–204.

25. Erwin F. Smith, "Synopsis of Researches of Erwin F. Smith in the United States Department of Agriculture (1886–1922)" in L. R. Jones, "Biographical Memoir of Erwin Frink Smith 1854–1927," *National Academy of Sciences of the United States of America, Biographical Memoirs,* vol. xxi: *First Memoir* (Washington, D.C.: National Academy of Sciences, 1939).

26. Erwin F. Smith, "Are There Bacterial Diseases of Plants," *Zentralblatt Fur Bakteriologie, Parasitenkunde Und Infektionskrankheiten, Bakteriologie II. Abt.* 5 (1899): 271–78, 810–17. Also see Alfred Fisher, "Vorlesungen Uber Backterien," trans. A. Coppen Jones, published as *Alfred Fisher: The Structure and Function of Bacteria* (Oxford: Clarendon Press, 1900).

27. Erwin F. Smith, "Recent Studies of the Olive-Tubercle Organism," *U. S. Department of Agriculture, Bureau of Plant Industry, Bulletin No. 131, Part IV* (Washington, DC: GPO, 1908).

28. Erwin F. Smith and C. O. Townsend, "A Plant-Tumor of Bacterial Origin," *Science* 25 (1907): 671–73. Smith was by no means the first investigator to talk of plant cancer. See, for example, W. Roger Williams, "Vegetable Neoplasms," in *The Principles of Cancer and Tumour Formation* (London: Bale & Sons, 1888), 69–100, 173–94.

29. Erwin F. Smith, Nellie A. Brown, and C. O. Townsend, *Crown-Gall of Plants: Its Cause and Remedy* (Washington, DC: GPO, 1911).

30. Smith et al., *Crown-Gall of Plants*, 157–77. For his lack of success with AACR members, see "American Association for Cancer Research," *ZFK* 11 (1912): 137–38 and 12 (1913): 435–36, 533–34; Erwin F. Smith, "On Some Resemblances of Crown-Gall to Human Cancer," *Science*, n.s. 35 (1912): 161–72; and "Resemblances of Plant and Tree Cancer to Human Cancer," *JAMA* 58 (1912): 872. Jensen of mouse tumor fame had argued that tumors in plants were in "an analogous position in the vegetable kingdom to that occupied by cancer in the animal kingdom." See "International Cancer Conference," 1267.

31. "Trace Cancer to Plants," *NYT*, February 4, 1911, 1; "Human Cancer in Plant Life," *Logansport [IN] Pharos*, February 11, 1911, 4; "Cancer in Plants," *The [IA] Homestead*, February 16, 1911, 17; "The Germ of Cancer Found?" *San Antonio Light and Gazette*, February 19, 1911, 38; and "Human Cancer in Plant Life," *Mansfield [OH] News*, March 1, 1911, 5.

32. Erwin F. Smith, "On Some Resemblances of Crown-Gall to Human Cancer," *Science* n.s. 35 (1912): 161–72.

33. Erwin F. Smith, Nellie A. Brown, and Lucia McCulloch, "The Structure and Development of Crown Gall: A Plant Cancer," *U. S. Department of Agriculture, Bureau of Plant Industry, Bulletin No. 255* (Washington, DC: GPO, 1912). Smith's 1911 and 1912 stimulated several physicians to claim that they had long been thinking along similar lines. See, for example, "Tree Cancer," *BMSJ* 165 (1911): 247–49; "Recent Progress in Cancer Research," *BMSJ* 165 (1911): 299–301; Jonathan Hutchinson, "Does Cancer Occur in Vegetables?," *Lancet* 1 (1912): 756; and "'Cancer' in Plants," *BMJ* 2 (1913): 462.

34. "Is Cancer Infectious?," *NYT*, August 11, 1912, 10; "Government Wages War on Plant Disease," *San Antonio Light*, June 9, 1912, 1; and "A Valuable Discovery," *Washington Post*, June 14, 1912, 6. Also see "Cancer Found in Plants," *NYT*, June 15, 1912, 1; and *Oxnard Courier*, January 31, 1913, 6.

35. Leonard Keene Hirshberg, "In Sight of the Cancer Cure," *Muskogee [OK] Times-Democrat*, February 29, 1912, 6.

36. "Plant Cancer," *BMJ* 2 (1912): 811. The AMA's action is mentioned in C. Lee Campbell, "Erwin Frink Smith—Pioneer Plant Pathologist," *Annual Review of*

Phytopathology 21 (1983): 25. Smith would serve as AACR president in 1925. Smith later reported that his trout experiments were inconclusive. See Erwin F. Smith, "Studies of the Crown Gall of Plants. Its Relation to Human Cancer," *Journal of Chemical Research* 1 (1916): 256. Doctors sometimes applied Smith's crown gall insights to human cancer. See D. A. Crow, "A Case of Chimney-Sweep's Cancer, and a Suggestion as to the Pathology of Cancer," *BMJ* 1 (1914): 413–14. Smith was by no means to discuss the transformation of the cancer parasite under different conditions. See, for instance, Dr. Abramowski, "Zur parasitären Krebstheorie," *ZFK* 9 (1910): 385–91.

37. "Is Cancer of Infectious Nature?" *JAMA* 59 (1912): 448; and "The Analogy of Animal and Vegetable Neoplasms," *BMSJ* 166 (1912): 260–61. Also see "Crown-Gall and Human Cancer," *Medical Record* 81 (1912): 472.

Chapter 7

1. "'606' As Malaria Cure," *NYT* October 3, 1910, 4; "Ehrlich's Remedy a Medical Wonder," *NYT*, September 11, 1910, 5; "Value of Ehrlich Remedy," *NYT*, August 14, 1910, C4; E. G. French, "A Report on Three Vases Treated With Ehrlich's Specific for Syphilis," *BMJ* 1 (1911): 361; "Discussion on Recent Developments in the Recognition and Treatment of Syphilis," *BMJ* 2 (1911): 673–79; "Salvarsan ('606')," *BMJ* 1 (1911): 226–27; and Edgar G. Ballenger and Omar F. Elder, "'606'; Its Administration 420 Times," *Southern Medical Journal* 5 (1912): 888–89.

2. Marcus, "From Ehrlich to Waksman," 266–83. For Ehrlich's laboratory and the identification of spirochetes and cancer, see "Deutsches Zentralkomitee zur Erforschung und Bekämpfung der Krebskrankheit, May 29, 1911," *ZFK* 11 (1912): 153–55. Traditional exegeses of Ehrlich's syphilis work include Paul De Kruif, *Microbe Hunters, 1926, 1954* (San Diego: Harcourt, 1996), 326–51; and John Parascandola, "The Theoretical Basis of Paul Ehrlich's Chemotherapy," *Journal of the History of Medicine and Allied Sciences* 36 (1981): 19–43. Newspaper reports include "A New School of Medicine," *NYT*, January 10, 1912, 16; Herman A. Metz, "Solving Medical Mysteries By Help of Animals," *NYT*, January 28, 1912, SM6; William J. Robinson, "Prof. Ehrlich's Salvarsan," *NYT*, February 11, 1912, 12; "Neo-Salvarsan," *NYT*, March 20, 1912, 12; " "Neo-Salvarsan is No. '914,'" *NYT*, April 28, 1912, C3; and "World Doctors Hail Ehrlich as Hero," *NYT*, August 9, 1913, 3.

3. "Finds a Specific for Blood Diseases," *NYT*, August 3, 1910, 5; "Metropolitan Counties Branch," *BMJ* 2 (1908): 229; "How Science Wars on the Infectious," *NYT*, March 18, 1911, 10; "Salvarsan," *NYMJ* 93 (1911): 437–38; and Hugo Schweitzer, "Ehrlich's Chemotherapy—A New Science," *Science*, n.s. 32 (1910): 809–23. Also see "Specifics for Organic Diseases," *NYT*, January 8, 1912, 12. Scientists also sought chemotherapeutic agents for tuberculosis and pneumonia. See, for example, "Chemotherapy of Pneumonia," *Medical Record* 81 (1912): 854; H. Gideon Wells and O. F. Hedenberg, "Studies on the Biochemistry and Chemotherapy of Tuberculosis," *Journal of Infectious Diseases* 11 (1912): 349–72; "Dead Germs Help To Fight Disease," *NYT*, July 21, 1912, C3; and "Chemotherapy in Tuberculosis," *Medical Record* 81 (1912): 995.

4. "Salvarsan With Cancer," *JAMA* 56 (1911): 1695–96; and "Salvarsan in Malignant Disease," *BMJ* 1 (1912): 1257–58. . For some confusion among

trypanosomes, spirochetes and the unidentified germ of cancer, see Carl H. Browning, "Experimental Chemotherapy in Trypanosome Infections," *BMJ* 2 (1907): 1405–9; Jonathan Hutchinson, "Experimental Syphilology," *BMJ* 2 (1908): 1215–16; and Henry B. Ward, "The Sleeping Sickness Bureau," *American Naturalist* 43 (1909): 124–27. Casimir Funk extended the analysis to see if arsenic, a primary ingredient of Salvarsan, was effective against Rous's chicken sarcoma. See Casimir Funk, "The Effect of Arsenic Compounds on the Rous Chicken Sarcoma," *JEM* 21 (1915): 574–76.

5. Dietrich Stolzenberg, "Scientist and Industrial Manager: Emil Fischer and Carl Duisberg," in *The German Chemical Industry in the Twentieth Century*, ed. John E. Lesch (Dordrecht: Kluwer Academic Publishers, 2000), 68; Ton Van Helvoort, "Scalpel or Rays? Radiotherapy and the Struggle for the Cancer Patient in Pre-Second World War Germany," *Medical History* 45 (2001): 42; and Frieder W. Lichtenthaler, "Emil Fischer: His Personality, His Achievements, and His Scientific Progeny," *European Journal of Organic Chemistry* (2002): 4100. For the report of the research and the later work, G. Klemperer, "Tagesordnung," *BKW* (1912): 130; Emil Fischer and G. Klemperer, "Über Eine Neue Klasse von Lipoiden Arsenverbindungen," *Therapie d. Gegenwart Berlin* 54 (1913): 1–3; and Georg Klemperer, *Der Jetzige Stand Der Krebsforschung* (Berlin: August Hirschwald, 1912). By 1914, its creators abandoned its cancer-fighting claims. See, for example, "Elarson," *BMJ* 1 (1914): 56.

6. For some of the speculation over the nature of chemotherapeutic and other drug action, see Cay-Rudiger Prull, Andreas-Holger Maehle, and Robert Francis Halliwell, *A Short History of the Drug Receptor Concept* (London: Palgrave Macmillan, 2009).

7. A. von Wassermann, Franz Keysser, and Michael Wassermann, "Beiträge zum Problem: Geschwülste von der Blutbahn aus therapeutisch zu beeinflussen Auf Grund chemotherapeutischer Versuche an Tumorkranken Tieren," *Deutsche Medizinische Wochenschrift* (1911): 2389–92; "Treatment of Cancer," *Daily Mail*, December 22, 1911, 1; "German Advance in Cancer Treatment," *NYT*, December 22, 1911, 1; "Cancer Cure Causes Stir," *NYT*, December 29, 1911, 1; "La Guerison Du Cancer Des Souris," *Paris Le Temps*, December 30, 1911, 4; "A Chemical Surgeon Has Been Evolved," *NYT*, January 8, 1912, 7; A. Wassermann and D. Hansemann, "Chemotherapeutische Versuche An Tumorkranken Tieren," *BKW* (1912): 4–10; "Berlin," *BMJ* 1 (1912): 50–51; "Our Berlin Letter," *Medical Record* 81 (1912): 78; "The New Wassermann Cancer Therapy," *Interstate Medical Journal* 19 (1912): 306–8; "Chemotherapy of Mouse Cancer," *Medical Record* 81 (1912): 235; A. Von Wassermann, Franz Keysser, and Michael Wassermann, "A Contribution to the Problem of the Therapeutic Treatment of Tumors Through the Circulation Based on Chemotherapeutic Experiments on Tumour-Bearing Animals," *Medical Times* 40 (1912): 29–31; and Eugene G. Kessler, "The Treatment of Carcinoma By Selenium," *Medical Record* 81 (1912): 1024–27. Soon after Wassermann's announcement, he went to Bashford's ICRF lab and worked with the scientists there. See "Our London Letter," *Medical Record* 81 (1912): 275–77. Others came to Berlin to work with Wassermann. See O. Kiliani, "Personal Observations of Wassermann's Experiments on Mouse Tumors," *Medical Record* 81 (1912): 789–91. Wassermann learned of absorption of

tellurium and selenium into living tissue from Bartolomeo Gosio, a turn-of-the-century Italian bacteriologist who published his work in German. For Gosio and Selenium and Tellurium, see Robert Bentley, "Batolomeo Gosio, 1863–1944. An Appreciation," *Advances in Applied Microbiology* 48 (2001): 238–39. The idea that animals perished because of tumor toxins unleashed by chemotherapeutic action persisted. See Angel H. Roffo, *Cancer Experimental* (Buenos Aires: Las Ciencias, 1914).

8. "The Application of Chemotherapy to Cancer," *JAMA* 58 (1912): 120; "Our London Letter," *Medical Record* 81 (1912): 275–76; "Tagesordnung," *BKW* (1912): 222–25; E. F. Bashford, *Review of Recent Cancer Research: Middleton Goldsmith Lecture to the New York Pathological Society, 1912* (Lancaster, PA: New Era Printing, 1914), 34; "The Non-Operative Treatment of Cancer," *BMJ* 2 (1912): 727–28; "University College, Dublin Medical Society," *Lancet* 1 (1912): 509; "Progress in Cancer Research," *BMSJ* 166 (1912): 180–81; and Pierre Delbet, "Traitement Des Cancers Par Le Selenium," *L'Étude* 6 (1913): 85–90. Spinoff experiments included R. Werner, "Zur Chemischen Imitation der Strahlenwirkung und Chemotherapie des Krebses," *DMW* 38 (1912): 1437; Herr Széci, "Wirkung Von cholinsalzen auf das Blut und über die beeinflussung von Mäusetumoren durch kolloidale Metalle," *DMW* 38 (1912): 1437; and William James Morton, "Some Problems in the Chemotherapy of Cancer," *NYMJ* 45 (1912): 524–26.

9. Articles discussing cancer laboratories and their directors started to appear with some frequency. Among the best was J. G. Adami, "The Cancer Research Institute," *NYMJ* 97 (1913): 1269–71.

10. "Ehrlich and Wassermann," *NYT*, January 30, 1912, 8; "Another Mouse Cancer Cure," *Medical Record* 81 (1912): 226; "Great Biologists Unite to seek a Cancer Cure," *NYT*, February 4, 1912, SM 6; "'Nigrosin,' Cancer Antidote," *NYT*, February 9, 1912; "Origin of 'Nigrosin,'" *NYT*, February 11, 1912, 1; "The Wassermann-Ehrlich Cancer Remedy," *Medical Record* 81 (1912): 322; "Prof. Kiliana Back with Cancer Cure," *NYT*, March 6, 1912, 7; "'Colossal,' Says Dr. Kilianai of German's Cancer Work," *NYT*, March 10, 1912, SM12; "Hope for Cancer Patients," *NYT*, March 10, 1912, 14; "Ehrlich Won't Risk Human Cancer Tests," *NYT*, March 26, 1912, 4; and "New Post for Wassermann," *NYT*, July 28, 1913, 3. The two denizens of German chemotherapy published a yearly volume detailing the new discoveries. See P. Ehrlich, F. Kraus, and A.V. Wassermann, *Zeitschrift Fur Chemotherapie Und Verwandte Gebiete* (Leipzig: Georg Thieme, 1912), especially 3–4, 262–72.

11. S. B. Wolbach and C. A. L. Binger, "A Contribution to the Parasitology of Trypanosomiasis," *JMR* (1912): 83–107; S. B. Wolbach and C. A. L. Binger, "Notes on a Filterable Spirochete from Fresh Water-Spirocheta Biflexa (New Species)," *JMR* (1914): 23–25; and J. L. Todd and S. B. Wolbach, "Concerning the Filterability of Spirocheta Duttoni," *JMR* (1914): 27–36.

12. "Medicine as a Science," *NYT*, January 14, 1912, 14; William James Morton, "Some Problems in the Chemotherapy of Cancer," *NYMJ* 95 (1912): 625–27; "Is Cancer Infectious?" *NYT*, February 14, 1912, 10; "Clue to Parasite as Cause of Cancer," *NYT*, February 14, 1912, 8; Simon Flexner, "The Huxley Lecture on Recent Advances In Science in Relation to Practical Medicine. Some Problems in Infection and Its Control," *BMJ* 2 (1912): 1261–68; and Simon Flexner and Hideyo Noguchi, "The Microorganism Causing Epidemic Poliomyelitis," *Science* 38 (1913):

504–6. In 1913, investigators identified an ultramicroscopic yellow fever germ and one causing hydrophobia. See "The Germ of Yellow Fever," *Journal of Southern Medicine* 6 (1913): 27; "Noguchi Isolates the Germ of Rabies," *NYT*, September 7, 1913, 1; and "Noguchi's Discovery of the Germ of Hydrophobia," *NYT*, September 7, 1913, 12. Some investigators even found bacteria to be filterable with some filters. See N. S. Ferry, "The Filterability of B. bronchiseptieus: With an Argument for a Uniform Method of Filtration," *Science* 39 (1915): 619–20.

13. C. Neuberg, W. Caspari, and H. Löhe, "Weiteres über Heilversuche an Geschwulst-Kranken Tieren mittels tumoraffiner Substanzen," *BKW* 49 (1912): 1405–12; "The Experimental Chemotherapy of Cancer," *BMJ* 2 (1912): 448–50; Charles Walker, "Theories and Problems of Cancer," *Science Progress in the Twentieth Century: A Quarterly Journal of Scientific Work and Thought* 7 (1912): 234–38; "Chemotherapy of Experimental Cancer," *JAMA* 59 (1912): 1230; and "Tumoraffin Substances," *Medical Record* 81 (1912): 524–25. Colloidal suspensions for medicinal purposes were generally made by the method described in the text. Of utility is Max Morse, "Inorganic Colloids and Protoplasm," *Science*, n.s., 37 (1913): 423–25.

14. Harvey R. Gaylord, "Ueber die therapeutische Wirkung der Metalle auf Krebs," *BKW* 30 (1912): 2017–19; "Therapeutic Action of Metals in Cancer," *NYMJ* 96 (1912): 1189; Charles E. Walker, "The Treatment of Cancer with Selenium," *Lancet* 1 (1912): 1337–38; and Eugene G. Kessler, "The Treatment of Carcinoma By Selenium," *Medical Record* 81 (1912): 1024–27.

15. J. Gaube du Gers, *De La Decancerisation* (Paris: Rousset, 1912); and J. Gaube du Gers, *La Cuprase Et Le Cancer: Cinquante Observations Nouvelles* (Paris: Jules Rousset, 1913); "Copper Cancer Cure," *Washington Post*, March 4, 1912, 2; "Finds Cure for Cancer," *Waukesha Freeman*, March 14, 1912, 2; and "Certain Cure For Cancer Is Found," *Oakland Tribune*, March 24, 1912, 4. A letter to the editor in *JAMA* referred to Gers as "promoter" of an "alleged cancer cure." See "An Alleged Cancer Cure (Colloid of Copper) and Its Promoter (Gaube du Gers)," *JAMA* 58 (1912): 1773. Two letters to *BMJ* discussed purchasing Gers's nostrum and its lack of effectiveness in battling cancer. See "The Cuprase Treatment of Cancer," *BMJ* 2 (1913): 156, 284. The *Medical Record* lists Gers as a Paris scientist. See "Tummoraffin Substances," 525.

16. Ernest W. Goodpasture, *Leo Loeb, 1869–1959: A Biographical Memoir* (Washington, DC: National Academy of Sciences, 1961). For some of Loeb's earlier efforts, see, for example, Leo Loeb, "Tumor Growth and Tissue Growth," *Proceedings of the American Philosophical Society* 47 (1908): 3–13.

17. Leo Loeb, C. B. McClurg, and W. O. Sweek, "The Treatment of Human Cancer with Intravenous Injections of Colloidal Copper," *Interstate Medical Journal* 19 (1912): 1015–22; "Colloidal Copper in the Treatment of Cancer," *BMJ* 1 (1913): 255; and Leo Loeb and Moyer S. Fleisher, "Intravenous Injections of Various Substances in Animal Cancer," *ZFK* 12 (1913): 542–46. The paper was presented to the Washington meeting of the AACR. Assessing the state of the art became a regular feature of the medical literature. See Moyer S. Fleisher, "Recent Advances in Cancer Research," *Interstate Medical Journal* 19 (1912): 627–32.

18. "See the Right Road to Cure of Cancer," *NYT*, December 22, 1912, 8; "Dr. Leo Loeb Makes Bold Experiments in Cancer Cases," *NYT*, December 29, 1912, 38;

"See the Right Road to Cure Cancer," *Journal-Tribune*, January 4, 1913, 7; "Colloidal Copper's Value in Cancer Confirmed," *NYT*, May 25, 1913, SM6; "Cancer is Being Cured," *MacLean's Magazine* 26 (1913): 134–35; and "New Treatment for Deadly Cancer May Bring Good Results," *Milford [IA] Mail*, August 28, 1913, 6.

19. Leo Loeb, "Further Observations on the Treatment of Human Cancer With Intravenous Injections of Colloidal Copper," *Interstate Medical Journal* 20 (1913): 9–16; Leo Loeb, Moyer S. Fleisher, W. E. Leighton, and O. Oshii, "The Influence of Intravenous Injections of Various Colloidal Copper Preparations Upon Tumors in Mice," *Interstate Medical Journal* 20 (1913): 16–18. Loeb presented his copper colloid work to the AACR. See "Scientists Talk of Research Results," *Nevada State Journal*, December 30, 1913, 3.

20. Leo Loeb, "Some Recent Results of Cancer Investigations," *Lancet-Clinic* 90 (1913): 667–68. A paper two years later confirmed Loeb's assessment. See C. B. McClurg, W. O. Sweek, H. N. Lyon, M. S. Fleisher, and Leo Loeb, "A Study of General and Localized Effects of Intravenous Injections of Colloidal Copper and Casein in Cases of Human Cancer," *Archives of Internal Medicine* 15 (1915): 974–1013. Numerous others experimented with chemotherapeutic cancer agents. See, for instance, "Paris," *BMJ* 1 (1912): 1215; "Potassium Iodine as a Reactive in Cancerous Growths and as a Therapeutic Agent, Together with Subcutaneous Administration of Sodium Arsenate in a Solution of Phenol," *NYMJ* 97 (1913): 1319; A. J. Gelarie, "The Influence of Copper Upon the Growth of Mouse Carcinoma," *BMJ* 2 (1913): 222–23; Keneth F. Junor, "Clinical Observations on Cancer: Its Treatment and Cure by Chemicals Alone," *NYMJ* 98 (1913): 966–70; "A New Internal Antiseptic," *BMJ* 2 (1913): 2; "Polonium as Medicine," *NYT*, November 26, 1913, 2; "Progress Reported in Cancer Research," *NYT*, November 22, 1914, C3; James Rae, "The Clinical Uses of Colloidal Metals," *BMJ* 1 (1914): 1016; G. L. Rohdenburg, "Colloidal Silver with Lecithin, In the Treatment of Malignant Tumors," *JMR* 31 (1915): 331–38; L. F. Ballester, "Chemical Therapy of Cancer," *NYMJ* 101 (1915): 751–52; Richard Weil, "Chemotherapeutic Experiments On Tumors," in Verhandlungen der Jahresversammlung Der American Association for Cancer Research am 1. April 1915 in St. Louis, *ZFK* 15 (1916): 449; and "Chemotherapy and Tumors," *NYMJ* 101 (1915): 913–14. As late as June 1914, English physicians were championing Gaube Du Gers and colloidal copper in their medical journals. See Lovell Drage, "The Chemical Treatment of Cancer," *Lancet* 1 (1914): 1651; and J. Leonard Joyce, "The Chemical Treatment of Cancer," *Lancet* 1 (1914): 1786.

Chapter 8

1. Henry Butlin, "Two Lectures on Unicellula Cancri: The Parasite of Cancer," *BMJ* 2 (1911): 1393–96, 1457–61, 1535–40. For another argument that adapted evolutionary theory, see C. J. Bond, "On Cancer," *Lancet* 2 (1911): 349–56; and "Cancer," *NYMJ* 94 (1911): 397–98.

2. "A Biological View of the Cancer Cell," *BMJ* 2 (1911): 1494–95; "The Cancer Cell," *Lancet* 2 (1911): 1566–67; William J. Collins, "The Cause of Cancer," *Lancet* 2 (1911): 1588; H. Charlton Bastian, "The Origin of Cancer and the Origin of Life," *Lancet* 2 (1911): 1658–59; J. Thomson Shirlaw, "The Nature and Origin of Cancer," *BMJ* 2 (1911): 1625 and 1 (1912): 163, 395, 811; "Unicellula Cancri," *NYMJ* 94 (1911):

1245, 1297–98; A. T. Brand, Arthur J. Brock, William P. Kennedy, and Alexander Haig, "The Nature and Origin of Cancer," *BMJ* 2 (1911): 1577; "Parasite of Cancer," *JAMA* 57 (1911): 2108–9; and John Bland-Sutton, "Unicellula Cancri," *Lancet* 1 (1912): 608–9. A third installment of Butlin's theory was published posthumously. See Henry Butlin, "A Third Lecture on Unicellula Cancri: The Parasite of Cancer," *BMJ* 1 (1912): 933–37.

3. Howard W. Novell [*sic*], "Experimentelle Krebsforschungen," *Zentralblatt für Allgemeine Pathologie Und Pathologische Anatomie* 24 (1913): 682–86; Howard W. Nowell, "An Etiological Factor in Carcinoma and its Possible Influence on Treatment," *BMSJ* 168 (1913): 838–42; "Etiological Factor in Carcinoma," *JAMA* 60 (1913): 1980; "Experimental Investigation in Cancer," *NYMJ* 98 (1913): 732; Van Buren Thorne, "Cause of Cancer Found At Last By Boston Scientist," *NYT*, April 20, 1913, SM3; "Cancer Alleviated By Nowell Serum," *NYT*, May 11, 1913, 3; "Extends Cancer Study," *NYT*, June 16, 1913, 9; and Ernst Fränkel and Wassa Klein, "Studien über die chemische Aetiologie des Carcinoms Nach Nowell," *ZFK* 15 (1916): 76–84.

4. See, for example, "Vitamines and Cancer," *BMJ* 2 (1913): 1551–52; Hastings Gilford, "On the Nature of Old Age and Of Cancer," *BMJ* 2 (1913): 1617–20; "Tumours Produced By Viruses," *BMJ* 1 (1914): 389–90; and Max Bürger, "Untersuchungen über das Hühnersarkom (Peyton Rous)," *ZFK* 14 (1914): 526–42. Rous published in Germany too. See Peyton Rous and James B. Murphy, "Beobachtungen an einem Hühnersarkom und seiner filterbaren Ursache," *BKW* (1913): 637–39; and Peyton Rous, "Histologische Variationen eines Hühnersarkoms mittels filterbarem Agens erzeugt," *BKW* (1914): 1265–66.

5. Robert Kilduffe, "Morphological Changes Observed in a Mouse Carcinoma in the Course of Long-Continued Transplantation, and the Influence of an Experimentally Produced Decrease in the Growth-Energy of the Tumors Upon Their Morphological Character," *JEM* 13 (1911): 234–38; "Inhibition of Tumor Growth," *JAMA* 56 (1911): 1298; "Cancer Research," *Lancet* 2 (1911): 391–92; George Thomas Beatson, "The Role of Fat in the Etiology and Progress of Cancer," *Lancet* 1 (1911): 1560–61; W. H. Woglom, "The Nature of the Immune Reaction to Transplanted Cancer in the Rat," *Proceedings of the Royal Society of London, Series B* 85 (1912): 197–200; "Imperial Cancer Fund," *BMJ* 2 (1912): 129–31; B. R. G. Russell, "The Manifestation of Active Resistance to the Growth of Implanted Cancer," *Proceedings of the Royal Society of London, Series B* 85 (1912): 201–13; "Resistance to Growth of Cancer," *NYMJ* 96 (1912): 393; E. E. Tyzzer, "Factors in the Production and Growth of Tumor Metastases," *JMR* 28 (1913): 309–32; "The Vaccination Treatment of Cancer," *BMJ* 1 (1914): 54–55; Albert Wilson, "Cases of Inoperable Cancer Treated with Goat Serum," *BMJ* 1 (1915): 155–56; and William N. Berkeley, "Some Comments on a New Antiserum for Cancer," *NYMJ* 102 (1915): 44–47.

6. Buffalo's Gaylord, St. Louis's Loeb and Columbia's Beebe attempted experiments with filtrates from rat or dog sarcomas similar to Rous's chicken sarcoma investigation. Each had mixed results. See Harvey R. Gaylord and Burton T. Simpson, "Filtration Experiments With Transplantable Sarcoma of the Rat," *ZFK* 11 (1912): 131–37. Gaylord's paper was presented at the Buffalo meeting of the

American Association for Cancer Research in 1911.

7. D. Hansemann, "Ueber Krebsprobleme," *DMW* 40 (1914): 1753–56. For a radically different proposition, see Frederic S. Lee, *Scientific Features of Modern Medicine* (New York: Columbia University Press, 1911), 110–32. Lee's piece was delivered to the public at the American Museum of Natural History.

8. See, for example, "Animal Experimentation," *JAMA* 56 (1911): 816–17; Charles E. Walker, "Progress in Cancer Research," *Lancet* 1 (1911): 1275–76; Edward H. Risley, "The Treatment of Cancer With Body Fluids and Cancerous Ascitic Fluid," *JAMA* 56 (1911) 1383–89; "Imperial Cancer Fund," *Lancet* 2 (1911): 315–19; Katharine Freytag, "Ueber Das Mäusecarcinom," *ZFK* 10 (1911): 155–67; G. Fichera, "The Action of the Products of Homogeneous Fetal Autolysis on Malignant Tumours in Man," *Lancet* 2 (1911): 1194–97; M. Beck, "Versuche Uber Mäusekrebs," *ZFK* 10 (1911): 149–54; R. A. Lambert, "On the Question of Immunization Against Transplantable Cancer By Injection of An Animal's Own Tissues," *Proceedings of Society for Experimental Biology and Medicine* 9 (1911–1912): 18–19; Isaac Levin, "Immunity and Specific Therapy in Experimental Cancer," *JAMA* 59 (1912): 517–21; Isaac Levin, "Tumor Inoculation Into Organs and the Analogy Between Human Cancer and the Tumors of White Mice and White Rats," *JEM* 16 (1912): 155–64; Francis Carter Wood, "Problem of Cancer," *JAMA* 60 (1913): 1250–52; Robert A. Lambert, "Comparative Studies Upon Cancer Cells and Normal Cells: II. The Character of Growth in Vitro with Special Reference to Cell Division," *JEM* 17 (1913): 499–510; William Henry Woglom, *Studies in Cancer and Allied Subjects: Pathology*, vol. 2 (New York: Columbia University Press, 1912); and Isaac Levin, The Cancer Problem and the Modern Methods of the Treatment of Malignant Tumors," *Interstate Medical Journal* 21 (1915): 683–91. Not surprising, Hansemann saw little relationship between experimental and human cancer. See D. Hansemann, "Ueber Krebsprobleme," *DMW* 40 (1914): 1753–56. Loeb remained diametrically opposed. See Leo Loeb, "Some Remarks on the Definition and Solution of the Cancer Problem," *Interstate Medical Journal* 19 (1912): 45–49.

9. "Editorial–The Cancer Problem," *Interstate Medical Journal* 16 (1909): 233–35; Henry T. Butlin, "Presidential Address Delivered at the Seventy-Eighth Annual Meeting of the British Medical Association," *BMJ* 2 (1910): 241–46; and Leo Loeb, "The Relationship Between Practitioner and Investigator in Medicine," *JAMA* 59 (1912): 594–97.

10. "A Preliminary Report on the Mortality of Cancer in the United States as Given by the Census of 1910," *JAMA* 56 (1911): 58; William Renner, "Cancer and the Creoles of Sierra Leone," *BMJ* 1 (1911): 110–11; J. S. Mackintosh, "The Cancer Problem," *BMJ* 1 (1911): 164; "Bath Clinical Society," *BMJ* 1 (1911): 202; "Cancer in the Coloured Race in the States," *BMJ* 1 (1911): 269–70; "Statistics of Cancer," *JAMA* 56 (1911): 1050; "Cancer Statistics in France," *Lancet* 1 (1911): 970–71; Munch Soegaard, "Die Relative Krebsimmunitat Der Leprakranken," *BKW* (1911): 1718–22; "Distribution of Tuberculosis and Cancer in Paris," *BMSJ* 165 (1911): 655; "The Cancer Hospital and the Causes of Cancer," *Lancet* 2 (1911): 1661; "Lessons from Cancer Research in Baden," *JAMA* 57 (1911): 1954; "Cancer in the Penal Institutions of Norway," *JAMA* 59 (1912): 1500; "Family Incidence of Malignant Tumors," *JAMA* 60 (1913): 863–64; W. Gordon and W. F. Thompson,

"The Distribution of Cancer Cases in Two Registration Districts of North-East Cornwall," *BMJ* 2 (1913): 546; "Geographical Distribution of Cancer," *JAMA* 61 (1913): 1580; "Statistics of the Geographical Distribution of Cancer," *NYMJ* 98 (1913): 930; Robert Behla, "Die Gesamtmortalitat An Tuberkulose mUnd Krebs In Preussen Im Jahre 1913," *BKW* (1913): 675; W. Gifford Nash, "Cancer Houses," *Lancet* 1 (1914): 1149; "Buyo Cheek Cancer," *BMJ* 2 (1915): 105–6; and "Cancer in Great Britain," *NYMJ* 102 (1915): 51–52. For Coley, see William B. Coley, "The Increase of Cancer," *Transactions of the Southern Surgical and Gynecological Society* 22 (1910): 536–50.

11. Percivall Pott, *Chirurgical Observations Relative to the Cataract, the Polypus of the Nose, the Cancer of the Scrotum, the Different Kinds of Ruptures, and the Mortification of the Toes and Feet* (London: T. J. Carney, 1775). As late as 1914, investigators were suggesting that Smith's work on crown gall suggested that scrotal cancer might be caused by a microbe. See D. A. Crow, "A Case of Chimney-Sweep's Cancer, and a Suggestion as to the Pathology of Cancer," *BMJ* 1 (1914): 413–14.

12. H. C. Ross, "The Vacuolation of the Blood-Platelets: An Experimental Proof of the Cellular Nature," *Proceedings of the Royal Society of London. Series B* 81 (1909): 351–53; H. C. Ross, "On a Combination of Substances Which Excite Amoeboid Movements in Leucocytes," *Lancet* 1 (1909): 152–56; H. C. Ross and C. J. Macalister, "On the Flagellation of Lymphocytes in the Presence of Excitants Both Artificial and Cancerous," *BMJ* 1 (1909): 206–8; Hugh C. Ross and Charles Macalister, "A Report on Cancer Research: An Investigation By 'In Vitro' Methods," *BMJ* 2 (1909): 1212–20; and H. C. Ross and J. W. Cropper, "The Gas-Works Pitch Industries and Cancer," *BMJ* 1 (1911): 884–85.

13. H. C. Ross, *Induced Cell Reproduction and Cancer* (London: John Murray, 1910); "Further Researches Into Induced Cell-Reproduction and Cancer," *Nature* 88 (1911): 174; R. J. Gibson, W. A. Herdman, B. Moore, J. Reynolds Green, and C. S. Sherrington, "Induced Cell Division and Cancer," *BMJ* 2 (1910): 2007; H. C. Ross, "Induced Cell Division," *BMJ* 2 (1910): 2052; Sir Ronald Ross, "Induced Division of Leucocytes and the Genesis of Tumours," *Proceedings of the Royal Society of Medicine*, Pathological Section (1911), 103–8; Ronald Ross, "Induced Division of Human Lymphocytes," *BMJ* 1 (1911): 163; and "Induced Action of Leucocytes," *Nature* 88 (1911): 231–32. A history of chemical carcinogenesis can be had at M. B. Shimkin and V. A. Triolo, "History of Chemical Carcinogenesis: Some Prospective Remarks," *Progress on Experimental Tumor Research* 11 (1969): 1–20.

14. Hugh Campbell Ross and John Westray Cropper, *Further Researchers Into Induced Cell-Reproduction and Cancer* (London: John Murray, 1911); C. E. W., "Cancer Problems," *Nature* 89 (1912): 601–2; "Notes on New Books," *Johns Hopkins Hospital Bulletin* 23 (1912): 95; H. T. K., "Further Researches Into Induced Cell Reproduction and Cancer," *American Journal of Medical Sciences* 145 (1913): 135–36; Ronald Ross, "The New Cell Proliferant," *BMJ* 1 (1912): 160; and Ronald Ross, "Further Researchers Into Induced Cell Reproduction and Cancer," *Nature* 90 (1913): 102.

15. "Blast Furnace Pitch and Cancer," *BMJ* 2 (1911): 393; "Gasworks Pitch Industries and Cancer," *BMJ* 1 (1913): 36–37, 511–513; Thomas Oliver, "A

Presidential Address on Some Industrial Accidents and Diseases," *Lancet* 1 (1913): 1575–78; "Cancer and the Manufacture of Patent Fuel," *BMJ* 2 (1913): 760–61; and Alfred Herbert Lush, *Second Report to His Majesty's Secretary of State For the Home Department on the Draft Regulations Proposed to be Made for the Manufacture of Patent Fuel (Briquettes) With the Addition of Pitch* (London: Darling and Son, 1913).

16. Charles Walker, "The New Cell Proliferant," *BMJ* 1 (1912): 582–83, 810–11; H. C. Ross, "The New Cell Proliferant," *BMJ* (1912): 393–94; Dorothy Norris, "A Note on the Bases of Gasworks Coal-tar which are believed to be the Predisposing Cause of Pitch Cancer, with Special Reference to their Action on Lymphocytes together with a Method for their Inactivation," *Biochemical Journal* 8 (1914): 253–60; H. C. Ross, "The Cancer Problem and Radio-Activity," *Nature* 95 (1915): 617–18; and H. C. Ross, "The Danger of Saccharine," *BMJ* 2 (1915): 552–53. For the McFadden effort, see "Gift for Cancer Research," *NYT*, March 23, 1913, C2.

17. Silas Palmer Beebe was exemplary in this regard. Most of his early career was in conjunction with Cornell's Huntington effort. There, he set out much of what was known of the chemistry of tumors. See, for example, S. P. Beebe, "The Chemistry of Malignant Growths. First Communication," *American Journal of Physiology* 11 (1904): 139–44; S. P. Beebe, "The Chemistry of Malignant Growths. Second Communication," *American Journal of Physiology* 12 (1904): 167–72; S. P. Beebe, ""The Chemistry of Malignant Growths. III. Nucleo-histon as a Constituent of Tumors," *American Journal of Physiology* 13 (1905): 341–49; S. P. Beebe and Phillip Shaffer, "The Chemistry of Malignant Growths. The Pentose Content of Tumors," *American Journal of Physiology* 14 (1905): 231–38; S. P. Beebe, "Cytotoxic Serum Produced by the Injection of Nucleoproteids," *JEM* (1905): 1–18; S. P. Beebe, "Artificial Immunity in Non-Bacterial Diseases," *JAMA* 55 (1910): 1712–17; and S. P. Beebe, "The Chemistry of Cancer," *NYMJ* 97 (1910): 1–6. Other efforts focused on the use of chemistry to diagnose malignancies. See, for example, W. Cramer and James Lochhead, "Contributions to the Biochemistry of Growth: The Lycogen-Content of the Liver of Rats Bearing Malignant New Growths," *Proceedings of the Royal Society of London. Series B* 86 (1913): 302–7; R. A. Kocher, "The Hexone Bases of Malignant Tumors, " *Journal of Biological Chemistry* (1915): 295–303; Frederic G. Goodridge and Max Kahn, "The Neutral-Sulfur and Colloidal-Nitrogen Tests in The Diagnosis of Cancer," *Biochemical Bulletin* 4 (1915): 118–26; and Casimir Funk, "Serum Diagnosis of Rous's Chicken Sarcoma, Based on Chemical Methods," *Biochemical Bulletin* 4 (1915): 24–29.

18. See, for example, Lafayette B. Mendel and William C. Rose, "Experimental Studies on Creatine and Creatinine," *Journal of Biological Chemistry* (1911): 213–53; Thomas B. Osborne and Lafayette B. Mendel, "Maintenance Experiments with Isolated Proteins," *Journal of Biological Chemistry* (1912): 233–76; E. V. McCollum and Marguerite Davis, "The Necessity of Certain Lipins in the Diet During Growth," *Journal of Biological Chemistry* (1913): 167–75; Lafayette B. Mendel and Robert C. Lewis, "The Rate of Elimination of Nitrogen As Influenced By Diet Factors," *Journal of Biological Chemistry* (1913): 19–53; Thomas B. Osborne and Lafayette B. Mendel, "The Relation of Growth to the Chemical Constituents of the Diet," *Journal of Biological Chemistry* (1913): 311–26; Thomas B. Osborne and Lafayette B. Mendel, "Amino-Acids in Nutrition and Growth," *Journal of Biological*

Chemistry (1914): 325–49; Thomas B. Osborne and Lafayette B. Mendel, "The Influence of Cod Liver Oil and Some Other Fats on Growth," *Journal of Biological Chemistry* (1914): 401–9; Thomas B. Osborne and Lafayette B. Mendel, "The Influence of Butter-Fat on Growth," *Journal of Biological Chemistry* (1914): 423–37; and Casimir Funk and Archibald Bruce Macallum, "Studies on Growth: II. On the Probably Nature of the Substance Promoting Growth in Young Animals," *Journal of Biological Chemistry* (1915): 413–21.

19. Alexander Haig, "Diet and Inoperable Cancer," *Lancet* 1 (1911): 127, 1033; John T. MacLachlan and E. Wardman-Wilbourne, "The Cancer Problem," *BMJ* 1 (1911): 282; James Davison, "Diet and Inoperable Cancer," *Lancet* 1 (1911): 902; Thomas J. Horder, "Diet and Inoperable Cancer," *Lancet* 1 (1911): 967–68; "Uric-Acid-Free Diet in Inoperable Cancer," *BMJ* 2 (1912): 81–83; "The Relation of Diet to Cancer," *NYMJ* 100 (1914): 47; "Diet and Cancer," *NYMJ* 101 (1915): 310; "Foods in Relation to Cancer," *Woman's Medical Journal* 25 (1915): 157–58; "Cancer and the Citizen's Daily Food," *NYMJ* 102 (1915): 523–24; and "Cause of Cancer," *American Medicine* 21 (1915): 788–89.

20. Peyton Rous, "The Influence of Diet on Transplanted and Spontaneous Mouse Tumors," *JEM* (1914): 431–51. Also see Peyton Rous, "The Influence of Dieting Upon the Course of Cancer," *Johns Hopkins Hospital Bulletin* 26 (1915): 146–48. For some of the studies Rous sought to counter, see, for example, Simon Duplay and Savoire, "Recherches Sur Les Modifications De La Nutrition Chez Les Cancereux," *Revue Des Maladies Cancereuses* 2 (1897): 89–92; J. E. Sweet, E. P. Corson-White, and G. J. Saxon, "On the Influence of Certain Diets Upon the Growth of Experimental Tumors," *Proceedings of the Society for Experimental Biology and Medicine* 10 (1912–1913): 175–76; J. E. Sweet, Ellen P. Corson-White, and G. J. Saxon, "Further Studies on the Relation of Diets to Transmissible Tumors," *Journal of Biological Chemistry* (1915): 309–18.

21. Peyton Rous, "The Influence of Underfeeding on Spontaneous Mouse Tumors," *Proceedings of the New York Pathological Society* 14 (1914): 126–29. Ewing's remarks followed on pages 129–30. Beebe and Van Alstyne had worked in this area earlier. See their "The Influence of Non-Carbohydrate Diet on the Growth of Transplantable Sarcoma," *ZFK* 12 (1913): 547–49. Rous was present at the Washington AACR meeting where the two authors presented their findings.

22. T. Brailsford Robertson and Theodore C. Burnett, "Preliminary Report on the Influence of Lecithin and Cholesterin Upon the Growth of Tumors," *Proceedings of the Society for Experimental Biology and Medicine* 10 (1912–1913): 59–60; T. Brailsford Robertson and Theodore C. Burnett, "The Influence of Lecithin and Cholesterin Upon the Growth of Tumors," *JEM* (1913) 344–52; and T. Brailsford Robertson and Theodore C. Burnett, "Preliminary Communication on the Part Played By Cholesterol in Determining the Incidence of Carcinoma," *Proceedings of the Society for Experimental Biology and Medicine* 10 (1912–1913): 140–43.

23. Eleanor Van Ness Van Alstyne and S. P. Beebe, "Diet Studies in Transplantable Tumors. I. The Effect of Non-Carbohydrate Diet Upon the Growth of Transplantable Sarcoma in Rats," *JMR* (1913) 217–32. Also see "The Effect of Diet in Experimental Cancer," *BMJ* 1 (1914): 496–97. A rejoinder was William H. Woglom, "Diet and Tumor Growth," *JEM* (1915): 766–79.

24. S. P. Beebe and Eleanor Van Alstyne, "The Influence of Diet on Transplantable Sarcoma," *Proceedings of the New York Pathological Society* 14 (1914): 124–26; and "Influence of Diet on Transplantable Sarcoma in Rats," *JAMA* 63 (1914): 191–92.

25. Casimir Funk, "The Transplantation of Tumors to Foreign Species," *JEM* 21 (1915): 571–73.

26. Casimir Funk, "Studien Uber Das Wachstum. I. Mitteilung. Das Wachstum-Auf Vitaminhaltiger Und Vitaminfreier Nahrung," *Zeitschrift für Physiologische Chemie* 88 (1913): 352–56; Casimir Funk, "Studies on Growth: The Influence of Diet on Growth, Normal and Malignant," reprinted from the *Lancet, British Veterinary Journal* (1914): 126–32; and Casimir Funk, "Results of Studies on Vitamins and Deficiency Diseases, During the Years 1913–1915," *Biochemistry Bulletin* 4 (1915): 304–65. The prominent New York City cancer physician, L. Duncan Bulkley, rejected all nutrition experiments as incomplete and misleading. He advocated diet modification as a cancer remedy. See L. Duncan Bulkley, *Cancer: Its Cause and Treatment* (New York: Paul B. Hoeber, 1915), 170–210.

27. T. Brailsford Robertson and Theodore C. Burnett, "The Influence of the Anterior Lobe of the Pituitary Body Upon the Growth of Carcinomata," *JEM* (1915): 280–87. Also see Seeeye W. Little, "A Study of Cancer," *BMSJ* 170 (1914): 126–30.

28. J. E. Sweet, Ellen P. Corson-White, and G. J. Saxon, "The Relation of Diets and of Castration to the Transmissible tumors of Rats and Mice," *Journal of Biological Chemistry* (1913): 181–91.

29. G. L. Rohdenburg, F. D. Bullock, and P. J. Johnston, "The Effects of Certain Internal Secretions on Malignant Tumors," *Archives of Internal Medicine* 7 (1911): 491–99; and "Effects of Internal Secretions of Malignant Tumours," *BMJ* 2 (1911): 8. Also of interest is "Biology of Tumors," *NYMJ* 97 (1913): 43–44.

30. Gary N. Calkins, Frederick D. Bullock, and George L. Rohdenburg, "The Effects of Chemicals on the Division Rate of Cells With Especial Reference to Possible Pre-Cancerous Conditions," *Journal of Infectious Diseases* 10 (1912): 421–39. Rohdenburg and Bullock backtrack a bit in G. L. Rohdenburg and F. D. Bullock, "Notes on Tumor Genesis," *NYMJ* 96 (1912): 222–26. The search for the appropriate chemical accelerator included "Nuclease in Carcinoma," *JAMA* 58 (1912): 1544; and Walter W. Hamburger, "Comparative Studies in Cancer and Normal Tissue Ferments," *JAMA* 59 (1912): 847–51.

31. Ferdinand Blumenthal, "Ueber Die Ruckbildung Bosartiger Geschwulste Durch Die Behandlung Mit Dem Eigenen Tumorextrakt (Autovaccine)," *ZFK* 11 (1912): 427–48; Ferdinand Blumenthal, "Bemerkungen Zur Behandlung Bosartiger Geschwulste Mit Extrakten Des Eigenen Bzw. Eines Analogen Tumors," *ZFK* 14 (1914): 491–500; "Auto-Vaccines in Treatment of Cancer," *JAMA* 59 (1912): 962; and "Autovaccines in Cancer," *JAMA* 59 (1912): 1437.

32. Dr. Lunckenbein, "Zur Behandlung Maligner Geschwulste," *Muenchener Medizinische Wochenschrift* 61 (1914): 18–21; Dr. Lunckenbein, "Die Behandlung Maligner Geschwure Mit Tumorextrakt," *Muenchener Medizinische Wochenschrift* 61 (1914): 1047–49; "New Views on the Treatment of Cancer," *International Journal of Surgery* (1914): 257–58; "The Autolysate Treatment of Cancer," *BMJ* 1 (1914): 7, 67–68; "Cancer Extracts in the Treatment of Cancer," *Medical Record* 88 (1915):

22–23; and "Non-Operative Methods of Treating Cancer," *Progressive Medicine* 2 (1915): 205–7. Other advocates of autolysates include Carl Lewin, F. Blumenthal, and C. Lewin, "Weitere Versuche über Behandlung von Sarkomratten mit den Extraktstoffen des eigenen Tumors," *Therapie Der Gegenwart* 55 (1914): 115–18.

33. G. Fichera, "The Action of the Products of Homogeneous Foetal Autolysis on Malignant Tumours in Man," *Lancet* 2 (1913): 1194–97; "Fichera's Method of Preparing Fetal Autolysates for the Treatment of Cancer," *JAMA* 60 (1913): 228; W. Wayne Babcock, "Fetal Products in the Treatment of Carcinoma (Fichera's Method)," *International Clinics* 2 (1913): 81–88; Ferdinand Blumenthal, "Bemerkungen Zu Dem Aufsatz Von G. Fichera 'Ausbau Der Theorie Des Onkogenen Gleichgewichtsmangels Usw,'" *ZFK* 14 (1914): 327–35; G. Fichera, "Aktive Immunisierung Oder Histogene Chemotherapie? Erwiderung An Die Professoren F. Blumenthal Und C. Lewin," *ZFK* 14 (1914): 566–77; and G. Fichera, "Ueber die biologische Onkotherapie. Antwort an Professor F. Blumenthal," *ZFK* 15 (1916): 184–91.

34. G. L. Rohdenburg and F. D. Bullock, "The Influence of Autolytic Products on Tumor Growth," *Medical Record* 88 (1915): 233–34; and "The Influence of Autolytic Products on Tumor Growth," *JAMA* 65 (1915): 740. Francis Carter Wood, the Crocker Laboratory's director, also complained about poor experimental practice in cancer research. See F. C. Wood and E. H. McLean, "The Effect of Phlorhizin on Tumors in Animals," *Proceedings of the Society of Experimental Biology and Medicine* 12 (1915): 135–36.

Chapter 9

1. Johannes Fibiger, "Ueber eine durch Nematoden (Spiroptera sp. n.) hervorgerufene papillomatöse und carcinomatöse Geschwulstbildung im Magen Der Ratte," *BKW* 50 (1913): 289–98; Johannes Fibiger, "Untersuchungen über eine Nematode (Spiroptera sp. n.) und deren Fähigkeit, papillomatöse und carcinomatöse Geschwulstbildungen im Magen der Ratte hervorzurufen," *ZFK* 13 (1913): 217–80; and "Animal-Parasite Cancer in Rats," *JAMA* 63 (1914): 1244, 1432. For Galeb's study, see Osman Galeb, *Recherches Sur Les Entozoaires Des Insectes Organisation Et Developpment Des Oxyurides* (Paris: C. Reinwald et Co., 1879).

2. "Cancer and the Cockroach," *NYMJ* 97 (1913): 358; "Nematodes in the Production of Cancer," *BMJ* 1 (1913): 400–402; "A Nematode in Rat Cancer," *BMJ* 1 (1913): 405–6; D. Hansemann, "Demonstration Von Präparaten des Herrn Fibiger zur künstlichen Erzeugung von Krebs," *BKW* (1913): 988–89; "Cancer Induced in Rats By Feeding With Parasites of Cockroaches," *JAMA* 60 (1913): 948–49; and "Animal Parasites in Tumor Formation," *JAMA* 60 (1913): 1077–78; "Cockroaches and Cancer," *Lancet* 1 (1913): 361; "Cockroaches as Carriers of Cancer," *American Medicine* 19 (1913): 281–82; "On a Papillomatous and Carcinomatous Tumor in the Stomach of Rats Caused by a Nematode," *American Journal of the Medical Sciences* 146 (1913): 601; and M. C. Marsh, "The Occurrence of Nematodes and Acarines in Normal and Spontaneous Tumor in Mice," *ZFK* 15 (1916): 383; "Verhandlungen der Jahresversammlung der American Association for Cancer Research am 9 April 1914 in Toronto," *ZFK* 15 (1916): 434. The press also followed the story. See "Professor Creates Cancer," *NYT*, January 11, 1913, 5; and "Starve the Scavengers,"

Literary Digest, June 1913, 1376. Gaylord managed to mix metaphors as he sought nematodes in the typhoid glands of dogs. See his "On the Presence of Nematodes in Experimental Hyperplasia of the Thyroid of Dogs," *ZFK* 12 (1913): 556–58. Gaylord presented this work to the AACR's meeting in Washington.

3. "Sur Un Travail De M. Le. Dr. A. Borrel, Intitule: Tumeurs Cancereuses Et Helminthes," *Bulletin De L Academie De Medecine* 2 (1906): 141; and "Special Correspondence. Paris," *BMJ* 2 (1906): 392.

4. M. Haaland, "Spontaneous Cancer in Mice," *Proceedings of the Royal Society of London. Series B, Containing Papers of a Biological Character* 83 (1911): 532–40; "Report of the Societies," *BMJ* 1 (1911): 756; and "Cancer Research," *BMJ* 2 (1911): 1307–1309. For Haaland's career, see "Magnus Haaland—En Pioner I Internasjonal Kreftforskning," *Tidsskr Nor Laegeforen* 121 (2001): 832–33.

5. A. Borrel, "Acariens Et Cancer Du Systeme Pilaire," *Compte Rendue Societie Biologie* 28 (1908): 486–88; A. Borrel, "Parasitisme et Tumeurs," *Annales de l' Institute Pasteur* 24 (1910): 778–88; and Haaland, "Spontaneous Cancer." For contemporary work on disease vectors, see F. G. Novy, "Disease Carriers," *Science*, July 5, 1912, 1–10.

6. Fibiger, "Ueber Eine Durch Nematoden."

7. Harvey R. Gaylord, "Annual Report of the Director of the State Institute for the Study of Malignant Disease to the Trustees, For the Year 1911–12, in State of New York," *Second Annual Report of the Trustees of the State Institute for the Study of Malignant Disease* (Albany: J. B. Lyon Company, 1912), 6–12.

8. E. F. Bashford, "Fresh Light on the Cause of Cancer," *Nature* 90 (1913): 701–2. Also see "Cancer Research," *Nature* 88 (1911): 158–60.

9. "Syphilis and Cancer of the Tongue," *BMJ* 1 (1913): 734–35. Also see "Danger in Clay Pipes," *Washington Post*, July 30, 1911, 12.

10. F. D. Bullock and G. L. Rohdenburg, "Cell Proliferation and Parasites in Rats," *JEM and Biology* 16 (1912), 527–31. A fine survey of this two pronged understanding and what German researchers had published was Georg Klemperer, *Der Jetzige Stand Der Krebsforschung* (Berlin: August Hirschwald, 1912).

11. "Czerny Uber Entstehung Und Vehandlung Des Krebses," *Muenchener Medizinische Wochenschrift* 60 (1913): 734–35; and "The Etiology of Cancer," *NYMJ* 97 (1913): 833. For a similar argument, see M. Goldzieher and E. Rosenthal, "Zur Frage Der Geschwulstdisposition," *ZFK* 13 (1913): 321–31.

12. William B. Coley, "Injury as a Causative Factor in Cancer," *Annals of Surgery* 53 (1911): 449–88, 615–50; "The Causal Relationship Between Injury and Cancer," *JAMA* 56 (1911), 142, and *NYMJ* 93 (1911): 497; "Injury as a Cause of Cancer," *NYMJ* 93 (1911): 851; and "Injury as Causative Factor in Cancer," *NYMJ* 93 (1911): 1053; and *JAMA* 56 (1911): 1683.

13. "Trauma in Origin of Cancer," *JAMA* 56 (1911): 1170; S. Löwenstein, "Zur Frage der Posttraumatischen Krebse," *Beitrage Zur Klinischen Chirurgie, Tubingen* 74 (1911): 715–43; Hermann Schoppler, "Einmaliges Trauma Und Carcinom," *ZFK* 10 (1911): 219–23; S. Lowenstein, "Zur Frage Der Posttraumatischen Krebse," *BKW* (1911): 1697; and "Single Trauma and Cancer," *JAMA* 57 (1911): 38. Orth took great pains to argue that trauma need not be mechanical. See J. Orth, "Pracarcinomatose Krankheiten Und Kunstliche Krebse," *ZFK* 10 (1911): 42–54; and "Deutsches

Zentralkomitee Fur Krebsforschung," *DMW* (1910): 1057–58.

14. "Liability for Results of Bruise Followed by Cancer," *JAMA* 57 (1911): 1158.

15. A. Theilhaber and S. Greischer, "Zur Aetiologie Der Carcinome," *ZFK* 9 (1910): 530–54; "Cancer Following Contusions," *JAMA* 57 (1911): 431; A. Theilhaber, "Die Beziehungen Von Chronischer Entzundung, Narbe, Trauma Und Den Fortpflanzungsvorgangen Zu Der Entstehung Von Tumoren," *DMW* 38 (1912): 264–67; and "Trauma and Irritation in Origin of Cancer," *JAMA* 58 (1912): 823. A popularized view of irritation theory was James J. Walsh, "Many Mysteries of Cancer Made Clear by Science," *Washington Post,* June 23, 1912, M8. A formalized mechanistic explanation of cancer from irritation was offered by Arthur Trumbull in his "On the Genesis of Cancer," *BMJ* 2 (1913): 905–6. By about 1914, it became common to link certain kind of cancers to certain specific industries. See, for instance, "Cancer in Relation to Fuel," *BMJ* 1 (1914): 266–67; Benjamin Franklin Davis, "Paraffin Cancer," *JAMA* 62 (1914): 1716–20; "Cancer in France in Relation to Fuel," *NYMJ* 101 (1915): 257–58; and "Philadelphia County Medical Society," *JAMA* 64 (1915): 275. At least one investigator tried to link cancer to the architectural elements of residences. See "Cancer Houses," *American Medicine* 19 (1913): 280–81.

16. "Influence of Heredity on the Occurrence of Cancer," *JAMA* 63 (1914): 1480–81. An interesting early paper on cancer and heredity among a group was Isaac Levin, "Cancer Among the American Indians and its Bearing Upon the Ethnological Distribution of the Disease," *ZFK* 9 (1910): 422–35. England's Royal Society of Medicine thought the relationship between disease and heredity so important that it held a symposium on the topic in 1908. It was published as W. S. Church, William Gowers, Arthur Latham, and E. F. Bashford, *The Influence of Heredity on Disease: With Special Reference to Tuberculosis, Cancer and Diseases of the Nervousa System: A Discussion* (New York: Longmans, Green and Co., 1909).

17. E. E. Tyzzer, "A Study of Heredity in Relation to the Development of Tumors in Mice," *JMR* 17 (1907): 199–211; E. E. Tyzzer, "A Series of Spontaneous Tumors in Mice With Observations on the Influence of Heredity on the Frequency of Their Occurrence," *JMR* 21 (1909): 479–518; E. E. Tyzzer, "A Study of Inheritance in Mice with Reference to Their Susceptibility of Transplantable Tumors," *JMR* 21 (1909): 519–73; and "Cancer and Heredity," *BMJ* 1 (1911): 516–17. For the state of the art, see P. Ledoux-Lebard, "Rapport Sur La Question De L'heredite Du Cancer," *L'Étude* 1 (1908): 92–112. For Tyzzer's career, see Thomas H. Weller, *Ernest Edward Tyzzer, 1875–1965* (Washington, DC: National Academy of Sciences, 1978).

18. E. F. Bashford, "Heredity and Cancer," *Proceedings of the Royal Society of Medicine, General Reports* (1909): 63–75; E. F. Bashford and J. A. Murray, "The Incidence of Cancer in Mice of Known Age," *Proceedings of the Royal Society of London, Section B, Containing Papers of a Biological Character* 81 (1909): 310–13; "Imperial Cancer Research Fund," *Lancet* 1 (1914): 248–50; and "Imperial Cancer Research Fund," *BMJ* 2 (1914): 189–90.

19. J. A. Murray, "Cancerous Ancestry and the Incidence of Cancer in Mice," *Proceedings of the Royal Society of London, Section B, Containing Papers of a Biological Character* 84 (1911): 42–48; "Cancer Research," *BMJ* 2 (1911): 171–74, 1307–1309; "Cancerous Heredity," *BMJ* 1 (1911): 1177; "Cancer Research," *Lancet* 2 (1911): 1345–

46; and "Imperial Cancer Research Fund," *Nature* 89 (1912): 531–32.

20. A. E. C. Lathrop and Leo Loeb, "The Incidence of Cancer in Various Strains of Mice," *Proceedings of the Society for Experimental Biology and Medicine* 11 (1913): 34–38; A. E. C. Lathrop and Leo Loeb, "The Influence of Pregnancies on the Incidence of Cancer in Mice," *Proceedings of the Society for Experimental Biology and Medicine* 11 (1913): 38–40; Leo Loeb, "Some Recent Results of Cancer Investigations," *Cincinnati Lancet-Clinic* 110 (1913): 664–68; Leo Loeb and Moyer S. Fleisher, "Heredity of the susceptibility to Inoculation with Cancer," *ZFK* 12 (1913): 434–36. Loeb and Fleisher presented the paper at the Philadelphia meeting of the AACR in 1912. A. E. C. Lathrop and Leo Loeb, "Some Factors Determining the Incidence of Cancer in Mice," a paper presented to the American Association for Cancer Research, April 9, 1914, *ZFK* 15 (1916): 421–22; and A. E. C. Lathrop and Leo Loeb, "Further Investigations on the Origin of Tumors in Mice," *JEM* (1915): 646–73. Other investigators recognized a group of Lathrop mice extremely resistant to cancer. See Joseph McFarland and Guthrie McConnell, "A Group of Mice With Exceptional Resistance to Mouse Carcinoma," *JMR* (1913): 437–43. For Loeb's career, see Ernest W. Goodpasture, *Leo Loeb, 1869–1959* (Washington, DC: National Academy of Sciences, 1961).

21. "American Association For Cancer Research," *JAMA* 60 (1913): 2020; "Verhandlungen Der Jahresversammlung Der American Association For Cancer Research AM 5 Mai 1913 in Washington," *ZFK* 12 (1913): 534–38; Maud Slye, "The Incidence and Inheritability of Spontaneous Cancer in Mice (Preliminary Report)," *ZFK* 13 (1913): 500–504; Maud Slye, "The Inheritability of Spontaneous Tumors in Mice," a paper presented to the American Association for Cancer Research, April 9, 1914, *ZFK* 15 (1916): 422–24; Maud Slye, "The Incidence and Inheritability of Spontaneous Tumors in Mice," *JMR* 30 (1914): 281–98; and 32 (1915): 159–200; Maud Slye, Harriet F. Holmes, and H. Gideon Wells, "The Primary Spontaneous Tumors of the Lungs in Mice," *JMR* 30 (1914): 417–42; and "Recent Work on Cancer," *JAMA* 64 (1915): 1326; Maud Slye, "The Influence of Heredity Upon the Occurrence of Spontaneous Cancer," *Interstate Medical Journal* 21 (1915): 692–721; and "Incidence and Inheritability of Spontaneous Cancers in Mice: Inheritability of Tumors of Specific Organs," *JAMA* 64 (1915): 1610.

22. Edward Reginald Morton, "The 'X'-Ray Treatment of Malignant Disease," *BMJ* 2 (1911): 901–4; Ernst Frankel and Friedrich Gumpertz, "Ueber Die Einwirkung Von Thorium X-Injektionen Auf Die Agglutinine," *BKW* (1914): 209–10; and Worthington Seaton Russell, "Radium in Cancer," *Woman's Medical Journal* 25 (1915): 148–51. The idea of employing radiant energy to cancer as a means to cure the disease was commonplace. Rous even tried ultraviolet radiation on the filterable agent of his chicken sarcoma. See Peyton Rous, "The Influence of Ultra-Violet Light on a Tumor Caused by a Filterable Agent," *ZFK* 12 (1913): 555–56.

23. "Review-Recherches Experimentales Sur Les Tumeurs Malignes," *Lancet* 1 (1911): 1647–48; Francis Hernaman-Johnson, "An Inquiry into the Causes of Failure of X-Ray Treatment in Deep Seated Cancer," *BMJ* 2 (1912): 377–79; "Discussion on Ray Therapeutics In Malignant Disease," *BMJ* 1 (1912): 373–77; "Radiotherapy of Cancer," *JAMA* 61 (1913): 2022; Van Buren Thorne, "The Plain Truth About the Radium Cancer Cure," *NYT*, January 4, 1914, SM1; "Give Up Use

of Radium," *Washington Post*, July 18, 1914, 6; "The Cancer Problem Discussed at the Annual Meeting of the American Surgical Association, Held in New York," *American Medicine* 20 (1914): 306–7; Frank Fowler, "The Place of X Rays un the Treatment of Cancer," *BMJ* 1 (1914): 1284–86; and "Roentgen Treatment of Cancer," *JAMA* 63 (1914): 1432.

24. "Radium in Malignant Disease," *BMJ* 1 (1911): 1138–39; "Dr. Douglas Fears Radium Monopoly," *NYT*, December 20, 1913, "Call Radium Experts," *Washington Post*, January 19, 1914, 2; "Real Cancer 'Cure,'" *Washington Post*, January 20, 1914, 2; "Offer to donate Radium Institute," *NYT*, January 27, 1914, 9; "The Government and Radium," *Washington Post*, January 22, 1914, 6. The acknowledged pioneer of radium usage was Louis Wickham, a Frenchman who introduced the technique in 1906. His magnum opus was Louis Wickham and Paul Degrais, *Radium*, trans. A. and A. G. Bateman (London: Adlard and Son, 1913); and Thomas Ordway, "The Use of Radium in Cancer and Allied Conditions at the Huntington Hospital—Illustrative Cases," *BMSJ* 171 (1914), 771–83.

25. "Our London Letter," *Medical Record* 81 (1911): 532–33; "Scientists to Test Powders of Radium," *Evening Post* (Frederick, MD), January 4, 1911, 8; "Manchester and District," *BMJ* 2 (1913): 1558; "A Philanthropic Radium Institute," *NYMJ* 98 (1913): 925; John M. Lee, "A Clinical Report of Cancer Cases Treated With Radium," *Buffalo Medical Journal* 70 (1915): 670–78; "The Board of Governors," *Science* 39 (1915): 720; Ehrlich and Hansemann both gave their blessing to radium. See "Ehrlich's View of Radium," *NYT*, February 2, 1914, 3; and "Berlin Letter," *JAMA* 63 (1914): 879–80.

26. For some of the extant labs, see, for example, "More Doubt About Radium," *NYT*, February 7, 1909, 20; "Our Energy Due to the Sun," *NYT*, May 15, 1911, 3; "Our London Letter," *JAMA* 58 (1912): 870; "Cancer Study at Harvard," *Lancet* 1 (1913): 1497; "Harvard Wages War on Cancer," *Indianapolis Sunday Star*, May 25, 1913, 26; "The Effect of Radium," *BMJ* 1 (1913): 1158; "Discussion on Radium and Radio-Therapeutics, chiefly in Malignant Growths," *BMJ* 2 (1913): 908–15; "Radium in Inoperable Cancer," *NYMJ* 99 (1914): 1247; "Radium's Use in Cancer, *NYT*, May 3, 1915. For the Crocker Institute and its radium connection, see, for instance, "Dr. Jacobi Cured of Cancer By Radium," *NYT*, December 29, 1913, 3; "Error in Radium Treatment," *NYT*, February 18, 1914, 1; "Use Radium on Mice in Cancer Inquiry," *NYT*, January 18, 1914, 16; "Radium in the Treatment of Cancer," *BMJ* 2 (1914): 1113; "The Plain Truth About the Radium Cancer Cure," *Galveston [TX] Daily News*, January 11, 1914, 24; "Radium 'Cure' is a Failure," *Burlington [IA] Hawkeye*, April 11, 1914, 1; "Cancer Research Fails to Find Cure," *NYT*, December 13, 1915, 11; "64,500 Animals Used in Cancer Research," *Atlanta Constitution*, December 14, 1915; and Henry Janeway, *Radium Therapy in Cancer at the Memorial Hospital New York–First Report 1915–1916* (New York: Paul B. Hoeber, 1917), 10. For scarcity, see "Radium Scarcity Prevents Test," *Waterloo [IA] Times-Tribune*, November 14, 1913, 6.

27. W. S. Lazarus-Barlow, "On the Electrical and Photographic Phenomena Manifested By Certain Substances That Are Commonly Supposed to be Aetiologically Association With Carcinoma," *Fifth Report Cancer Research Laboratory, Middlesex Hospital* (hereafter CRL,MH) 7 (1906): 189–217; W. S.

Lazarus-Barlow, "The Influence of Carcinomatous and Non-Carcinomatous Tissues Upon Electroscopic Leak," *Eighth Report CRL,MH* 15 (1909): 118–44; W. S. Lazarus-Barlow, "On Retardation of Electroscopic Leak By Means of Recognized Radio-Active and Certain Other Substances," *Eighth Report CRL,MH* 15 (1909): 145–46; W. S. Lazarus-Barlow and Victor Bonney, "The Influence of Radio-Activity on the Division of Animal Cells," *Eighth Report CRL,MH* 15 (1909): 147–55; H. MacCormac, "Preliminary Communication on the Power of Certain Micro-Organisms to Affect a Photographic Plate in the Dark," *Eighth Report CRL,MH* 15 (1909): 177–81; W. S. Lazarus-Barlow, "The Croonian Lectures on Radio-Activity and Carcinoma: An Experimental Inquiry," *BMJ* 1 (1909): 1536–44; and "Radioactivity and Carcinoma," *Medical Record* 76 (1909): 233–34. Lazarus-Barlow's notoriety persisted through the decade. See Thorpe Lee, "No More Mysteries in Medicine," *London Daily Mail*, February 26, 1914, 6.

28. S. Russ, "A Comparison of X-Ray and Radium Measurements for Biological Purposes," *Eleventh Report CRL,MH* 27 (1912): 13–23; C. R. C. Lyster, "The Clinical Use of the Active Deposit of Radium," *Eleventh Report CRL,MH* 27 (1912): 24–28; Helen Chambers and S. Russ, "The Bactericidal Action of Radium Emanation," *Eleventh Report CRL,MH* 27 (1912): 29–45; B. H. Wedd and S. Russ, "The Effect of Rontgen and Radium Radiations Upon the Vitality of the Cells of Mouse Carcinoma," *Eleventh Report CRL,MH* 27 (1912): 50–62; H. A. Colwell, "The Effects of X-Rays Upon Various Organic Substances," *Eleventh Report CRL,MH* 27 (1912): 63–70; W. S. Lazarus-Barlow, "On the Use of Electroscopes for the Measurement of Radio-Activity," *Eleventh Report CRL,MH* 27 (1912): 71–90; W. S. Lazarus-Barlow, "On the Presence of Radium in some Carcinomatous Tumours and Other Tissues," *Eleventh Report CRL,MH* 27 (1912): 91–107; W. S. Lazarus-Barlow, "On the Presence of Radium in some Gallstones and On a Correlation of This With the Frequence of Gallstone Occurrence in Carcinoma," *Eleventh Report CRL,MH* 27 (1912): 108–27; Sommerville Hastings, "On the Action of the Secondary X-Rays From Copper on the Development of the Ova of Ascaris Megalocephala," *Eleventh Report CRL,MH* 27 (1912): 154–56; W. S. Lazarus-Barlow, "On the Presence of Radium in some Carcionomatous Tumours," *Proceedings of the Royal Society of London, Series B* 85 (June 14, 1912): 170–73; "Etiology and Pathology of Cancer," *BMJ* 2 (1913): 373–74; W. S. Lazarus-Barlow, "Comparative Observations on Changes in Columnar and in Squamous Epithelium and in Sub-Epithelial Tissues Induced by the Gamma Rays of Radium," *Thirteenth Report CRL,MH* 33 (1914): 34–55; S. Russ, "Measurements of Radium Rays as Used Clinically," *Thirteenth Report CRL,MH* 33 (1914): 60–70; E. H. Lepper, "Experiments to Determine Whether Variations in Temperature Influence the Effects Produced When Malignant Cells are Irradiated By Radium Bromide," *Thirteenth Report CRL,MH* 33 (1914): 77–84; W. S. Lazarus-Barlow, "On Retardation of Electroscopic Leak Following Estimation of Radium Emanation of the Order 10^{-7} Millicurie," *Thirteenth Report CRL,MH* 33 (1914): 91–109; A. C. Morson, "Changes Which Occur in Malignant Tumours on Exposure to the Gamma Rays of Radium," *Thirteenth Report CRL,MH* 33 (1914): 110–22; H. Beckton, "Some Experiments on the Action of Beta and Gamma Rays Upon Animal Tissues," *Thirteenth Report CRL,MH* 33 (1914): 123–25; and W. S. Lazarus-Barlow, "Experiments Upon the Influence of Platinum Screens

With a View to Determining Their Value in the Radium Treatment of Malignant Disease," *Thirteenth Report CRL,MH* 33 (1914): 131–40. Also see "The Scourges of Man," *London Daily Mail,* August 9, 1913, 5–6; and "Abstracts of Reports," *XVIIth International Congress of Medicine, London, 1913,* (London: Lancet, 1913), 7.

29. W. S. Lazarus-Barlow, "A Lecturer on the Cause and Cure of Cancer Viewed in the Light of Recent Radio-Biological Research," *BMJ* 1 (1914): 1001–1006; Lazarus-Barlow, "The Croonian Lectures,"; "Cancer Germs," *Jamaican Gleaner,* September 2, 1909, 12; "Radium Cause of Cancer?" *NYT,* April 24, 1914, 7; "Cancer Research," *Indianapolis Medical Journal* 17 (1914): 28–29; "The Cause of Cancer," *Lancet-Clinic* 112 (1914): 2; J. Joly, "Radio-Therapy: Its Scientific Basis and Its Teachings," *Nature,* June 10, 1915, 409–41. Lazarus-Barlow made this cancer theory known to the 17th International Medical Congress in 1913. See "Etiology and Pathology of Cancer," *BMJ* 2 (1913): 373–74. For other immunity studies produced by radiation, see B. H. Wedd, A. C. Morson, and S. Russ, "On the Immunity Conferred Upon Mice by Radium-Irradiated Mouse Carcinoma," *Thirteenth Report CRL,MH* 33 (1914): 71–76; and James B. Murphy and John J. Norton, "The Effect of X-Ray on the Resistance to Cancer in Mice," *Science* 42 (1915): 842–43.

30. Alfred Pearce Gould, "An Address on Radium and Cancer," *BMJ* 1 (1914): 1–6; "Radium Checks Cancer in London," *NYT,* January 8, 1914, 1; "Cancer and Radium," *London Daily Mail,* January 9, 1914, 3; "Radium and Cancer," *London Daily Mail,* January 9, 1914, 4; "Don't Claim Cancer Cures," *NYT,* January 10, 1914, 6; "Radium and Cancer," *BMJ* 1 (1914): 160–61; "Radium and Cancer," *Lancet* 1 (1914): 188–89; and "Radium Supersedes Knife For Cancer," *NYT,* August 16, 1914, 12.

31. Lazarus-Barlow's cancer theory failed to generate extensive support. Yet its lack of success did not seem to hurt his career. For a brief recapitulation of his work, see "Obituary—W. S. Lazarus-Barlow," *BMJ* 1 (1950): 253.

Chapter 10

1. E. F. Bashford, "Cancer, Credulity, and Quackery," *BMJ* 1 (1911): 1221–30. The statements in question were published in Robert Bell, *Health at Its Best vs. Cancer* (London: T. Fisher Unwin, 1908). A similar literature was found in America. See, for example, Eli G. Jones, *Cancer: Its Causes, Symptoms and Treatment* (Boston: Therapeutic Printing Co., 1911), passim.

2. "Cancer Fighters Baffled," *NYT,* July 21, 1911, 5; "Cancer Treatment," *London Daily Mail,* January 31, 1912, 6; "'Cure for Cancer' Case," *Lloyd's Weekly News,* May 19, 1912, 3; "The Cure of Cancer," *London Daily Mail,* May 20, 1912, 12; "Great Medical Dispute," *London Daily Mail,* June 12, 1912, 8; "Special Law Reports," *London Daily Mail,* June 13, 1912, 8; "Our London Letter," *Medical Record* 82 (1912): 73–74; "Differ About Cancer Remedies," *Letheridge Daily Herald,* June 14, 1912, 10; "Cancer Increased With Meat Eating," *Manitoba Free Press,* June 15, 1912, 10; "Special Law Reports," *London Daily Mail,* June 15, 1912, 6; "Called Quack, Gets $10,000," *NYT,* June 15, 1912, 5; L2,000 Damages for Cancer Libel," *Lloyd's Weekly News,* June 16, 1912, 6; "The Cancer Libel Suit," *NYT,* June 16, 1912, 16; and "A Cancer Wrangle," *Indianapolis Star,* July 6, 1912, 8. Bell continued

eschewing surgery after the verdict. See T. J. Allen, "London Controversy Over Cancer," *Washington Post*, August 12, 1912, 5; and "Dr. Bell's Success With Cancer," *Washington Post*, January 6, 1913, 4.

3. "Warns of Cancer Quacks," *NYT*, October 3, 1912, 22; and "One Woman in Seven," *Wabash Daily Plain Dealer*, October 19, 1912, 5. Bashford continued his campaign against quackery after the judgment. See, for example, "Cancer Cures," *BMJ* 2 (1913): 512–13. Also see E. F. Bashford, *Review of Recent Cancer Research* (Lancaster, PA.: New Era Printing, 1912).

4. "A Lecture," *Nature* 90 (1912): 89–90; "The Treatment of Cancer," *BMJ* 2 (1912): 807; "Professor Von Czerny's Resignation," *NYMJ* 95 (1912), 447; and "Praises American Sanitary Triumphs," *NYT*, February 8, 1914, 27. Also of note is Koenigsfeld, "Probleme Der Experimentellen Krebsforschung," *DMW* 1 (1915): 180. Orth, in the name of the German Comite, also claimed that the cause of cancer was not likely to be discovered in the near future. See "Verhandlungsschrift Der Mitgliederversammlung Des Deutschen Zentralkomitees Zur Erforschung Und Bekampfung Der Krebskrankheit," *ZFK* 14 (1914): 336–48.

5. F. C. Wood, "Advances in Our Knowledge and Treatment of Cancer in the Last Thirty Years," *NYMJ* 102 (1915): 159; James Ewing, "The Cancer Research Hospital," *NYMJ* 98 (1913): 1241–47; and "Dr. Rous Expects A Cure for Cancer," *NYT*, November 4, 1912, 1; Ewing offered an apologia almost as stark a year earlier. See James Ewing, "The Treatment of Cancer on Biological Principles," *NYMJ* 96 (1912): 773–79; and "Treatment of Cancer," *JAMA* 59 (1912): 1654. Bashford reiterated his thoughts several times. See "The Imperial Cancer Research Fund," *NYMJ* 100 (1914): 630. State of the art assessments, depressing as they were, were commonplace. See E. F. Bashford, "Das Krebsproblem," *DMW* 39 (1913): 4–8, 55–59; and Leo Loeb, "The Present State of Cancer Research," *Popular Science* 84 (1914): 17–38.

6. Joseph Louis Ransohoff, "Cancer," *Lancet-Clinic* 109 (1913): 55–56; "Cancer Research," *American Medicine* 20 (1914): 435; Samuel Squire Sprigge, "Cancer Death-Rates: A Statistical Study," *Lancet* 1 (1911): 525; "Berlin Letter," *JAMA* 63 (1914): 879–80; and "Gemeinsame Sitzung Des Deutschen Zentralkomitees Zur Erforschung Und Bekampfung Der Krebskrankheit E.V. Mity Den Deutschen Landeskomitees Fur Krebsforschung," *ZFK* (1913): 200–216. Also see, for example, "The Status of the Cancer Question," *NYMJ* 97 (1913): 989–90; and "Imperial Cancer Research Fund," *BMJ* 2 (1913): 256–59; "Cancer," *Buffalo Medical Journal* 70 (1915): 687–90.

7. Roswell Park, "Recent Views Concerning the Nature and Treatment of Cancer," *Transactions of the Southern Surgical and Gynecological Association* 23 (1911): 346–62.

8. "Antitrypsin Reaction in Diagnosis of Cancer," *JAMA* 56 (1911): 463; "Deviation of Complement With Cancer," *JAMA* 56 (1911): 1429; Leo A. Juhnke, "The Meiostagmin Reaction: A Review of the Literature," *Interstate Medical Journal* 5 (1911): 233–37; "Trytophan Test for Cancer," *JAMA* 57 (1911): 1305; "Specific Cancer Reactions," *JAMA* 57 (1911): 1412; "The Serological Diagnosis of Cancer," *BMJ* 1 (1912): 1030, 1081–82, 1138–39; J. L. Jacque and R. T. Woodyatt, "The Peptolytic Power of Gastric Juice and Saliva With Special Reference to the

Diagnosis of Cancer," *Archives of Internal Medicine* 6 (1912): 560–76; "Certain Reactions of the Blood in Carcinoma, With Suggestions on Treatment," *JAMA* (1912): 486; "Reaction of Carcinoma," *NYMJ* 96 (1912): 245; "Cancer Cured By Serum," *Washington Post*, April 4, 1912, 4; "Serodiagnosis of Cancer," *JAMA* 60 (1913): 1116; "Hema-Uro-Chrome," *JAMA* 61 (1913): 59–60; J. Louis Ransohoff, "Anaphalaxis in the Diagnosis of Cancer," *JAMA* 61 (1913): 8–10; W. H. Burmeister, "The Meiostagmin and Epiphanin Reactions in the Diagnosis of Carcinoma," *Journal of Infectious Diseases* 12 (1913): 459–71; Isaac Levin, "The Importance of the Subjective Symptoms for the Early Recognition of Cancer," *Archives of Diagnosis* 7 (1914): 1–8; Elizabeth T. Fraser, "The Meiostagmin Reaction in the Diagnosis of Cancer," *Lancet* 1 (1914): 643–44; "Serodiagnosis of Malignant Tumors," *NYMJ* 100 (1914): 191; "A Simple Diagnostic Reaction for Malignant Tumors," *NYMJ* 100 (1914): 285; Albert Robin, "L'acide Urique et Les Corps Puriques Chez Les Cancereux Leurs Rapports A L'acide Phosphorique Urinaire Total," *Academe De Medicine* (1913): 259–75; W. P. Semenow, "Ueber Die klinische Bedeutung der Bestimmung des Kolloidalstickstoffes Im Harn nach der Methode von Salkowski und Kojo zur Diagnostizierung des Carcinoms der inneren Organe," *BKW* (1913): 1436–1437; Albert Robin, "Recherches Sur Les Troubles Des Echanges Chez Des Cancereux. L'azote Ammoniacal et L'amino-acidurie," *Academe De Mediceine* (1914): 761–63; and "The Meiostagmin Reaction for Cancer," *JAMA* 65 (1915): 468.

9. E. Salkowski, "Ueber Die Verwertung des Harnbefundes zur Carcinomdiagnose," *BKW* 47 (1910): 1746–47, 2297–98; W. D. Robbins, "Sulphur Reaction in the Urine of Cancer Patients," *JAMA* 56 (1911): 1593; Edward H. Risley, "The Hemolytic Skin Reaction in Carcinoma," *BMSJ* 165 (1911): 127–28; "Methylene Blue Test of Urine of Cancer Patients," *JAMA* 57 (1911): 1642; "Sulphur Reaction in the Urine of Cancerous Patients," *NYMJ* 95 (1912): 351; "Sulphur Reaction in the Urine as Sign of Cancer," *JAMA* 59 (1912): 492; Frank P. Underhill and Lorande Loss Woodruff, "Protozoan Protoplasm as an Indicator of Pathological Changes. II. In Carcinoma," *Journal of Biological Chemistry* 14 (1913): 401–14; and "A New Indicator of Pathologic Tissue Changes," *JAMA* 61 (1913): 1720–21.

10. R. Paltauf, "Die Klinische Diagnostik Des Krebses," *Wiener Kliniasche Wochenschrift* 33 (1910): 1623–30; "Clinical Diagnosis of Cancer," *JAMA* 56 (1911): 82–83; "Serodiagnosis of Cancer," *JAMA* 57 (1911): 691; Ernst Freund and Gisa Kaminer, "Zur Chemie Der Pradilektionsstellen Fur Karzinom," *Wiener Klinische Wochenschrift* 25 (1912): 1698–99; "Freund and Kaminer," *BMJ* 2 (1912): 1760; Ernest Freund, "Chemistry of Cancer 'Soil'" *Medical Record* 82 (1912): 1128; "Ueber Chemische Grundlagen Fur Karzinomtherapie," *Wiener Klinische Wochenschrift* 26 (1913): 2108–2110; Ugo Mello, "Etude DuSerum De Chevaux Porteurs De Tumeurs Malignes Par La Methode De Freund Et Kaminer,"*CRSB* 1 (1913): 231–33; "Chemical Bases for Treatment of Cancer," *JAMA* 62 (1914): 340–42; and Ernst Freund and Gisa Kaminer, "Ueber Beziehungen Sterischer Atomgruppierung Zum Karzinom," *Wiener Klinische Wochenschrift* 27 (1914): 357–58.

11. The English translation of Abderhalden's classic 1911 work is Emil Abderhalden, *Defensive Ferments of the Animal Organism*, trans. J. O. Gavronsky and W. F. Lanchester (London: John Bale, Sons & Danielsson, 1914). Also see Emil Abderhalden, "Studien Uber Den Stoffwechsel Von Geschwulstzellen," *ZFK* 9

(1910): 266–74. For discussions of the techniques suitability for detecting cancer and pregnancy, see, for example, "Abderhalden's Biologic Test for Cancer," *JAMA* 60 (1913): 1585–86; "Serodiagnosis of Pregnancy," *JAMA* 60 (1913): 1586; "The Biological Diagnosis of Pregnancy," *American Journal of Obstetrics and Diseases of Women and Children* 68 (1913): 143; N. Markus, "Untersuchungen über die Verwertbarkeit der Abderhalden'schen Fermentreaktion bei Schwangerschaft und Carcinom," *BKW* (1913): 776–77; "The Application of Abderhalden's Ferment Reaction in Pregnancy and With Carcinoma," *American Journal of Obstetrics and Diseases of Women and Children* 68 (1913): 581; Otto Lowy, "A Serum Reaction as an Aid in the Diagnosis of Cancer," *JAMA* 62 (1914): 437–38; Eugen Weiss, "Beitrag zur Karzinomfrage," *DMW* 40 (1914): 66–67; "Serodiagnosis of Cancer," *JAMA* 62 (1914): 1056; Ernst Frankel, "Ueber Die Verwendung Der Abderhalden'schen Reaktion Bei Carcinom Und Tuberkulose," *BKW* (1914): 356–58; C. F. Ball, "Abderhalden's Test in the Diagnosis of Cancer," *JAMA* 62 (1914): 1169–1172; Jean Benech, "Essai De La Sero-Reaction D' Abderhalden Dans Le Cancer (Methode De La Dialyse)," *CRSB* 1 (1914): 361–63; Henry Schwarz, "Value of Abderhalden's Biologic Reactions to the Obstetrician and the Gynecologist," *JAMA* 63 (1914): 371–75; R. Freund and C. Brahm, "Weitere Erfahrungen Mit Der Abderhaldenschen Reaktion Allein Und Im Vergleich Mit Der Antitrypsin Methode," *Munchener Medizinische Wochenschrift* 61 (1914): 1662–65; "Serodiagnosis of Pregnancy," *JAMA* 63 (1914): 1142; "Serodiagnosis of Cancer," *JAMA* 63 (1914): 1143; Isaac Levin, "The Value of the Abderhalden Test for Cancer," *NYMJ* 100 (1914): 621–23; and Isaac Levin and Donald D. Van Slyke, "Results of Applying a Quantitative Method to the Abderhalden Serum Test for Cancer," *JAMA* 65 (1915): 945–46.

12. "Cancer Statistics in Bavaria," *JAMA* 56 (1911): 827; "Cancer Statistics in Bavaria," *JAMA* 56 (1911): 827–28; "Cancer," *JAMA* 57 (1911): 767; Ira S. Wile, "Cancer Statistics and Their Meaning," *NYMJ* 94 (1911): 1169–72; "The Incidence of Cancer in Finland," *Lancet* 1 (1912): 446; J. Clunert, "Le Cancer Au Maroc," *L'Étude* 5 (1912): 167–68; "Cancer Statistics: A Lesson in Delay," *NYMJ* 95 (1912): 999–1000; E. Jeanselme and A. Barbe, "Etude Statistique Sur Les Cas De Cancer Traits A L'hopital Tenon Pendant La Periode Sexennale, 1901–1906," *L'Étude* 5 (1912): 363–89; "London Letter," *JAMA* 60 (1913): 1893–95 and 64 (1915): 1776–77, 2152–53; "Cancer Statistics," *JAMA* 61(1913): 774–75; R. Hinston Fox, "Progress of Life Assurance Medicine," *Lancet* 1 (1914): 159–61; "Cancer Death Rate in New England," *JAMA* 65 (1915): 868; and "Cancer Statistics," *NYMJ* 102 (1915): 1249–50. Also of interest was the independently compiled Rollo Russell, *Preventable Cancer: A Statistical Research* (London: Longmans, Green, 1912).

13. Bashford's attack was printed as E. F. Bashford, "Fresh Alarms on the Increase of Cancer," *Lancet* 1 (1914): 379–82. He was responding in good measure to the comments of Frederick Hoffman, statistician of the Prudential Insurance Company of America. Hoffman's comments were printed as "The Menace of Cancer," in "Transactions of the New York Academy of Medicine," *American Journal of Obstetrics and Diseases of Women and Children* 68 (1913): 88–91, and *JAMA* 60 (1913): 1735–36. Also see U.S. Census Bureau, *Mortality for Cancer and Other Malignant Tumors in the Registration Area of the United States, 1914* (Washington,

DC: GPO, 1916); "The Prevalence of Cancer in the United States," *Lancet* 1 (1914): 47–48. Bashford's and Hoffman's papers engendered considerable debate in Britain. See, for instance, Frederick L. Hoffman, "'The Menace of Cancer' And American Vital Statistics," *Lancet* 1 (1914): 1079–83; Horst Oertel, "'The Menace of Cancer' and American Vital Statistics," *Lancet* 1 (1914): 1150–52; Anglo-American, "'The Menace of Cancer' and American Vital Statistics," *Lancet* 1 (1914): 1360; and Benjamin G. Brock, "The Menace of Cancer," *Lancet* 1 (1914): 1650–51.

14. John B. Deaver, "Malignant Disease as a Problem of Modern Surgery," *American Journal of Surgery* 25 (1911): 245–51; and "Malignant Disease," *NYMJ* 94 (1911): 446. Also see, for example, Alfred C. Wood, "On the Prevention of Cancer," *NYMJ* 100 (1914): 122–26.

15. Charles E. De M. Sajous, "The Status of the Cancer Problem," *NYMJ* (1913): 989–90. Also of interest is "The Cancer Problem," *Southern Medical Journal* 8 (1915): 642.

16. Charles H. Castle, "The War Against Cancer," *Lancet-Clinic* 114 (1915): 2; and W. A. Bryan, "The Cancer Problem," *Southern Medical Journal* 6 (1913): 770–75.

17. Joseph C. Bloodgood, "Cancer Control: Precancerous Lesions," *Northwest Medicine* 6 (1914): 111–12; Joseph C. Bloodgood, "The Cancer Problem From the Standpoint of the Laity, the General Practitioner and the Expert Surgeon," *Southern Medical Journal* 7 (1914): 20–29; Sajous, "The Status"; and Deaver, "Malignant Disease as a Problem."

18. William J. Mayo, "The Prophylaxis of Cancer," *Annals of Surgery* 59 (1914): 805–14; "Presidential Address," *NYMJ* 99 (1914): 952; "Prophylaxis of Cancer," *JAMA* 63 (1914): 350; and James Alexander Lindsay, "The Threshold of Disease," *BMJ* 2 (1914): 955–59. Also of interest was Southgate Leigh, "The Importance of Educating the Public in Regard to Cancer," *American Journal of Surgery* 25 (1911): 10–13.

19. Deaver, "Malignant Disease as a Problem." For the consequences of this approach, see Ellen Leopold, *A Darker Ribbon: Breast Cancer, Women, and Their Doctors in the Twentieth Century* (Boston: Beacon Press, 1999), 41–80.

20. Pennsylvania was early involved in the education campaign and persisted well after the ASCC's creation. See, for instance, "Proceedings-Medical Society of Pennsylvania," *JAMA* 57 (1911): 1560; "Report of the Commission on Cancer," *Pennsylvania Medical Journal* 15 (1912): 529–31; "Organizing to Fight Cancer," *The Survey* 30 (1913): 164; "Control of Cancer—Read and Teach Statements," *Indianapolis Medical Journal* 17 (1914): 123–24; A. M. Hetherington, "Public Education of the Cancer Question," *Indianapolis Medical Journal* 17 (1914): 154–56; "A Nation Wide Cancer Movement," *Pennsylvania Medical Journal* 18 (1915): 475; "The Prevention and Control of Cancer," *BMSJ* 173 (1915): 99–101; and "The Cancer Decalogue," *Pennsylvania Medical Journal* 18 (1915): 765–844. For Missouri, see B. T. Quigley, "Medical Society of the Missouri Valley," *JAMA* 60 (1913): 1101–1103. See also Southgate Leigh, "The Importance of Educating the Public in Regard to Cancer," *American Journal of Surgery* 25 (1911): 10–13; "TriState Medical Association of the Carolinas and Virginia," *JAMA* 56 (1911): 1063–64; and Curtis E. Lakeman, "The

Organization of National and Local Forces in the Campaign Against Cancer," *BMSJ* 173 (1915): 107–9. For the *JAMA* quote, see "Anticancer Fight," *JAMA* 61 (1913): 208. ASCC physicians were not shy about their agenda. They took their plans to the professional group most affected by their new effort. See "Verhandlungen Der Jahresversammlung Der American Association for Cancer Research Am 5. Mai 1913 in Washington," *ZFK* 12 (1913): 532–33. ASCC physicians took the matter to the public. See "Cancer Claims Many Thousands of Lives," *Fort Wayne Daily News*, November 14, 1913, p. 4. For a retrospective practitioner history, see Victor A. Triolo and Michael B. Shimkin, "The American Cancer Society and Cancer Research Origins and Organization: 1913–1943," *Cancer Research* 29 (1969): 1615–41. The German Central Committee, in league with the insurance industry, had adopted this approach earlier. See ""Verhandlungen des Deutschen Zentralkomitees zur Erforschung und Bekämpfung der Krebskrankheit," *ZFK* 10 (1911): 365–82. For the British complement, see Ornella Moscucci, "The British Fight Against Cancer: Publicity and Education, 1900–1948," *Social History of Medicine* 23 (2009): 356–73. The ASCC took the campaign against tuberculosis as its model and inspiration. For tuberculosis, for instance, see S. Adolphus Knopf, *A History of the National Tuberculosis Association: The Anti-Tuberculosis Movement in the United States* (New York: National Tuberculosis Association, 1922). An attempt by practitioners to assess what had been done in the early years of the cancer control movement worldwide was *Cancer Control: Report of An International Symposium Held Under the Auspices of the American Society for the Control of Cancer* (Chicago: Surgical Publishing Co., 1927); and John W. Spies, "Cancer Organizations in France, Belgium, England, Germany and Sweden," *Yale Journal of Biology and Medicine* 3 (1931): 533–46. For racial bias in the early control campaign, see Keith Wailoo, *How Cancer Crossed the Color Line* (Oxford: Oxford University Press, 2011).

21. Rollo Russell, *Preventable Cancer. A Statistical Research* (Longmans, Green and Co., 1912); and Rollo Russell, *The Reduction of Cancer* (Longmans, Green and Co., 1907). For the twin pillars of prevention and early detection in various countries, see David Cantor, "Introduction: Cancer Control and Prevention in the Twentieth Century," *Bulletin of the History of Medicine* 81 (2007): 1–38; Stephen Snelders, Frans J. Meijman, and Toine Pieters, "Cancer Health Communication in the Netherlands 1910–1950: Paternalistic Control or Popularization of Knowledge," *Medical History Journal* 41 (2006): 271–89; and Ornella Moscucci, "The Emergence of Cancer as a Public Health Concern," *American Journal of Public Health* 95 (2005): 1312–21.

22. "Cancer Research," *Lancet-Clinic* 106 (1911): 299.

23. J. G. Adami, "The Cancer Research Institute," *JAMA* 60 (1913): 1911–1912. The French tried to remain relevant by offering a prize for the best work on the pathogenesis of cancer. See "Bouchard Prize," *JAMA* 61 (1913): 209.

24. Francis Carter Wood, "Surgery is Sole Cure For Bad Varieties of Cancer," *NYT*, April 19, 1914, SM6; "The Questionable Character of Much of Our Data on Cancer," *American Medicine* 21 (1915): 728–29; Francis Carter Wood, "Cancer and the Public Health," *American Journal of Public Health* 6 (1916): 118–23; and "Urges Collection of Data on Cancer," *NYT*, September 10, 1915, 12.

25. "Better Knowledge of Cancer Desired," *JAMA* 61 (1913): 216.

26. "Reminiscence of the II. International conference for Cancer Research Paris 1–5 October 1910," *Cancer: International Monthly Review* (hereafter *C:IMR*) 2 (1910): 156; "Protocol of the Meeting of the Committee on Business of the International Association for Cancer Research," *C:IMR* 2 (1910): 167; and "Protocol of the Meeting of the Board of Directors of the International Association for Cancer Research," *C:IMR* 2 (1910): 167–71. The German Central Committee wrote its own history on its tenth anniversary and presented the IACI as an almost appendage. See George Meyer, "Bericht Uber Die Zehnjahrige Wirksamkeit Des Deutschen Zentralkomitees fur Krebsforschung," *ZFK* 10 (1911): 8–33.

27. "Protocol of the Meeting of the Board of Directors;" and "International Hygienic Exposition in Dresden 1911," *C:IMR* 3 (1911): 28. Also see Harvey R. Gaylord, "Annual Report of the Cancer Laboratory," in the *Thirty-First Annual Report of the State Department of Health, State of New York, 1911*, 364–65, for the United States display.

28. "Proposals for Changement [*sic*] of the Statutes," *C:IMR* 3 (1911): 99–100; "Protocol of the Meeting of the Committee on Business of the International Association for Cancer Research, August 7, 1911," *C:IMR* 3 (1911): 130–33; "Protocol of the Meeting of Members of the International Association for Cancer Research, August 7, 1911," *C:IMR* 3 (1911): 134–37; and "French Association for Cancer Research," *C:IMR* 3 (1911): 185–88.

29. "Sketch of a Question-Form for International Cancer-Statistics," *C:IMR* 3 (1911): 82–83.

30. "Program of the Meeting of the International Association for Cancer Research, Dresden, August 7, 1911," *C:IMR* 3 (1911): 97.

31. "French Association"; and "Verhandlungsschrift Der Mitgliederversammlung Des Deutschen Zentralkomitees Zur Erforschung Und Bekampfung Der Krebskrankheit E.V.," *ZFK* 12 (1913): 1–16.

32. "XVIIth International Congress of Medicine," *C:IMR* 4 (1912): 21–25; and "The XV International Congress on Hygiene and Demography," *C:IMR* 4 (1912): 38–40. Also see George Meyer, "Report on the Work of the International Association for Cancer Research by the General Secretary Professor George Meyer at the International conference for Cancer Research since August 1911," *C:IMR* 5 (1913): 117–22.

33. "Proceedings of the Meeting of the Committee On Business on Business of the International Association for Cancer Research, October 19, 1912," *C:IMR* 4 (1912): 156–58. Also see "A National League," *BMJ* 1 (1913): 919; and "Uterine Cancer," *JAMA* 63 (1914): 1145.

34. "Proceedings of the Meeting, October 19, 1912"; "The Third International Congress on Cancer Research," *BMJ* 1 (1913): 993; "International Conference for Cancer Research," *Medical Record* (1913): 23; "3rd International Conference for Cancer Research at Brussels," *C:IMR* 5 (1913): 38–39. The two additional questions were published in May, 1913, a few short months before the conference.

35. "Programme of the Third International Conference of Cancer Research, Brussels, August 1 to 5, 1913," *C:IMR* 5 (1913): 58–61, 90–92; and "Tagesgeschichtliche Notizen," *BKW* (1913): 1096.

36. The full proceedings were published as *Travaux De La Troisieme*

Conference International Pour L'Étude Du Cancer Tenue A Bruxelles August 1–5, 1913 (Bruxelles: Misch et Thron, 1914). Also see A. Pinkuss and Dr. Kloninger, "Zur Vaccinationstherapie des Krebses," *BKW* (1913): 1941–42; and Ferdinand Blumenthal, "Der Gegenwärtige Stand der Behandlung der bösartigen Geschwulste," *BKW* (1913): 1942–44; and Ferdinand Blumenthal, "Der Gegenwartige Stasnd Der Behandlung Der Bosartigen Geschwulste," *BKW* (1913): 1942–44. The Germans knew the meeting would be a disaster before it was held. See ""Gemeinsame Sitzung des Deutschen Zentralkomitees zur Erforschung und Bekämpfung der Krebskrankheit E.V. mit den deutschen Landeskomitees für Krebsforschung," *ZFK* 13 (1913): 200–216.

37. "Protocol of the Meeting of Members of the International Association for Cancer Research, August 5, 1913," *C:IMR* 5 (1913): 141–43; and "The International Commission for the Nomenclature of Tumors," August 4, 1913," *C:IMR* 5 (1913): 148–49.

38. Meyer, "Report on the Work of the International Association." A few American papers published a few lines about the meeting. See "Cure for Cancer," *Lowell [MA] Sun*, August 22, 1913, 11.

39. "Minutes of the Council Meeting of the AACR, Toronto, April 9, 1914," *Minute Books of the AACR*, housed at the headquarters of the AACR, Philadelphia, PA.

40. For the ICRF's experimental animals being shipped to the United States for safekeeping, see "Mice Are Saved From Zeppelins," *Los Angeles Times*, May 19, 1916, 12; "Mice Moved to Safety to Escape Bomb Raids," *Atlanta Constitution*, May 19, 1916, 2; and "Mice Here to Dodge Bombs," *Washington Post*, May 20, 1916, 6. The idea of an international cancer union was revived some decades later. See J. H. Maisin, *L'Union Internationale Contre Le Cancer De Sa Fondation a Nos Jours* (Geneva: D. De Buren, 1966).

41. "Imperial Cancer Research Fund," *BMJ* 2 (1915): 141–42; G. M. Findlay, "James Alexander Murray, 1873–1950," *Obituary Notices of Fellows of the Royal Society* 7 (1951): 444–52; "Obituary-Ernest Francis Bashford, O.B.E., M.D.," *BMJ* 2 (1923): 440–41; and "Dr. E. F. Bashford, O.B.E.," *Nature* (1923): 481.

42. "See Hope in New Cancer Remedy," *NYT*, May 16, 1915, SM 16; "New Cancer Cure Called a Success," *Oakland Tribune*, May 30, 1915, 28; and "Upholds Horovitz Cancer Treatment," *NYT*, June 24, 1915, 12.

43. "Dr. Paul Ehrlich, Scientist, Is Dead," *NYT*, August 21, 1915, 7; "Obituary-Professor Paul Ehrlich," *BMJ* 2 (1915): 349–50; and "August V. Wassermann, M.D." *BMJ* 1 (1925): 638.

44. Dorthea Liebermann-Meffert, Hubert J. Stein, and Harvey White, "Vinzenz Czervy (1842–1915): Grand Seigneur of Oncological Surgery—Life, Influence, and Work of the Second Congress President of the ISS/SIC," *World Journal of Surgery* 24 (2000): 1589–98; "Professor Von Leyden," *JAMA* (1902): 1372.

45. See, for example, "The Campaign Against Cancer in New England," *Long Island Medical Journal* 9 (1914): 303–4; and Wood, "Cancer and the Public Health." For Wood's career, see Wilhelmina F. Dunning, "Francis Carter Wood, 1869–1951," *Cancer Research* (1951): 296.

46. "The Cancer Problem," *Maryland Medical Journal* 58 (1915): 180–82; and Commission on Cancer of the Medical Society of the State of Pennsylvania, "Why We Should Have A War Against Cancer," *Maryland Medical Journal* 58 (1915): B–C.

47. Jacob Wolff, *Die Lehre Von Der Krebskrankheit Von Den Altesten Zeitsen Bis Zur Gegenwart* (Jena: Gustav Fischer, 1907); and John Thomas, *Le Cancer*, 2nd ed. (Paris: A. Maloine, 1910). Of a similar vein was P. Menetrier, *Cancer: Nouveau Traite De Medecine Et De Therapeutique* (Paris: J. B. Bailliere Et Fils, 1908).

48. William H. Woglom, *Studies in Cancer and Allied Subjects: The Study of Experimental Cancer. A Review* (New York: Columbia University Press, 1913); and "An American Cancer Research Fund," *BMJ* 1 (1914): 714–15. For Woglom's career, see Milton J. Eisen, "Obituary: William H. Woglom (1879–1953)," *Cancer Research* 14 (1954): 155–56.

49. William Seaman Bainbridge, *The Cancer Problem* (New York: Macmillan, 1914); and "The Cancer Problem," *American Medicine* 21 (1915): 3–4. Newspapers offered a summary.

50. Bainbridge, *Cancer Problem*, 452–53. Bainbridge was not alone. See, for instance, M. S. F., "The Cancer Problem," *Interstate Medical Journal* 22 (1915): 635–38.

51. Harvey R. Gaylord, "Etiology of Cancer in the Light of Recent Cancer Research," *JAMA* 64 (1915): 968–72; and "Etiology of Cancer in the Light of Recent Cancer Research," *NYMJ* 101 (1915): 700. Moyer S. Fleisher offered a much less sophisticated view at about the same time. Bacteriologist at St. Louis University, a colleague of Loeb's and the longtime cancer editor for the *Interstate Medical Journal*, he suggested simply that the debate among those who sought an external agent and those who believed cancer was an internal process could be resolved by believing that cancer could be caused by either a pathogen or bodily process. He argued that research sustained both, so both were true. If adopted, Fleisher's bifurcated model would simply have propagated the problems it sought to resolve. Researchers would then have two separate causes to chase after. Fleisher's cancer would have been unique in that it would have had two separate causes for the same disease. See Moyer S. Fleisher, "The Cancer Problem," *Interstate Medical Journal* 21 (1915): 635–38. Gaylord's cancer work soon switched to radium and continued until his death. For a good summary of his career, see Burton T. Simpson, "Harvey R. Gaylord, M.D.," in *Fourteenth Annual Report of the Trustees of the State Institute for the Study of Malignant Disease (1924)* (Albany: J. B. Lyons, 1925), 4–7.

52. James Ewing, "Pathological Aspects of some Problems of Experimental Cancer Research," *Journal of Cancer Research* 1 (1916): 71–86. For the entirety of Ewing's career, see James B. Murphy, *James Ewing, 1866–1943* (Washington: National Academy of Sciences, 1951).

Epilogue

1. Frederick L. Hoffman, *The Mortality From Cancer Throughout the World* (Newark, NJ: The Prudential Press, 1915). Hoffman had been making a similar argument for several years. See "Educational Value of Cancer Statistics to Insurance Companies," *Medical Record* 84 (1913): 1002.

BIBLIOGRAPHY

Ackerknecht, Edwin. *Rudolf Virchow: Doctor, Statesman, Anthropologist.* Madison: University of Wisconsin, 1953.

Allen, Garland. *Life Science in the Twentieth Century.* New York: Wiley, 1975.

Ausoker, Joan. *A History of the Imperial Cancer Fund, 1902–1986.* Oxford: Oxford University Press, 1988.

Baldwin, Peter. *Contagion and the State in Europe, 1830–1930.* Cambridge: Cambridge University Press, 1999.

Bäumler, Ernst. *Paul Ehrlich: Scientist for Life.* Trans. by Grant Edwards. New York: Holmes & Meier, 1984.

Becsei-Kilborn, Eva. "Scientific Discovery and Scientific Reputation: The Reception of Peyton Rous' Discovery of the Chicken Sarcoma Virus." *Journal of the History of Biology,* 43 (2010): 111–57.

Bignold, L. P., Brian L. D. Coghlan, and Hubertus P. A. Jersmann, *David Paul Von Hansemann: Contributions to Oncology.* Basel: Birkhauser Verlag, 2007.

Brock, Thomas D. *Robert Koch: A Life in Medicine and Bacteriology.* Raleigh, NC: Science Tech Publishing, 1988.

Brown, Richard. *Rockefeller Medicine Men: Medicine and Capitalism in America.* Berkeley: University of California Press, 1979.

Bruton, Deborah, ed. *Medicine Transformed: Health, Disease and Society in Europe, 1800–1930.* Manchester: Bath Press, 2004.

Bulloch, William. *A History of Bacteriology.* Oxford: Oxford University Press, 1938.

Bynum, W. E. *Science and the Practice of Medicine in the Nineteenth Century.* Cambridge, UK: Cambridge University Press, 1994.

Campbell, C. Lee. "Erwin Frink Smith—Pioneer Plant Pathologist." *Annual Review of Phytopathology* 21(1983): 25.

Cancer Control: Report of an International Symposium Held under the Auspices of the American Society for the Control of Cancer. Chicago: Surgical Publishing Company, 1927.

Canguilhem, Georges. "What is Scientific Ideology." In *Ideology and Rationality in the History of the Life Sciences.* Translated by Arthur Goldhammer. Cambridge: MIT Press, 1990.

Cantor, David. "Cancer." In *Companion Encyclopedia of the History of Medicine,* Vol. 1. Edited by W. F. Bynum and Roy Porter. London: Routledge, 1993.

———. "Introduction: Cancer Control and Prevention in the Twentieth Century." *Bulletin of the History of Medicine* 81 (2007): 1–38.

Carpenter, Kenneth J. *Beriberi, White Rice, and Vitamin B: A Disease, A Cause, and A Cure.* Berkeley: University of California Press, 2000.

Carter, K. Codell. *The Rise of Causal Concepts of Disease: Case Histories*. Burlington, VT: Ashgate Publishing, 2003.

———. "Edwin Kleb's Grundversuche." Bulletin of the History of Medicine 75 (2001): 771–81.

———. "Koch's Postulates in Relation to the Work of Jacob Henle and Edwin Klebs." *Medical History* 29 (1985): 353–74.

Chase, Marilyn. *The Barbary Plague: The Black Death in Victorian San Francisco*. New York: Random House, 2004.

Clow, Barbara. *Negotiating Disease: Power and Cancer Care, 1900–1950*. Montreal, McGill-Queens University Press, 2001.

Clowes, G. H. A. "Cancer Research Fifty Years Ago and Now." *Cancer Research* 16 (1956), 1–4.

Creager, Angela N. H. *The Life of A Virus: Tobacco Mosaic Virus as an Experimental Model, 1930–1965*. Chicago: University of Chicago Press, 2002.

Cunningham, Andrew, and Perry Williams, eds. *The Laboratory Revolution in Medicine*. Cambridge: Cambridge University Press, 1992.

Daston, Lorraine, and Peter Galison, eds. *Objectivity*. New York: Zone Books, 2010.

De Kruif, Paul. *Microbe Hunters, 1926, 1954*. San Diego: Harcourt, 1996.

Dear, Peter. "Science is Dead; Long Live Science." *Osiris* 27 (2012): 37–55.

Dubos, Rene J. *Louis Pasteur: Freelance of Science*. Boston: Little, Brown, and Company, 1950.

Dunning, Wilhelmina F. "Francis Carter Wood, 1869–1951." *Cancer Research* 11 (1951): 296.

Eckart, Wolfgang U., ed. *100 Years of Organized Cancer Research*. Stuttgart: Georg Thieme, 2000.

Ehrlich, Paul. Publications. http://www.pei.de/EN/institute/paul-ehrlich/publications/publications-of-paul-ehrlich-node.html

Ellis, Jack D. *The Physician-Legislators of France: Medicine and Politics in the Early Third Republic, 1870–1914*. New York: Cambridge University Press, 1990.

Evans, Alfred S. *Causation and Disease: A Chronological Journey*. New York: Plenum Medical, 1993.

Febvre, Lucien. *The Problem of Unbelief in the 16th Century: The Religion of Rabelais*. Cambridge: Harvard University Press, 1985.

Finnegan, Dairmid A. "The Spatial Turn: Geographic Approaches in the History of Science." *Journal of the History of Biology* 41 (2008): 369–88.

Fleck, Ludwik. *Genesis and Development of a Scientific Fact*. Translated by Thaddeus J. Trenn and Robert K. Merton. Chicago: University of Chicago, 1979.

Foucault, Michel. *The Archaeology of Knowledge and the Discourse on Language*. New York: Vintage, 1982.

Gardner, Kirsten E. *Early Detection: Women, Cancer, and Awareness Campaigns in the Twentieth-Century United States*. Chapel Hill: University of North Carolina, 2006.

Gaudilliere, Jean-Paul. "Cancer." In *The Cambridge History of Science*. Vol 6: *The Modern Biological and Earth Sciences*. Edited by Peter Bowler and John Pickstone. Cambridge: Cambridge University Press, 2009.

Geertz, Clifford. *The Interpretation of Cultures: Selected Essays*. New York: Basic

Books, 1973.

Geison, Gerald. *The Private Science of Louis Pasteur.* Princeton: Princeton University Press, 1995.

Geison, Gerald L. *Professions and the French State, 1700–1900.* Philadelphia: University of Pennsylvania Press, 1984.

Gerbi, Antonello. *The Dispute of the New World: The History of a Polemic, 1750–1900.* Translated by Jeremy Moyle. Pittsburgh: University of Pittsburgh Press, 1973.

Gradmann, Christoph. "Spirit of Scientific Rigour: Koch's Postulates in Twentieth-Century Medicine." *Microbes and Infection* 16 (2014): 885–92.

———. *Laboratory Disease: Robert Koch's Medical Bacteriology.* Translated by Elborg Foster. Baltimore: Johns Hopkins University Press, 2009.

Grafe, Alfred. *A History of Experimental Virology.* Translated by Elvira Reckendorf. Berlin: Springer, 1991.

Hahn, Roger. *The Anatomy of a Scientific Institution: The Paris Academy of Sciences, 1666–1803.* Berkeley: University of California, 1971.

Hallyn, Fernand, ed. *Metaphors and Analogies in the Sciences.* Amsterdam: Springer Netherlands, 2000.

Hamlin, Christopher. "Providence and Putrefaction: Victorian Sanitarians and the Natural Theology of Health and Disease." *Victorian Studies* 28 (1985): 381–411.

Harden, Victoria A. "Koch's Postulates and the Etiology of Rickettsial Diseases." *Journal of the History of Medicine and Allied Sciences* 42 (1987): 277–95.

Hempel, Sandra. *The Strange Case of the Broad Street Pump: John Snow and the Mysteries of Cholera.* Berkeley: University of California Press, 2007.

Hughes, Sally Smith. *The Virus: A History of the Concept.* New York: Science History Publications, 1977.

Hunter, Michael. *Establishing the New Science: The Experience of the Early Royal Society.* Woodbridge, UK: Boydell Press, 1989.

"Julius Cohnheim (20 July 1839–15 August 1884) and His Work. Papers from a Festschrift." *Zentralblatt für allgemeine Pathologie und pathologische Anatomie* 130 (1985): 281–347.

Kevles, Daniel J. *The Physicists: The History of a Scientific Community in Modern America.* New York: Vintage, 1979.

Knopf, S. Adolphus. *A History of the National Tuberculosis Association: The Anti-Tuberculosis Movement in the United States.* New York: National Tuberculosis Association, 1922.

Kohler, Robert E. "Lab History: Reflections." *Isis* 99 (2008): 761–68.

———. "Practice and Place in Twentieth-Century Field Biology: A Comment." *Journal of the History of Biology* 45 (2012): 579–86.

Lakatos, Imre. "Falsification and the Methodology of Science Research Programmes." In *Criticism and the Growth of Knowledge.* Edited by Imre Lakatos and Alan Musgrove. Cambridge, UK: Cambridge University Press, 1965.

Lakatos, Imre, and Paul Feyerabend. *For and Against Method, Including Lakatos's Lectures on Scientific Method and the Lakatos-Feyerabend Correspondence.* Edited by Matteo Motterlini. Chicago: University of Chicago Press, 1999.

Latour, Bruno, and Steve Woolgar. *Laboratory Life: The Construction of Scientific*

Facts. 2nd ed. Princeton: Princeton University Press, 1986. First published 1979 by Sage Publications, Inc.

Latour, Bruno. *Science in Action*. Cambridge: Harvard University Press, 1987.

———. *The Pasteurization of France*. Translated by Alan Sheridan and John Law. Cambridge, MA: Harvard University Press, 1988.

Lechevalier, Hubert A., and Morris Salotorovsky. *Three Centuries of Microbiology*. New York: McGraw-Hill, 1965.

Lederer, Susan E. *Subjected to Science: Human Experimentation in America Before the Second World War*. Baltimore: Johns Hopkins University Press, 1995.

Lewis, R. A. *Edwin Chadwick and the Sanitary Movement, 1832–1854*. London: Longmans, Green and Co., 1952.

Liebermann-Meffert, Dorthea, Hubert J. Stein, and Harvey White. "Vinzenz Czervy (1842–1915): Grand Seigneur of Oncological Surgery—Life, Influence, and Work of the Second Congress President of the ISS/SIC." *World Journal of Surgery* 24 (2000): 1589–98.

Linton, Derek S. *Emil Von Behring: Infectious Disease, Immunology, Serum Therapy*. Philadelphia: American Philosophical Society, 2005.

Livingstone, David N., and Charles W. J. Withers, eds. *Geographies of Nineteenth-Century Science*. Chicago: University of Chicago Press, 2011.

Lowood, Henry E. *Patriotism, Profit, and the Promotion of Science in the German Enlightenment: The Economic and Scientific Societies, 1760–1815*. New York; Garland, 1991.

Maisin, J. H. *L'Union Internationale Contre Le Cancer De Sa Fondation a Nos Jours*. Geneva: D. De Buren, 1966.

Marcus, Alan I. *Plague of Strangers: Social Groups and the Origins of Municipal Services, Cincinnati, 1819–1870*. Columbus: Ohio State University Press, 1991.

———. "From Individual Practitioner to Regular Physician: Cincinnati Medical Societies and the Problem of Definition among Mid-Nineteenth Century Americans." In *Technical Knowledge in American Culture: Science, Technology, and Medicine in America Since the Early 1800s*, edited by Hamilton Cravens, Alan I Marcus, and David M. Katzman. Birmingham: University of Alabama Press, 1996.

———. "From Ehrlich to Waksman: Chemotherapy and the Seamed Web of the Past." In *Beyond History of Science: Essays in Honor of Robert E. Schofield*, edited by Elizabeth Garber, 266–83. Bethlehem: Lehigh University Press, 1990.

———. "Professional Revolution and Reform in the Progressive Era: Cincinnati Physicians and the Elections of 1897 and 1900." *Journal of Urban History* 5 (1979): 183–207.

———. "Setting the Standard: Fertilizers, State Chemists and Early National Commercial Regulation, 1880–1887." *Agricultural History* 61 (1987): 47–73.

———. "When Numbers Failed: Social Scientists, Modernity and the New Cities of the 1920s and 1930s." In *Great Depression: People and Perspectives*, edited by Hamilton Cravens, 165–84. Santa Barbara: ABC-CLIO, 2009.

———. *Agricultural Science and the Quest for Legitimacy: Farmers, Agricultural Colleges and Experiment Stations, 1870–1890*. Ames: Iowa State University Press, 1986.

Marks, Harry M. "'Until the Sun of Science . . . the True Apollo of Medicine Has Risen': Collective Investigation in Britain and America, 1880–1910." *Medical History* 50 (2006): 147–66.

———. *The Progress of Experiment. Science and Therapeutic Reform in the United States, 1900–1990.* Cambridge, UK: Cambridge University Press, 1997.

Maulitz, Russell. "Rudolf Virchow, Julius Cohnheim and the Program of Pathology." *Bulletin of the History of Medicine* 52 (1978): 162–82.

Mazumdar, Pauline M. H. *Species and Specificity. An Interpretation of the History of Immunology.* Cambridge, UK: Cambridge University Press, 1995.

McClellan III, James E. *Science Reorganized: Scientific Societies in the Eighteenth Century.* New York: Columbia University Press, 1985.

McConaghey, R. M. S. "The BMA and Collective Investigation." *BMJ* (1956): 2666–71.

Mirand, Edwin A. *Legacy and History of Roswell Park Cancer Institute, 1898–1998.* Virginia Beach, VA: Donning, 1998.

Mitrus, Iwona, Ewa Bryndza, Aleksander Sochanik, and Stanislaw Szala. "Evolving Models of Tumor Origin and Progression." *Tumor Biology* 33 (2012): 911–17.

Moscucci, Ornella. "The British Fight Against Cancer: Publicity and Education, 1900–1948." *Social History of Medicine* 23 (2009): 356–73.

———. "The Emergence of Cancer as a Public Health Concern." *American Journal of Public Health* 95 (2005): 1312–21.

Moss, Ralph W. "The Life and Times of John Beard, DSc (1858–1924)." *Integrative Cancer Therapies* 7 (2008): 229–51.

Mukherjee, Siddhartha. *The Emperor of All Maladies: A Biography of Cancer.* New York: Scribners, 2010.

Murphy, Caroline C. S. "From Friedenheim to Hospice: A Century of Cancer Hospitals." In *The Hospital in History,* edited by Lindsay Granshaw and Roy Porter, 221–41. London: Routledge, 1989).

Olson, James S. *The History of Cancer: An Annotated Bibliography.* Westport: Greenwood Press, 1989.

Parascandola, John. "The Theoretical Basis of Paul Ehrlich's Chemotherapy." *Journal of the History of Medicine* 36 (1981): 19–43.

Passler, Jann. *Composing the Citizen: Music as Public Utility in Third Republic France.* Berkeley: University of California Press, 2009.

Patterson, James T. *The Dread Disease: Cancer and Modern American Culture.* Cambridge, MA: Harvard University Press, 1987.

Peller, Sigismund. *Cancer Research Since 1900.* New York: Philosophical Library, 1979.

Pickstone, John V. "Sketching Together the Modern Histories of Science, Technology, and Medicine." *Isis* 102 (2011): 122–33.

Pinell, Patrice. "Cancer." In *Medicine in the Twentieth Century,* edited by Roger Cooter and John V. Pickstone, 671–86. Amsterdam: Harwood Academic, 2000.

———. *The Fight Against Cancer: France 1890–1940.* Translated by David Madell. London: Routledge, 1992.

Poovey, Mary. *A History of the Modern Fact: Problems of Knowledge in the Sciences of Wealth and Society.* Chicago: University of Chicago, 1998.

Porter, Theodore M. *Karl Pearson: The Scientific Life in a Statistical Age*. Princeton: Princeton University Press, 2005.

———. *The Rise of Statistical Thinking, 1820–1900*. Princeton: Princeton University Press, 1986.

———. *Trust in Numbers: The Pursuit of Objectivity in Science and Public Life*. Princeton: Princeton University Press, 1995.

Prull, Cay-Rudiger, Andreas-Holger Maehle, and Robert Francis Halliwell. *A Short History of the Drug Receptor Concept*. London: Palgrave Macmillan, 2009.

Rader, Karen. *Making Mice: Standardizing Animals for American Biomedical Research, 1900–1955*. Princeton: Princeton University Press, 2004.

Rather, L. J., Patricia Rather, and John B. Frerichs. *Johannes Muller and the Nineteenth-Century Origins of Tumor Cell Theory*. Canton, MA: Science History Publications, 1986.

Reich, Leonard S. *The Making of American Industrial Research. Science and Business at GE and Bell, 1876–1926*. London: Cambridge University Press, 1985.

Rettig, Richard. *Cancer Crusade: The Story of the National Cancer Act of 1971*. Princeton: Princeton University Press, 1977.

Robinson, Victor. *The Life of Jacob Henle*. New York: Medical Life Company, 1921.

Ross, Karen Deane. "Making Medicine Scientific: Simon Flexner and Experimental Medicine at the Rockefeller Institute for Medical Research, 1901–1945." PhD diss., University of Minnesota, 2006.

Ross, Walter Sanford. *Crusade: The Official History of the American Cancer Society*. New York: Arbor House, 1987.

Salomon-Bayet, Claire, ed. *Pasteur Et La Revolution Pastorienne*. Paris: Payot, 1986.

Shapiro, Henry D. "Daniel Drake's 'Sensorium Commune' and the Organization of the Second American Enlightenment." *Cincinnati Historical Society Bulletin* 27 (1969): 42–62.

Shaughnessy, Donald F. "The Story of the American Cancer Society." PhD diss., Columbia University, 1957.

Shimkin, Michael B. *Contrary to Nature*. Washington, DC: GPO, 1977.

Silverstein, Arthur M. *Paul Ehrlich's Receptor Immunology: The Magnificent Obsession*. San Diego: Academic Press, 2002.

Smith, Murphy D. *A Museum: The History of the Cabinet of Curiosities of the American Philosophical Society*. Philadelphia: American Philosophical Society, 1996.

Snelders, Stephen, Frans J. Meijman, and Toine Pieters. "Cancer Health Communication in the Netherlands 1910–1950: Paternalistic Control or Popularization of Knowledge." *Medical History Journal* 41 (2006): 271–89.

Spies, John W. "Cancer Organizations in France, Belgium, England, Germany and Sweden." *Yale Journal of Biology and Medicine* 3 (1931): 533–46.

Stapleton, Darwin H., ed. *Creating a Tradition of Biomedical Research: Contributions to the History of the Rockefeller University*. New York: Rockefeller University Press, 2004.

Stolzenberg, Dietrich. "Scientist and Industrial Manager: Emil Fischer and Carl Duisberg." In *The German Chemical Industry in the Twentieth Century*, edited by John E. Lesch, 57–90. Dordrecht: Kluwer Academic Publishers, 2000.

Suckow, Mark A., Steven H. Weisbroth, and Craig L. Franklin. *The Laboratory Rat*. Waltham, MS: Academic Press, 2005.

Tomes, Nancy J., and John Harley Warner. "Introduction to Special Issue on Rethinking the Reception of the Germ Theory of Disease: Comparative Perspectives." *Journal of the History of Medicine and Allied Sciences* 52 (1997): 7–16.

Tomes, Nancy. *The Gospel of Germs: Men, Women, and the Microbe in American Life*. Cambridge, MA: Harvard University Press, 1998.

Triolo, Victor A. "Nineteenth Century Foundation of Cancer Research: Advances in Tumor Pathology, Nomenclature, and Theories of Oncogenesis." *Cancer Research* 25 (1965): 75–106.

———. "Nineteenth Century Foundations of Cancer Research. Origins of Experimental Research." *Cancer Research* 24 (1964): 4–27.

Triolo, Victor A., and Ilse L. Riegel. "The AACR, 1907–1940: Historical Review." *Cancer Research* 21 (1961): 137–42.

———. "The American Association for Cancer Research, 1907–1940: A Historical Review." *Cancer Research* 21 (1961): 143–44.

Triolo, Victor A., and Michael B. Shimkin. "The American Cancer Society and Cancer Research Origins and Organization: 1913–1943." *Cancer Research* 29 (1969): 1615–41.

Tsoucalas, G., K. Laios, M. Karamanou, V. Gennimata, and G. Androutsos. "The Fascinating Germ Theories on Cancer Parthogenesis." *JBUON* 19 (2014): 319–23.

Turner, James. *Without God, Without Creed: The Origins of Unbelief in America*. Baltimore: Johns Hopkins University Press, 1986.

Van Helvoort, Ton. "Scalpel or Rays? Radiotherapy and the Struggle for the Cancer Patient in Pre-Second World War Germany." *Medical History* 45 (2001): 42.

Vetter, Jeremy. "Introduction." *Knowing Global Environments: New Historical Perspectives on the Field Sciences*. New Brunswick: Rutgers University Press, 2010.

———. "Introduction: Lay Participation in the History of Scientific Observation." *Science in Context* 24 (2011): 259–80.

———. "Labs in the Field? Rocky Mountain Biological Stations in the Early Twentieth Century." *Journal of the History of Biology* 45 (2012): 587–611.

Wagner, Gustav, and Andrea Mauerberger. *Krebsforschung in Deutschland. Vorgeschichte Und Geschichte Des Deutschen Krebsforschungszentrums*. Berlin: Springer-Verlag, 1989.

Wailoo, Keith. *How Cancer Crossed the Color Line*. Oxford: Oxford University Press, 2011.

Weisz, George. *The Medical Mandarins. The French Academy of Medicine in the Nineteenth and Early Twentieth Centuries*. Oxford: Oxford University Press, 1995.

Weller, Thomas H. *Ernest Edward Tyzzer, 1875–1965*. Washington: National Academy of Sciences, 1978.

Witkowski, Jan A. "Experimental Pathology and the Origins of Tissue Culture: Leo Loeb's Contribution." *Medical History* 27 (1983): 269–88.

Wolff, Jacob. *The Science of Cancerous Disease from Earliest Times to the Present*. Translated by Barbara Ayoub. Canton, MA: Science History Publications, 1987. Originally published as *Die Lehre von der Krebskrankheit von den Ältesten Zeiten Bis Zur Gegenwart* (Jena: G. Fischer, 1907).

Worboys, Michael. *Spreading Germs: Disease Theories and Medical Practice in Britain, 1865–1900*. Cambridge, MA: Cambridge University Press, 2000.

INDEX